CHRONIC PAIN MANAGEMENT

GUIDELINES FOR MULTIDISCIPLINARY PROGRAM DEVELOPMENT

PAIN MANAGEMENT

1. Ethical Issues in Chronic Pain Management, *edited by Michael E. Schatman*
2. Chronic Pain, *Gary W. Jay*
3. Chronic Pain Management: Guidelines for Multidisciplinary Program Development, *edited by Michael E. Schatman and Alexandra Campbell*

CHRONIC PAIN MANAGEMENT

GUIDELINES FOR MULTIDISCIPLINARY PROGRAM DEVELOPMENT

EDITED BY

MICHAEL E. SCHATMAN
Consulting Clinical Psychologist
Bellevue, Washington, USA

ALEXANDRA CAMPBELL
American Academy of Pain Management
Sonora, California, USA

FOREWORD BY
JOHN D. LOESER

informa
healthcare

New York London

Informa Healthcare USA, Inc.
52 Vanderbilt Avenue
New York, NY 10017

Printed in Great Britain by CPI Antony Rowe, Chippenham, Wiltshire
10 9 8 7

International Standard Book Number-10: 1-4200-4512-1 (Hardcover)
International Standard Book Number-13: 978-1-4200-4512-3 (Hardcover)

Library of Congress Cataloging-in-Publication Data

Chronic pain management : guidelines for multidisciplinary program development / edited by Michael E. Schatman, Alexandra Campbell.
p.; cm. – (Pain management; 3)
Includes bibliographical references and index.
ISBN-13: 978-1-4200-4512-3 (hb : alk. paper)
ISBN-10: 1-4200-4512-1 (hb : alk. paper)
1. Chronic pain – Treatment. 2. Pain clinics. I. Schatman, Michael E. II. Campbell, Alexandra, PhD. III. Series.
[DNLM: 1. Pain–therapy. 2. Chronic Disease. 3. Combined Modality Therapy. 4. Pain–rehabilitation. 5. Pain Clinics–organization & administration. 6. Patient Care Team. WL 704 C5585 2007]

RB127.C4963 2007
616′.0472 – dc22 2007012048

Visit the Informa Web site at
www.informa.com

and the Informa Healthcare Web site at
www.informahealthcare.com

Foreword

The idea that chronic pain is a medical problem was born with the pioneering work of John J. Bonica, M.D., at the end of World War II. Chronic pain entered the world of academic medicine when Dr. Bonica was appointed the founding Chairman of Anesthesiology at the University of Washington in 1960. The term, multidisciplinary pain clinic (MPC), was invented by Dr. Bonica, originally to describe an approach to the diagnosis and treatment of chronic pain patients by a group of physicians who interacted with each other as well as with the patients. In the 1960's, also at the University of Washington, Wilbert Fordyce, a psychologist in the Department of Rehabilitation Medicine, recognized that a behavioral approach to the treatment of chronic pain patients could be more successful than injections, pills or surgery. He started a behavioral pain management service in Rehabilitation Medicine and brought his principles of pain management into the multidisciplinary pain clinic. Other psychologists broadened the Fordyce approach to include cognitive-behavioral strategies and increased its effectiveness. In 1983, Dr. Fordyce and I started a 20-bed inpatient and outpatient multidisciplinary pain clinic that was independent of any single academic department. This served as the prototype for multidisciplinary pain clinics throughout the world, in part because of our active teaching programs and openness to visitors. Physicians of many specialties, psychologists, nurses, physical and occupational therapists and vocational counselors were all integral members of our team.

Many other health care providers also played important roles in the development of multidisciplinary pain management; the Commission on Accreditation of Rehabilitation Facilities (CARF) adopted our model as the accreditation standard for multidisciplinary pain clinics. Multidisciplinary pain clinics were developed throughout the world, often with varying content and emphasis to fit the needs of the patients they treated and the providers they had available. In countries with rational health care systems, this form of patient diagnosis and treatment seems to have prospered, as it has been recognized as more effective, less hazardous, and less costly than traditional approaches to treating chronic pain patients. Based squarely upon a biopsychosocial model rather than the prevalent biomedical model, multidisciplinary pain management has been seen as a threat to biomedicine and the industry's imperative to consume expensive health resources.

In the United States, with a non-system of health care and the dramatic intrusion of economic factors into health care decisions, MPCs have not fared as well and the number of programs has decreased steeply in the past ten years. There are many factors that have contributed to the relative demise of MPCs. First, a labeling issue: Any group of two or more health care providers can call themselves a multidisciplinary pain clinic and is capable of deceiving the public as to what they offer insofar as diagnostic and treatment options. This is a common occurrence and has brought considerable disrepute to *bona fide* MPCs. Second, decisions about what forms of health care are to be offered are not made uniquely by doctors and their patients. Instead, insurance companies and large hospitals and academic medical centers ignore both the moral imperatives to treat chronic pain and the available outcomes data on treatment efficacy and often will not fund MPCs. For large, American hospitals, especially those associated with a medical school, revenue generation is the major determinant of what services the institution will offer. MPC is not seen as a value compared to cosmetic surgery. Third, payment to providers is skewed in favor of procedures and surgeries, putting great economic pressures on those who provide a personal service without a procedural intervention. Fourth, proceduralists have done a much better job lobbying funding agencies and the public as to the utility of their interventions than have those who run MPCs. Fifthly, there is no single optimal plan for how to run an MPC and what its content, duration of treatment and team members should be. This has made it difficult for funding agencies to evaluate programs and compare costs and efficacy. Finally, organized medicine has never accepted the validity of multidisciplinary pain management and there are many impediments to its implementation in the medical community.

This book is designed to combat many of the problems that confront multidisciplinary pain management in the United States today. A stellar group of contributors has addressed the problems of building and maintaining a multidisciplinary pain clinic. The emphasis is upon outcomes, not personal anecdotes. Multidisciplinary pain care is the best treatment we now have for the rehabilitation and relief of suffering of chronic pain patients. Chronic pain patients always have psychosocial factors that influence their disability and suffering; pills and surgery do not address these at all. This volume will be an important tool in the restoration and continued development of multidisciplinary pain management in the United States and the remainder of the developed world.

John D. Loeser, M.D.
Professor of Neurology and Anesthesiology
University of Washington Medical School
Seattle, Washington, U.S.A.

Preface

Chronic pain of benign origin results in staggering costs, to society as a whole as well as to the individual sufferer. Although it is impossible to accurately determine the total economic cost of chronic pain to society, its combined direct and indirect annual cost in the United States was estimated in 2001 to be almost $300 billion (1). A huge proportion of the economic cost associated with chronic pain consists of fees for treatments which have not been found to be particularly efficacious. These were estimated in 2001 to be about $125 billion annually (2). It should be noted that both of these figures are conservative, as neither has been adjusted for inflation.

Of greater *moral* importance, however, is the overwhelming non-economic cost of chronic pain to the people that it afflicts. Those affected include not only the person who experiences the pain directly, but loved ones as well. Losses experienced by patients with chronic pain include not only the physical, but vocational, financial, social, sexual, recreational, emotional, and spiritual. A recent qualitative study found that in addition to socioeconomic losses and financial hardships, people with chronic pain experienced decreases in self-worth, positive expectations for the future, and hope (3). Other studies (4)–(8) have identified increases in feelings of despair, loss of meaning of life, losses of freedom/independence, threat to integrity, role loss, and disorganization of the patient's "being in the world" as the worst consequences of chronic pain conditions. Chronic pain is clearly a disease of the *person*, not simply of the *body*.

Despite the fact that traditional medical approaches to treating chronic pain such as surgery, medications and other invasive interventions, do little, if anything, to restore the chronic pain sufferer's *overall quality of life*, these traditional approaches continue to be considered the first line of offense against chronic pain. This is particularly disheartening given the lack of empirical support for the clinical efficacy of these approaches in terms of long-term pain relief, much less for their ability to impact the myriad indirect negative effects of the chronic pain experience. The good news is that for many years, pain practitioners have possessed a treatment model that can help people with chronic pain restore their lives. The bad news is that the health insurance industry, as a whole, is becoming progressively less willing to fund this treatment approach. As is discussed throughout this textbook, comprehensive multidisciplinary chronic pain management has been empirically demonstrated, *beyond a doubt*, to be a clinically effective and cost-efficient approach to the treatment of chronic pain of benign origin. The ethical failure of the insurance industry, however, has led to a dramatic decrease in the availability of such programs over the past decade (9), (10).

We appreciate the inspiration of the American Academy of Pain Management in our decision to produce this book which we hope will serve two purposes. The first is to arm the multidisciplinary pain practitioner with a concise resource that powerfully presents overwhelming evidence regarding the efficacy and cost-efficiency of multidisciplinary chronic pain management, particularly in comparison to the traditional and ineffective approaches that continue to be overutilized in the treatment of chronic pain. We have enlisted the participation of leading authorities in the world of multidisciplinary chronic pain management to contribute chapters on this topic. Our second purpose is to provide a "how-to" manual for multidisciplinary chronic pain management program development. We have been fortunate to obtain the participation of chronic pain clinicians/academicians who are certainly experts in this area.

Chronic Pain Management: Guidelines for Multidisciplinary Program Development is divided into 5 sections. Following a Foreword by John Loeser, one of the eminent pioneers in the field, the first section covers the history and empirical support of multidisciplinary chronic pain management. This section includes a chapter on the history of the multidisciplinary approach to chronic pain (Marcia Meldrum), an in depth analysis of the clinical efficacy and cost-efficiency of the multidisciplinary approach in comparison to "traditional" approaches (Dennis Turk and Kimberly Swanson), and a presentation of the literature on problems associated with "carving out" specific services from programs that need to be offered as coherent wholes (Robert Gatchel, Nancy Kishino, and Carl Noe). For those of us who have practiced pain management from a multidisciplinary approach and have seen the problems associated with efforts that treat the "pain" but not the "person," the superiority of the multidisciplinary approach is very obvious. For those whose understanding of chronic pain is more limited, however, the chapters in this section serve to erase any doubt regarding the efficacy of the more "person-centered" approach to chronic pain treatment.

The second section of this text covers the *need* for multidisciplinary chronic pain management given the countless problems associated with other approaches. This section includes a chapter on multidisciplinary treatment as an alternative to chronic opioid therapy (Jane Ballantyne) and spinal surgery (Richard Guyer and Andy Block), both of which have been heavily criticized as overutilized and of questionable efficacy. This section also includes chapters on the use of approaches that have been empirically demonstrated to be of limited efficacy when provided in a unimodal fashion, but which can be valuable components of a comprehensive chronic pain management program. Chapters are provided on complementary and alternative medicine (CAM) (Gabriel Tan and Mark Jensen) and on interventional approaches (Mike Hatzakis and Michael Schatman).

The next section of the book focuses on people who are actually treated through multidisciplinary chronic pain management programs, as well as on those who are sometimes not treated at all. We were fortunate to have a patient (Debra Benner) who experienced first-hand the benefits of being treated in a program that was developed by the book's first editor (MES) and whose training and work as a hospital chaplain provide unique insights into pain management that few are fortunate enough to experience. Additionally, a chapter in this section by one of the great champions of vulnerable populations (Ray Tait) allows the reader to consider issues of distributive justice in the field of chronic pain management.

The fourth section of the textbook looks at clinical elements of a comprehensive pain management program that make it truly "multidisciplinary." The section includes a broad chapter on the "nuts and bolts" of putting together a comprehensive interdisciplinary/multidisciplinary treatment team, delineating the functions of all of the members (Steven Stanos). This chapter is of great importance, as it outlines the need for communication and cooperation between various types of healthcare professionals whose training may not necessarily be based on the same underlying assumptions about illness and disease. The other chapter in this section discusses the role of psychological assessment in multidisciplinary chronic pain management (Allen Lebovits). As these programs place a heavy emphasis on the psychological sequelae of chronic pain as well as upon the patient's nociceptive experience, the value of psychologists providing other treatment team members with an understanding of a patient's psychodynamics as they relate to his or her pain is essential if the patient is to achieve success.

The fifth and final section of this book is the longest, dealing with the administrative/financial aspects of developing a multidisciplinary chronic pain management program. At present, it is not the clinical efficacy of multidisciplinary chronic pain programs that is in question; rather, it is the ability of these programs to remain effective in the rapidly changing economic climate while maintaining financial viability. The first chapter in this section addresses strategies for developing strong policies and procedures, which are likely to contribute to the consistency of treatment that is provided to chronic pain patients (Paula Spoonhour and Michael Schatman). While each multidisciplinary program is likely to have its own unique qualities, internal consistency is essential if referral sources and third party payors are to consider a program seriously. The next chapter addresses the importance of outcomes measurement and data collection in multidisciplinary chronic pain management as a means of documenting and improving the quality of programs (Kevin Vowles, Rick Gross, and Lance McCracken). The third chapter in this section speaks to pain program accreditation (Alexandra Campbell). While any licensed health care professional can claim to provide chronic pain management services, meeting the standards necessary for accreditation can contribute significantly to a program's legitimacy, both in the eyes of the insurance industry and potential referral sources. The next chapter provides strategies for obtaining reimbursement for the provision of multidisciplinary chronic pain management (Ron Kulich and Michael Adolph), the necessity of which is obvious if this treatment model is to continue to be viable. The authors take the perspective that programs need to be run like businesses if they are to survive in a health care industry climate that considers cost-containment and profitability to be more important than the welfare of those who suffer from chronic pain. The final chapter in the book discusses the very successful model for multidisciplinary chronic pain management that has been developed and nurtured in one of the nation's largest and best known health maintenance organizations, Kaiser Permanente (Bill McCarberg).

We are highly appreciative of all of the authors who contributed their time and effort to write chapters for what we believe to be an important and timely volume. A wide variety of healthcare professionals are represented among the authors but they share the common thread of *believing* in multidisciplinary chronic pain management, and have dedicated their professional lives to practicing and/or furthering the field. In a presentation at the Eighth World Congress of the International

Association for the Study of Pain, John Bonica was referred to as the "world champion of pain" (11). All of the authors who contributed to this textbook were influenced by Dr. Bonica, and all of them embody his spirit in continuing to serve as "champions of pain" through their efforts to practice and promote multidisciplinary chronic pain management.

Michael E. Schatman
Alexandra Campbell

REFERENCES

1. National Academies of Sciences and Institute of Medicine. Musculoskeletal disorders and the workplace: low back pain and upper extremities. Washington, DC: National Academies Press, 2001.
2. Okifuji A, Turk DC, Kalauoklani D. Clinical outcome and economic evaluation of multidisciplinary pain centers. In: Block AR, Kremer EF, Fernandez E, eds. Handbook of Pain Syndromes: biopsychosocial perspectives. Mahwah, NJ: Lawrence Erlbaum Associates, 1999:77–97.
3. Walker J, Sofaer B, Holloway I. The experience of chronic back pain: accounts of loss in those seeking help from pain clinics. Eur J Pain. 2006; 10:199–207.
4. Bowman JM. The meaning of chronic low back pain. AAOHN J. 1991; 39:381–384.
5. Hellstrom C, Carlsson SG. The long-lasting now: disorganization in subjective time in long-standing pain. Scand J Psychol. 1996; 37:416–423.
6. Soderberg S, Ludman B, Norberg A. Struggling for dignity: the meaning of women's experiences of living with fibromyalgia. Qual Health Res. 1999; 9:575–587.
7. Harris S, Morley S, Barton SB. Role loss and emotional adjustment in chronic pain. Pain. 2003; 105:363–370.
8. Sorajjakool S, Thompson KM, Aveling L, Earl A. Chronic pain, meaning, and spirituality: A qualitative study of the healing process in relation to the role of meaning and spirituality. J Pastoral Care Counsel. 2006 Winter; 60(4):369–78.
9. Schatman ME. The demise of multidisciplinary pain management clinics? Practical Pain Manage. 2006; 6:30–41.
10. Schatman ME. The demise of the multidisciplinary chronic pain management clinic: bioethical perspectives on providing optimal treatment when ethical principles collide. In: Schatman ME, ed., Ethical Issues in Chronic Pain Management. New York: Informa Healthcare. 2007; 43–62.
11. Liebeskind JC, Meldrum ML. John J. Bonica, world champion of pain. In: Jensen TS, Turner JA, Wiesenfeld-Hallin Z, eds. Proceedings of the 8th World Congress in Pain Research and Management, Vol. 8. Seattle, WA: IASP Press. 1997:19–32.

Contents

Contributors

Michael Adolph Pain and Palliative Medicine Service, James Cancer Hospital and Solove Research Institute, Ohio State University Medical Center, Columbus, Ohio, U.S.A.

Jane C. Ballantyne Division of Pain Medicine, Department of Anesthesia and Critical Care, Massachusetts General Hospital and Harvard Medical School, Boston, Massachusetts, U.S.A.

Debra E. Benner Hershey Medical Center, Hershey, Pennsylvania, U.S.A.

Andrew R. Block Texas Back Institute, Plano, Texas, U.S.A.

Alexandra Campbell The American Academy of Pain Management, Sonora, California, U.S.A.

Robert J. Gatchel The University of Texas at Arlington, Arlington, Texas, U.S.A.

Richard T. Gross Columbia Health Centre, Dartmouth, Nova Scotia, Canada

Richard D. Guyer Texas Back Institute, Plano, Texas, U.S.A.

Michael Hatzakis, Jr. Bellevue Rehabilitation Associates, Bellevue, Washington, U.S.A.

Mark P. Jensen Department of Rehabilitation Medicine, University of Washington, Seattle, Washington, U.S.A.

Nancy D. Kishino West Coast Spine Restoration Center, Riverside, California, U.S.A.

Ronald J. Kulich Massachusetts General Hospital Pain Center, Wang Ambulatory Care Center; Department of General Dentistry, Tufts School of Dental Medicine; and Departments of Psychiatry and Anesthesia, Harvard Medical School, Boston, Massachusetts, U.S.A.

Allen H. Lebovits Neurology and Integrative Pain Medicine ProHealth Care Associates, LLP, Lake Success, New York, U.S.A.

Bill H. McCarberg Kaiser Permanente San Diego and University of California, San Diego, San Diego, California, U.S.A.

Lance M. McCracken Pain Management Unit, Royal National Hospital for Rheumatic Diseases and University of Bath, Bath, U.K.

Marcia L. Meldrum John C. Liebeskind History of Pain Collection, University of California, Los Angeles, California, U.S.A.

Laura Miller Saint Louis University School of Medicine, St. Louis, Missouri, U.S.A.

Carl Noe Baylor Medical Center, Dallas, Texas, U.S.A.

Michael E. Schatman Consulting Clinical Psychologist, Bellevue, Washington, U.S.A.

Paula Spoonhour Pinnacle Health Rehab Options, Harrisburg, Pennsylvania, U.S.A.

Steven P. Stanos Chronic Pain Care Center, Rehabilitation Institute of Chicago, and Department of Physical Medicine and Rehabilitation, Northwestern University Medical School, Feinberg School of Medicine, Chicago, Illinois, U.S.A.

Kimberly Swanson Department of Anesthesiology, University of Washington, Seattle, Washington, U.S.A.

Raymond C. Tait Saint Louis University School of Medicine, St. Louis, Missouri, U.S.A.

Gabriel Tan Michael E. DeBakey VA Medical Center, and Departments of Anesthesiology, and Physical Medicine and Rehabilitation, Baylor College of Medicine, Houston, Texas, U.S.A.

Dennis C. Turk Department of Anesthesiology, University of Washington, Seattle, Washington, U.S.A.

Kevin E. Vowles Pain Management Unit, Royal National Hospital for Rheumatic Diseases and University of Bath, Bath, U.K.

1 Brief History of Multidisciplinary Management of Chronic Pain, 1900–2000

Marcia L. Meldrum
John C. Liebeskind History of Pain Collection, University of California, Los Angeles, California, U.S.A.

THE PROBLEM OF LESIONLESS PAIN, 1900–1945

Chronic pain might have been considered an orphan in the early 1900s, in that none of the medical disciplines that had emerged in the previous century were anxious to claim the problem as their own. This had not always been the case. In the early years of pathological anatomy studies, when European physicians began to follow the example of the Paris School, in linking bedside observations of signs and symptoms to postmortem findings, there was much interest in chronic pain that could not be linked to a lesion at autopsy. What was the meaning, and what was the physiology behind "lesionless" pain? The French pathologist François J.V. Broussais described chronic pain as a neural malfunction in 1826. The English physician Sir Benjamin Brodie in the 1830s made the analogy to inflammation or irritation, one buried within the spinal cord. The great German neurophysiologist Johannes Müller, whose concept of "specific nerve energies" (in his *Handbüch der Physiologie* in 1840) was adapted by the field of neurophysiology to describe very specific cellular responses to different stimuli, also proposed a systemic disorder in which a person lost the ability to interpret physical sensations, which he called *Gemeingefühl* or *cenesthesis* from the Greek. Throughout the century, however, as neurologists, pathologists, and other physicians became increasingly skilled at diagnosis, syndromes with clear physiological etiologies became the hallmark of disciplinary expertise. Lesionless pain that remained unexplained was simply uninteresting (1).

Perhaps, after all, it was unnecessary to explain pain as new anesthetics and analgesics were developed by enterprising physicians and industrial chemists. The introduction of ether and chloroform into surgery in 1846–1848, the isolation of morphine in 1805 and the development of the hypodermic syringe for its controlled administration in 1854–1855, the demonstration of cocaine as a topical anesthetic in 1884 and the synthesis of procaine in 1905, and the marketing of aspirin in 1899, an easily tolerated salicylate drug, all eased suffering that had once been the everyday lot of many. Headache, toothache, arthritis, childbirth, the pain of injuries and wounds—all these ancient miseries could be safely and effectively relieved. By 1900, the risk that a patient might develop "the morphia habit" from overuse of the drug was clear, but many scientists and physicians thought this problem would prove to have a laboratory solution as well. In 1929, after morphine and other narcotics had come under federal regulation, the Harvard pharmacologist Reid Hunt proposed that "a thorough study of the morphine molecule might show a possibility of separating the analgesic from the habit-forming property," and under his leadership, the National Research Council organized a Drug Addiction Committee to oversee research toward this objective (2).

Not all chronic pain patients responded to the available analgesics. For these "pariahs," as the sympathetic French surgeon René Leriche called them (3), the alternatives were drastic or disabling neurosurgical procedures to ligate the neural pathways that conveyed sensation to the brain, or the psychiatrist's office. Many physicians saw the patient with persistent unexplained pain as beyond the purview of any discipline. The Boston surgeon John Homans reflected the perception of many when he wrote in 1940 of causalgia not directly linked to an injury, "That there is something basically at fault about the nervous system of certain of the individuals affected, is probable. Some are insurance problems. Others have grudges against the world, or are perhaps stupid, or even criminal" (4).

During 1900–1945 chronic lesionless pain did not in fact fit within the principles of any of the newly established medical disciplines. The clinical evidence contradicted the knowledge of the laboratory.

Laboratory Models

Animal experiments suggested that each of the four types of stimuli— touch, heat, cold, and pain—used to trigger responses in exposed animal nerves followed a specific neural pathway to the higher centers; this was called "specificity," a concept historically traceable to Müller and Descartes. The neurophysiological evidence was compelling. Max von Frey had identified distinct cellular skin "spots," or receptors, that responded differentially to each stimulus in Leipzig in 1894 (5). The Nobel laureates Joseph Erlanger and Herbert Gasser demonstrated the different conduction speeds of nerve fibers that responded to touch (fast) and pain (slow) with an oscillograph in St. Louis in the 1920s; this work was continued by their students, James O'Leary, Peter Heinbecker, and George H. Bishop (6). A number of physiologists, including Sir Charles Sherrington, had suggested that the brain might integrate this highly specific information based on frequency, location, or other data for a more complex understanding, but there was no experimental support for these hypotheses (7).

The implication was that "real pain" was by definition a straightforward proportionate response to a measurable stimulus, an assumption supported by the Cornell experiments of James D. Hardy, Harold G. Wolff, and Helen Goodell on human volunteers in the 1940s. These researchers used a *dolorimeter* invented by Hardy, a physicist and physiologist, to focus a beam of radiant heat at one spot on the volunteer's skin—usually on the hand or forehead. This technique seemed unlikely to cause permanent harm, and it permitted Hardy and his colleagues to measure and control the exact temperature of the stimulus and the area and duration of skin exposure (8,9).

The subjects reported their initial sensation of pain (threshold) and maximum tolerance of the stimulus to establish their baselines and then were tested under aspirin, morphine, codeine, and other analgesics. Changes in threshold and tolerance under analgesia were measured in terms of stimulus intensity and duration. The dolorimeter method made it possible to develop quantitative and graphic comparisons of the available analgesics. However, many of the volunteers need to go through a series of trials to learn how to best report changes in perceived sensation: "untrained subjects, even of high intelligence, cannot be used successfully" in such experiments (10–12).

The Cornell experiments suggested that, although human pain could only be measured through self-report, "real pain" was indeed proportionate to measurable stimuli and could readily be quantified in the way that other symptoms such as heart rate and body temperature were measured. Hardy and his associates developed the "dol scale," calibrated in units of just noticeable difference or "jnd," the point at which the subject perceives and reports a difference in intensity. The jnd is then equated to the appropriate level of stimulus intensity and duration, and two jnds equal one "dol." When the subject's tolerance is at maximum, however, there is no perceivable difference in pain, even if the stimulus intensity is increased; therefore, the scale will range from 0 to this maximum dol level (9).

The work of Hardy, Wolff, and Goodell thus provided behavioral support for the animal evidence and validated the assumption that real pain was not a problem requiring disciplinary analysis, but an easily definable and routine response.

Clinical Reports

The clinical reports of patients with persistent and chronic pain disorders were so inconsistent with this laboratory picture that physicians cannot, perhaps, be blamed for doubting their veracity. Of these, the classic accounts of nerve injuries and phantom pain written by S. Weir Mitchell after the Civil War remain the iconic examples. Mitchell wrote of causalgia, the burning pain that developed in an extremity after the original bullet wound had apparently healed, that it was "the most terrible of all tortures ... Under such torments... the most amiable grow irritable, the soldier becomes a coward, and the strongest man is scarcely less nervous than the most hysterical girl" (13). Soldiers suffering from such pain could not bear to be touched or bathed, barely to be spoken to; many of Mitchell's staff considered them to be near insanity. He relieved the pain of some with morphine, but 30 years after the war, many reported that they still suffered from the inexplicable pain (14).

Rene Leriche described similar syndromes among the wounded of World War I (3); but they appeared in the clinical literature as well under names such as algodystrophy, reflex dystrophy, shoulder-hand syndrome, and Sudeck's atrophy (15). Added to these were the accounts of patients who suffered from recurrent headache or low back pain, the enigmatic facial pain called *tic douleureux*, arthritis, sciatica, or the catchall description, neuralgia. Some of these were lifelong ailments, while others developed after an accident or other trauma. But few could be linked to an observable lesion.

The number of cases seemed to multiply in the United States after many states passed workers' compensation laws between 1902 and 1920. When the employee making a claim appeared not to have any residual disability, but stated that he or she was prevented from working because of "pain and suffering," the employer or the state insisted on further medical review—not by a pain specialist, since there were none, but usually by young general practitioners seeking to supplement small practice incomes.

One of these young men was a surgeon in Oregon, William K. Livingston. He saw many such patients in the 1930s, who suffered from conditions variously described as posttraumatic headache, bad back, painful scars, painful feet, or whiplash of the neck. The original injury had sometimes been handled badly but had usually healed without apparent complication. But pain remained in one or more sites, pain which the patients talked about as "blazing," "stabbing," "vise-like," "a thousand needles," language which seemed absurdly "out of proportion to the original injury." The patient would not move the affected hand, foot, arm, or leg, often resulting in a loss of circulation, atrophy of the muscles, numbness of the skin, but the pain remained constant and severe. Often it spread further along an extremity or appeared in the opposite limb. Livingston described his patients as often "argumentative and touchy." Most had been through a series of medical examinations and claims reviews, repeatedly described as neurotics, hysterics, and malingerers (16).

The sensations described in such cases were disproportionate to any past or present stimulus; they did not follow specific pathways but appeared almost at random in different body parts or caused other physiological responses, such as nausea or sensitivity to light. The problem of chronic lesionless pain fit within no disciplinary boundaries; in fact, according to the accepted understanding of the sensory nervous system, it could not really be pain.

IDEAS IN FERMENT, 1945–1965

The Maturation of Anesthesiology and the First Pain Clinics

The clinical discipline which might have laid an early claim to the problem of pain was anesthesiology, but this field was still in the process of professionalization and maturation in the first half of the twentieth century. In the early years of surgical anesthesia, ether and other gases were administered by assistant surgeons, interns, medical students, or nurses—almost anyone with a free pair of hands in the operating room might be asked to do so. A small number of physicians realized that greater safety and technical skills were necessary and began to specialize in anesthesia, or to train nurses as anesthetists, in the early 1900s. The medical specialty developed under the influence of Gaston Labat at the Mayo Clinic, Ralph Waters at the University of Wisconsin, and Emery Rovenstine at Bellevue in the 1920s and 1930s. In addition to improving the delivery and monitoring of general anesthesia, these pioneers developed the practice of regional anesthesia or nerve blocks for localized medical and surgical procedures (17).

Alcohol blocks were used to relieve trigeminal neuralgia in the early 1900s and chronic chest pain in the 1920s (18). Rene Leriche is generally credited with developing the first procaine blocks for his nerve-injured soldiers in World War I. He hypothesized that their persistent pain was the result of interconnections between the periarterial sympathetic and peripheral sensory fibers as the nerves regenerated and combined nerve blocks with a meticulous resection of the arteries and nerves. If there was no reduction in the pain, he then suggested ligation of the sympathetic fibers or sympathetic ganglia (3). Other surgeons in the 1920s used the procaine block as a diagnostic tool; if the block was successful, they proceeded with the neural ligation (18).

William Livingston first saw procaine blocks used by a football coach to relieve players' pain and later studied the work of Leriche. In the 1930s, he began using serial anesthetic blocks with the difficult pain patients referred to him by the Oregon State Industrial Commission and by other physicians. On finding that one injection often left the patient free of pain for several weeks or months, he would try a second, then a third, continuing for up to 2 years, until the patient reported that the pain was gone or reduced to a tolerable level (19). Rovenstine opened the first nerve-block clinic for the relief of chronic pain at Bellevue in 1936 (20). Blocking techniques were further developed during World War II, and a number of anesthesiologists started pain clinics in the United States and the United Kingdom in the 1950s; these included Duncan Alexander in Texas and Mark Swerdlow in Manchester (21,22).

It was Henry K. Beecher, however, who made the strongest claim for anesthesiology as the sole discipline of pain, not only of pain management but of pain research as well. Beecher had planned to be a surgeon but was convinced by his Harvard mentor, Edward Churchill, to move into anesthesiology and take on the challenge of developing a research program in the field. He set up the Anesthesia Research Laboratory at Massachusetts General, where he examined the chemical structure and physiological activity of the anesthetic gases. This work gained him an endowed chair, the Isaac Dorr Professorship of Anesthesiology at Harvard in 1941 (23).

Beecher's initial interest in pain as a research problem was heightened during his service as an army consultant during World War II. When he spoke to gravely wounded men on the beachheads awaiting medical assistance and evacuation, he found that few of them asked for morphine, or reported high levels of pain, while many were content with water or a cigarette (24). This behavior contrasted so strongly with that of trauma and postoperative patients he had worked with at Massachusetts General that it demanded explanation. Beecher developed an idea originally proposed by the psychologist Charles Strong in the 1890s that pain was not merely a sensory phenomenon, but a compound of sensory, cognitive, and affective factors (25). Thus, the soldier's relief at survival and anticipation of convalescence in a safe location reduced his distress and the perceived intensity of his pain. But in the hospital, the patient's pain was perceived as *more* severe because of the individual's anxiety and fear over the outcome of the injury or illness (26). Because each person's situation, history, and present expectations were different, Beecher argued, human pain had to be understood as a complex phenomenon that was "different for each individual." He bluntly challenged the findings of Hardy, Wolff, and Goodell, contending that the neatly graphed pain reports given by their subjects were functions of the experimental milieu and experience, as much as of simple sensation. For Beecher, clinical pain had to be understood in relation to the individual patient; it could never be a laboratory problem, but belonged within the purview of clinical research, and specifically, of anesthesiology (27).

Throughout the 1950s, Beecher studied the problem of pain measurement and the evaluation of analgesic efficacy. Although he collaborated with colleagues from internal medicine, pharmacology, and psychology in these studies (28), he remained focused on anesthesiology as the discipline of pain management. But others would find in the complexity of pain a compelling argument for a multidisciplinary approach.

Pioneer Multidisciplinary Pain Clinics in the Northwest

The tragic suffering of many wounded men in World War II played a pivotal role in the development of pain management by giving physicians the unique opportunity to treat multiple complex pain syndrome cases in organized teams. For both William Livingston and John Bonica, the war was a turning point in their careers.

Livingston, who had no neurosurgical training, was posted to a general surgery ward at Oak Knoll Naval Hospital in Oakland, California, in 1942, an assignment he initially found monotonous and "frustrating." But as his interest in nerve injuries and puzzling pain problems became known, more and more of these cases were transferred to him, including causalgia, phantom limbs, and many variants of neuropathic pain. He was put in charge of another ward, then two more, and assigned additional nurses, surgeons, psychiatrists, and neurologists. He found this collaborative experience so "exciting and profitable" that he was eager to continue it in peacetime. When offered the chairmanship of surgery at the University of Oregon School of Medicine in 1947, he accepted on condition that he would be able to assemble an interdisciplinary team to integrate patient care with laboratory and clinical research. The "Pain Project," where Ronald Melzack among others served an apprenticeship, had a strong research focus on elucidating the mechanisms of pain, but for 10 years, it also provided an opportunity for surgeons, anesthesiologists, psychologists, neurologists, and others to consult on the treatment of pain patients. Livingston found pain a great and complex puzzle, the unraveling of which would require the insights of both "philosophy and physiology," and which eluded him to the end of his life. But of the clinician's responsibility, he had no doubt: "don't ever give up attempts to lessen a patient's burden of pain," using the resources of every discipline (19).

John Bonica made the long trip from New York to the newly built Madigan Army Hospital in Washington State in 1944, expecting to begin his first position as an attending anesthesiologist. He was surprised to find himself the chief of anesthesia, with responsibility for training his own assistants, staffing 11 operating rooms, running the blood bank and the inhalation therapy program, and, almost as an afterthought, overseeing pain management. Working nonstop and staying up at night to read the available literature, he taught himself and his corpsmen and nurses how to administer regional nerve blocks with procaine and pontocaine. Bonica was startled to find how little information there was on how to treat complex "lesionless" pain problems, the ones that persisted after the wounds had healed. He referred his patients to other Madigan doctors—a neurologist, an internist, an orthopedic surgeon, a psychiatrist—and was also startled to find that "they knew less than I did. I had at least read these things." Time, moreover, was at a premium, with new platoons of wounded men arriving daily. Therefore he proposed that he and his colleagues meet a couple of times a week for lunch to talk over the pain cases (29).

The success of this ad hoc consultation made a deep impression on Bonica. After the war, as chief of anesthesiology at Tacoma General Hospital, as the author of the comprehensive *The Management of Pain* (1953) (30), and then as chair at the University of Washington in Seattle (1960), he became the champion of the multidisciplinary approach to pain, which he described as "the most complex human experience, in my view." His own Multidisciplinary Pain Clinic, which included specialists from eight disciplines, was intended to be a model for others. He was also recognized as a leader in regional and obstetrical anesthesia and worked hard "to sell the specialty" and to refine the techniques, which were exported around the world through Bonica's Seattle-based training programs. Anesthesiologists respected and applied his expertise in diagnostic and therapeutic techniques in treating chronic pain, but in single-modality pain clinics. By the mid-1960s, even Bonica was "about to give up" on trying to develop a multidisciplinary pain movement (29). Treatment options for chronic pain remained limited: There were the opioids, still mostly restricted only to short-term use in trauma or at the very end of life; there were a few suggested alternatives, such as the new antidepressants for chronic headache (31); there were anesthetic blocks; there was neurosurgery; and there was psychiatry. To most clinicians, these different options were mutually exclusive. What would a multidisciplinary program really mean in practice?

Part of the answer came from Seattle in the late 1960s, not from Bonica's clinic, but from a group of psychologists working in the Physical Medicine and Rehabilitation Department at the University Hospital. Wilbert Fordyce had found that known techniques in psychology often were unsuccessful with the disabled patients there, many of whom were incapacitated by severe pain, dependent on heavy medication, and reluctant to engage in the physical and occupational therapies offered. He picked up on a comment from a visiting behaviorist about the importance of social reinforcement and suggested to his colleagues that they stop giving attention to pain complaints, that they simply ignore them and instead give positive reinforcement to patients' attempts to exercise, interact socially, and deal with their pain. He himself thought it was a "harebrained idea . . . just crude." But it proved surprisingly effective (32). With his colleague Roy Fowler and resident Barbara DeLateur, Fordyce developed a program of gradually increased "quotas" of exercise, successful completion of which was rewarded with rest and social feedback; "therapist attention remained contingent upon performance." At the same time, medication was given on a timed schedule, in gradually decreasing dosages, to wean the patient from overdependence (33,34).

Bonica quickly realized the importance of Fordyce's work, invited him to become a participant in the Multidisciplinary Pain Clinic, and began referring patients to his program, although it remained part of Rehabilitation Medicine and was not incorporated into the pain clinic until 1978 (35). Fordyce's methods were adapted and employed by other psychologists, however, within the context of clinical pain programs that also provided medication, analgesic blocks, and traditional psychotherapy. The emphasis in these programs of the 1970s was less on pain eradication than on teaching an individual patient ways to control and maintain the pain at a tolerable level within the complexities of his or her life. As Livingston and Bonica had proposed, this approach usually required collaborative development of a multifaceted program. By offering a pragmatic, patient-centered therapeutic method that integrated with other disciplines, Fordyce and his fellow psychologists completed the conceptual shift from *what real pain ought to be* to *what real pain actually is and does.* Real pain as defined by the patient could now be understood as a legitimate concern of many disciplines.

"Total Pain" and the "Whole Human Being"

While the contributions of Beecher, Livingston, Bonica, and Fordyce were central to a new understanding of pain and pain management in this period, they were by no means alone. There were many other researchers and clinicians, often working in relative isolation in disparate fields, whose insights helped to reformulate the problem. As this is a brief essay focused on the development of multidisciplinary pain clinics, we will take the time to note only two examples, from oncology and from palliative medicine, which provided evidence of the need to treat pain as a complex problem "different for each individual."

Internist Raymond Houde and his nurse assistant Ada Rogers conducted a long series of analgesic trials from 1951 until 1970 at Memorial Sloan-Kettering in New York. Extended studies were initially possible because cancer patients often spent a long time on the wards with little hope of treatment; as chemotherapy and radiotherapy became more advanced, Houde found himself limited to short-term trials in postoperative cases. But he and Rogers had by then become general pain consultants for the institution (36,37). From their careful comparative studies on the onset of effect, duration of action, toxicity of each drug, and the differences in patient response and tolerance, they created a highly flexible, individualized approach to treatment. As Rogers wrote, "There is no one drug or combination of drugs ... that will suffice in every patient .... The patient expects to be treated as a whole human being; ... Our aim ... is an understanding of his suffering and, through understanding, relief" (38). Neurologist Kathleen Foley became the first Pain Fellow at Sloan-Kettering in 1971; she later developed the first classification of "cancer pain syndromes," demonstrating the complexity of pain suffering even in this major organic disease (39).

In the United Kingdom, Cicely Saunders qualified as a physician in 1957 and devoted the next 10 years to developing plans and raising funds for St. Christopher's, the first modern hospice for the care of the dying, which opened in London in 1967. From her earlier work in traditional religious hospices, Saunders had developed an analgesic philosophy based on regular opioid medication doses scheduled to keep the patient pain-free so that he never had to request or spend agonized moments waiting for relief. She insisted that pain management had to include more than the administration of drugs; the patient's suffering involved the "physical, psychological, social, and the spiritual need for safety, security, to be herself, and *that's* pain" (40). The hospice clinician had to find effective ways to address all these aspects of what Saunders called "total pain" (41).

REALIZATION: 1965–1990

The Challenge of Gate Control and the Birth of the Pain Field

While clinical evidence and theories continued to support the reality and complexity of "lesionless pain," the support for sensory specificity remained strong among neurophysiologists, although there were a few countervailing voices raised. In 1965, however, physiologists Patrick Wall and Ronald Melzack published their famous paper presenting the "gate control model," suggesting a spinal cord mechanism which ensured that minor noxious stimuli would usually be blocked from transmission to the brain by the plethora of normal sensory inputs constantly arriving from the periphery—but that stimuli of sufficient intensity and frequency would force open "the gate" and focus central attention on what the body would now perceive as *pain* (42). While incorrect in several of its assumptions, Melzack and Wall's article suggested cogently that the puzzling phenomena of clinical pain syndromes should and would prove to have physiological substrates, if researchers found the right ways to look at the evidence; patient behavior could be understood in terms of neural activity. Their challenging hypothesis was debated, indeed shouted down, at many conferences in the late 1960s (43), but the very heat of the protests illuminated the problem of pain with a new light. Apparently, there was new territory here for several disciplines.

The gate control theory did suggest one new therapeutic possibility: The use of electrical counterstimulation, of the peripheral nerves, at the spinal cord level or transcutaneously (TENS), to "close the gate" and reduce the perception of pain. The initial studies of peripheral nerve stimulation were carried out by Wall in collaboration with the Harvard neurosurgeon William Sweet in the late 1960s (44); Norman Shealy introduced spinal cord stimulation at about the same time and claimed a very high success rate, while a number of researchers were experimenting with TENS (45). With increasingly sophisticated equipment and experience, clinicians found that TENS was often effective for nociceptive, stimulus-related pain, while spinal cord stimulation is now recommended for neuropathic and vascular pain (46).

John Bonica, the indefatigable champion of the multidisciplinarity of pain, took heart at the new interest generated by the gate control method. Since 1960, he had influenced a generation of young anesthesiologists, who were trained as fellows at the University of Washington and took his ideas back to their homes in Australia, Canada, Europe, Japan, and Latin America, as well as to many parts of the United States. He also collected the names of researchers and clinicians interested in pain and had begun correspondences with many of them. Between 1969 and 1975, this evangelical work bore fruit, when Bonica was invited by the Japanese Ministry of Health and by corresponding agencies in several European and Latin American nations to consult on the development of pain clinics and facilities (47). In May 1973, he brought 350 pain researchers together in the Seattle suburb of Issaquah for 3 days of papers and discussion and gained the group's approval to launch an international, interdisciplinary professional organization devoted to pain research and management. The International Association for the Study of Pain (IASP) was formally incorporated the following year, and the first issue of the journal *Pain*, under Patrick Wall's editorship, was sent to members in January 1975 (21).

IASP membership grew to just under 2000 by the end of the decade and was mirrored in the proliferation of clinical facilities for the management of pain. By 1979, a survey by the American Society of Anesthesiologists found 426 pain clinics around the world, 278 (65%) of these in the United States. More than a third (38%) were based in anesthesiology departments, 10% in neurosurgery, and another 10% in rehabilitation medicine. While 39% of the clinics offered a single primary modality, such as analgesic blocks or TENS, and 21% were dedicated to the management of specific syndromes, such as low back pain or reflex sympathetic dystrophy, 172 (40%) were comprehensive or multidisciplinary pain clinics, although not all of these adhered to a collaborative, truly *inter*disciplinary model (48).

The Multidisciplinary Clinic Model

In 1982, neurosurgeon John Loeser took over the directorship of the Multidisciplinary Pain Center founded by his mentor John Bonica at the University of Washington, and instituted a structured inpatient program built around Fordyce's behavior modification program and a team concept of care. Many of the patients seen there had suffered from pain for many years, had left the workplace, endured multiple surgeries, and become heavily dependent on opiates or tranquilizers. All were evaluated by a physician, psychologist, and vocational counselor; the course of treatment included medication management, physical and psychological conditioning, patient education and rehabilitation with the goal of return to active work, and family re-education. Loeser has written eloquently that the high success rate of the program was not due to any particular treatment offered, but to the "magic ... in the interactions between the providers" (35).

Similar clinics were founded based on this model in the 1970s and 1980s: City of Hope near Los Angeles (Benjamin Crue), San Diego (Richard Sternbach), Denver (Richard Steig), Atlanta (Steven Brena), Boston (Gerald Aronoff), Rochester, Minnesota, and Adelaide, Australia are only a few of the leading exemplars. Pain clinic teams included physicians, nurses, psychologists, physical and occupational therapists, social workers, and vocational counselors. Complementary therapists, such as acupuncturists or biofeedback trainers, might also be available at the clinic or through referrals. The principal changes in the therapies used at multidisciplinary pain clinics in this period were the ongoing debate over the optimal use of opioid therapy for noncancer pain and the replacement of Fordyce's operant conditioning model with cognitive behavioral therapy (CBT). Although opioids are highly effective in relieving pain, and studies have shown that substance abuse is rare in chronic pain patients, chronic use often leads to reduced cognition and functionality contrary to the goal of most multidisciplinary programs (49,50).

Fordyce's program had proved helpful to many patients, but was criticized for its determinist emphasis on observable behavior and disregard of the fact that patients are "active information processors," and that their behavior is not merely a response to learned cues but shaped by cognitive processes, such as expectations of increasing pain or anxieties about physiological harm (51). The revised therapeutic programs developed in response to these criticisms drew on overlapping models linking health behavior to patient beliefs that new skills can be mastered that will improve control and coping with pain. Thus, the new therapeutic programs, the most widely practiced of which are CBT and coping skills training, seek to mediate behavioral change through cognitive relearning (52). There is considerable evidence, although of varying levels of rigor, for the efficacy of this approach; a 1992 meta-analysis found multidisciplinary programs including behavioral therapies superior to no treatment and to single-modality treatment—medical or physical therapy—in decreasing pain and impairment, improving mood, promoting return to work, and decreasing health-service utilization. "Even at follow up, patients ... are functioning better than 75%" of control groups; the findings of efficacy are "quite impressive" (53). With the development of CBT, the multidisciplinary pain clinic was seen by many as the culmination of the work of Bonica, Livingston, and other pain pioneers, and the best hope of the chronic pain patient.

ISSUES UNRESOLVED: 1990–2006

There were three dichotomies that have prevented the development of the multidisciplinary pain clinic as the recognized standard of care in the United States and have indeed contributed to a decline in numbers and in adherence to the Seattle model since 1990. By 2004, only 125 programs were still accredited by the Commission on Accreditation of Rehabilitation Facilities, down from a high of 200 in 1998 (35). The first dichotomy is between disciplinary collaboration and the discipline-segmented organization of major medical centers, the second is between the collaborative care model and the fee-for-service financing model standard in the United States, and the third is between the rehabilitative treatment program focused on individualized assessment and patient behavior change and the technological curative model of modern biomedicine.

Historically, pain clinics had developed under the aegis of departments of anesthesiology; however multidisciplinary they were in name or in concept, most institutions regarded them as cost centers and training units within that department. As third-party payer reimbursement structures changed in the 1980s and 1990s, financial survival became more and more dependent on "billable procedures," in preference to programs that integrated several therapeutic tools. Resident training programs also required procedural quotas to maintain accreditation. Anesthesiologists opted out of collaborative pain programs or competed against them with clinics offering the latest refinement in analgesic blocks. At the same time, insurance premiums rose, and individuals and employers often had to cut back on coverage. Reimbursement was linked to diagnosis and procedure, and a multiple-modality program was less likely to be fully covered. Inpatient reimbursement was rationed for shorter stays. In particular, fewer plans paid for the psychological and behavioral therapy essential to the multidisciplinary pain-treatment programs. (Parenthetically, it should be noted that financial issues are not a problem in the United States alone; in the United Kingdom, for example, programs such as St. Christopher's Hospice and the Pain Relief Foundation in Liverpool cannot be supported by the National Health Service and must rely on private support.)

Chronic pain patients themselves may reject therapies predicated on their own behavior change. Often such patients have spent years seeking a passive medical "fix," being offered diagnosis after diagnosis, drug after drug, surgery after surgery. They may have become depressed and disillusioned to the point where they no longer believe relief is possible; they may believe that opioids would provide the best help, if they could only get a long-term prescription; or they may simply believe that they have not yet found the right doctor, with the right diagnosis, drug, or treatment. But, for many, a major cognitive shift is necessary for them to see their own behavior as the agent of change in improving function and obtaining pain relief. Those patients who can successfully make the shift will often benefit from a multidisciplinary program; but, for others, the curative promise of modern biomedicine, even where it has failed, discourages them from making the investment required.

Pain management has evolved historically from a problem outside of disciplinary interest to a special interest of one discipline, to a complex problem that demands the involvement of many fields, but will not fit neatly within the dominant American medical model, with its clear disciplinary boundaries and investment in technologically passive patient therapies. The multidisciplinary pain clinic has proven to be beneficial for many who suffer from chronic pain, but has yet to establish itself as an essential part of the health-care system in the twenty-first century.

REFERENCES

1. Hodgkiss A. From Lesion to Metaphor: Chronic Pain in British, French, and German Medical Writings. Amsterdam: Editions Rodopi B. V., 2000.
2. Eddy NB, May EL. The search for a better analgesic. Science 1973; 181:407–414.
3. Leriche R, Young A, trans and ed. The Surgery of Pain. London, England: Baillière, Tindall, and Cox, 1939.
4. Homans J. Minor causalgia: A hyperesthetic neurovascular syndrome. N Engl J Med 1940; 222:870–874.
5. Von Frey M. Untersuchungen über die sinnesfunctionen der menschlichen haut; druckempfindung und schmerz. Abhandlungen der Mathematisch-Physichen Classe der K. Sächsichen Gesellschaft der Wissenschaft 1897; 13:169–266.
6. Heinbecker P, Bishop GH, O'Leary J. Pain and touch fibers in peripheral nerves. Arch Neurol Psychiatry 1933; 29:771–789.
7. Bonica JJ. Pain theories. In: Management of Pain, 2nd edn. Philadelphia, PA: Lea and Febiger, 1990:7–11.

8. Hardy JD, Wolff HG, Goodell H. Studies on pain. A new method for measuring pain threshold: Observations on spatial summation of pain. J Clin Invest 1940; 19:649–657.
9. Hardy JD, Wolff HG, Goodell H. Pain Sensations and Reactions. Baltimore, MD: Williams and Wilkins, 1952.
10. Hardy JD, Wolff HG, Goodell H. Studies on pain. Measurement of the effect of morphine, codeine, and other opiates on the pain threshold and an analysis of their relation to the pain experience. J Clin Invest 1940; 19:659–670.
11. Wolff HG, Hardy JD, Goodell H. Measurement of the effect on the pain threshold of acetylsalicylic acid, acetanilid, acetophenetidin, aminopyrine, ethyl alcohol, trichloroethylene, a barbiturate, quinine, ergotamine tartrate and caffeine: An analysis of their relation to the pain experience. J Clin Invest 1940; 20:63–80.
12. Beecher HK. Limiting factors in experimental pain. J Chronic Dis 1956; 4:11–19.
13. Mitchell SW. Injuries of Nerves and their Consequences. Philadelphia, PA: Lippincott, 1872.
14. Cervetti N. S. Weir Mitchell: The early years. Am Pain Soc Bull 2003; 13:7–9, 19.
15. Stanton-Hicks M, Janig W, Hassenbusch S, et al. Reflex sympathetic dystrophy: Changing concepts and taxonomy. Pain 1995; 63:127–133.
16. Livingston WK. Case descriptions. William K. Livingston Papers, MS Coll 136, John C. Liebeskind History of Pain Collection. Louise M. Darling Biomedical Library, UCLA, unpublished.
17. Volpitto PP, Vandam LD. The Genesis of Contemporary American Anesthesiology. Springfield, IL: Charles C. Thomas, 1982.
18. Swerdlow M. The development of chronic pain management. Roy. Coll. Anaesthe. Newslett. 1999; 47:165.
19. Livingston WK. Pain and Suffering. (Fields HK, ed.) Seattle, WA: IASP Press, 1998.
20. Rovenstine EA, Wertheim HM. Therapeutic nerve block. J Am Med Assoc 1941; 117:1599–1603.
21. Liebeskind JC, Meldrum ML. John J. Bonica, world champion of pain. In: Jensen TS, Turner JA, Wiesenfeld-Hallin Z, eds. Proceedings of the Eighth World Congress on Pain. Progress in Pain Research and Management, Vol. 8. Seattle, WA: IASP Press, 1997:19–32.
22. Swerdlow M. Oral history interview. John C. Liebeskind History of Pain Collection. Louise M. Darling Biomedical Library, UCLA, 1996.
23. Bunker JP, Henry K. Beecher. In: Volpitto PP, Vandam LD, eds. The Genesis of Contemporary American Anesthesiology. Springfield, IL: Charles C. Thomas, 1982:105–119.
24. Beecher HK. Pain in men wounded in battle. Ann Surg 1946; 123:95–105.
25. Strong CA. The psychology of pain. Psychol Rev 1895; 2:329–347.
26. Beecher HK. Pain and some factors that modify it. Anesthesiology 1951; 12:633–641.
27. Beecher HK. The measurement of pain: Prototype for the quantitative study of subjective responses. Pharmacol Rev 1957; 9:59–209.
28. Beecher HK, Keats AS, Mosteller F, et al. The effectiveness of oral analgesics (morphine, codeine, acetylsalicylic acid) and the problem of placebo 'reactors' and 'nonreactors'. J Pharmacol Exp Ther 1953; 9:393–400.
29. Bonica JJ. Oral history interview. John C. Liebeskind History of Pain Collection. Louise M. Darling Biomedical Library, UCLA, 1993.
30. Bonica JJ. The Management of Pain, with Special Emphasis on the Use of Analgesic Block in Diagnosis, Prognosis, and Therapy. Philadelphia, PA: Lea and Febiger, 1953.
31. Lance JW, Curran DA. Treatment of common tension headache. Lancet 1964; 1:1236–1239.
32. Fordyce WE. Oral history interview. John C. Liebeskind History of Pain Collection. Louise M. Darling Biomedical Library, UCLA, 1993.
33. Fordyce WE, Fowler RS, Jr, DeLateur B. An application of behavior modification technique to a problem of chronic pain. Behav Res Ther 1968; 6:105–107.

34. Fordyce WE, Fowler RS, Jr, Lehmann JF, et al. Operant conditioning in the treatment of chronic pain. Arch Phys Med Rehab 1973; 54:399–408.
35. Loeser JD. Multidisciplinary pain management. In: Merskey H, Loeser JD, Dubner R, eds. The Paths of Pain 1975–2005. Seattle, WA: IASP Press, 2005:503–511.
36. Houde RW. Oral history interview. John C. Liebeskind History of Pain Collection. Louise M. Darling Biomedical Library, UCLA, 1995.
37. Rogers AG. Oral history interview. John C. Liebeskind History of Pain Collection. Louise M. Darling Biomedical Library, UCLA, 1995.
38. Rogers AG. Sociological and nursing aspects of cancer pain. In: Bonica JJ, Ventafridda V, eds. Proceedings of the Symposium on Pain in Advanced Cancer, May 24–27, 1978. Advances in Pain Research and Therapy, Vol. 2. New York: Raven Press, 1979:108–116.
39. Foley KM. Cancer pain syndromes. In: Bonica JJ, Ventafridda V, eds. Proceedings of the Symposium on Pain in Advanced Cancer, May 24–27, 1978. Advances in Pain Research and Therapy. Vol. 2. New York: Raven Press, 1979:59–75.
40. Saunders CM. Oral history interview. John C. Liebeskind History of Pain Collection. Louise M. Darling Biomedical Library, UCLA, 1993.
41. Clark D. "Total pain", disciplinary power, and the body in the work of Cicely Saunders, 1958–67. Soc Sci Med 1999; 49:727–736.
42. Melzack R, Wall PD. Pain mechanisms: A new theory. Science 1965; 150:971–979.
43. Melzack R. Oral history interview. John C. Liebeskind History of Pain Collection. Louise M. Darling Biomedical Library, UCLA, 1993.
44. Wall PD, Sweet WH. Temporary abolition of pain in man. Science. 1967; 155:108–109.
45. Loeser JD, Black RD, Christman RN. Relief of pain by transcutaneous stimulation. J Neurosurg 1975; 42:308–314.
46. Meyerson BA, Linderoth B. Therapeutic electrical neurostimulation from a historical perspective. In: Merskey H, Loeser JD, Dubner R, eds. The Paths of Pain 1975–2005. Seattle, WA: IASP Press, 2005:313–327.
47. Bonica JJ. The ideal pain centre/clinic. In: Hyodo M, Oyama T, Swerdlow M, eds. The Pain Clinic IV, Proceedings of the Fourth International Symposium, November 18–21, 1990. Utrecht, The Netherlands: VSP BV, 1992:175–181.
48. Brena SF. Pain control facilities: Patterns of operation and problems of organization in the USA. Clin Anesthesiol 1983; 3:183–195.
49. Moulin DE. Opioids in chronic nonmalignant pain. In: Stein C, ed. Opioids in Pain Control: Basic and Clinical Aspects. New York: Cambridge University Press, 1999:295–308.
50. Portenoy RK. Opioid therapy for chronic nonmalignant pain: Current status. In: Fields HL, Liebeskind JC, eds. Pharmacological Approaches to the Treatment of Chronic Pain: New Concepts and Critical Issues. Seattle, WA: IASP Press, 1994:247–287.
51. Turk D, Meichenbaum D, Genest M. Pain and Behavioral Medicine: A Cognitive-Behavioral Perspective. New York: Guildford Press, 1983.
52. Turk D. A cognitive-behavioral perspective on treatment of chronic pain patients. In: Turk D, Gatchel R, eds. Psychological Approaches to Pain Management: A Practitioner's Handbook. New York: Guilford Press, 2002:138–158.
53. Flor H, Fydrich T, Turk DC. Efficacy of multidisciplinary pain treatment centers: A meta-analytic review. Pain 1992; 49:221–230.

2 Efficacy and Cost-Effectiveness Treatment for Chronic Pain: An Analysis and Evidence-Based Synthesis

Dennis C. Turk and Kimberly Swanson
Department of Anesthesiology, University of Washington, Seattle, Washington, U.S.A.

As we review and summarize the evidence of the prevalence and for the clinical effectiveness and cost-effectiveness of treatments for chronic pain patients, it is important to offer a caveat. Often diverse pain syndromes, sample characteristics, and interventions are compared on a spectrum of outcome measures that each has its own distinctive properties. Moreover, studies are conducted in different countries with unique medical, labor, compensation, and legal systems. This combination of factors will have important impacts on the prevalence estimate and outcomes, and likely influence the results of the efficacy of dissimilar treatments.

Throughout this chapter, we will convert all financial data to U.S. currency. We will correct all cost estimates for inflation conservatively estimated at 7% per year, unless noted.

PREVALENCE OF CHRONIC PAIN

Chronic and recurring pains are significant problems for a substantial portion of the world population. The majority of surveys have been conducted in the more developed countries. It is important to note that the figures cited must be viewed with some caution, as response to mail and telephone surveys will impact the estimates of the prevalence of symptoms.

Verhaak et al. (1) reviewed 15 epidemiological studies and noted that in the adult population, chronic pain ranges from 2% to 40%. They concluded that the median point prevalence (reports of pain at the time of survey and therefore not dependent on recollection) of 15% of the adult population reported chronic pain. Volinn (2) identified seven epidemiological studies conducted in Britain, Belgium, Germany, and Sweden that reported specifically on the point prevalence of low back pain, perhaps the most commonly reported pain. Weighting the percentages by the sample size and aggregating across studies reveals that the rates of back pain in these countries average approximately 34%.

Several epidemiological studies have been published since the Verhaak et al. (1) and Volinn et al. (2) reviews. In a large-scale telephone survey conducted in Australia, approximately 17% of males and 20% of females reported the presence of some form of chronic pain and 6.8% of the general adult population reported that the presence of chronic pain interfered significantly with their activities of daily living (3). The Welsh Health Survey found that over 30% of respondents reported that they experienced back pain and 25% of the adults indicated that they had pain associated with arthritis (4). In a mail survey conducted in Sweden, 34.5% of the population indicated the presence of persistent pain for at least 3 months (5). A survey conducted in Scotland found that over 50% of respondents reported that they experienced some form of chronic pain (6). Recently, a national survey conducted in the United States indicated that more than 25% of adults interviewed reported that they had experienced lower back pain and 15% had a migraine or severe headache in the previous 3 months (6).

The wide range (6.8–50%) of reported chronic pain may be partially due to the sampling methods used, definition of chronicity, type of measure, focus on specific body locations, phrasing of the questions, and the sample size included. Despite the discrepancies, there seems no question that when asked, a significant proportion of the populations in the most developed countries indicate that they experience chronic pain.

In comparison, epidemiological studies in lower-income countries (i.e., Nepal, India, Nigeria, China, Indonesia, and the Philippines) indicate comparable point prevalence rates of 18.5% overall, but almost half the rate for back pain reported in more developed countries (2). Overall, the World Health Organization estimates that 20% of individuals worldwide have some form of chronic pain (www.who.int, accessed on 10/21/06).

Beyond the absolute numbers, it is important to consider the behavioral impact of symptoms for those who report they have chronic pain. In particular, are those who report chronic pain impaired or disabled by their symptom? The results of the Australian survey mentioned above noted that approximately 35% of those who specified that they experienced chronic pain reported that pain interfered with their daily activities (3).

Back pain is one of the most common sources of disability as well as pain. According to the U.S. Labor Bureau of Labor Statistics, lower-back injuries were the leading occupational injury during 2005 in the United States (www.bls.gov, accessed on 11/3/06). The international literature regarding the incidence of disabling lower back pain reports it as an even greater problem in Canada, Great Britain, the Netherlands, and Sweden in comparison to the United States and Germany (7). Specifically, the days absent from work each year per patient ranged from 9 days in the United States, to 10 days in West Germany, to 20 days in Canada, to 25 days in The Netherlands, to 30 days in Great Britain, and to 40 days in Sweden (7). In the Netherlands, over 10,000 new cases of work-related disabilities are reported annually (8). In the United Kingdom, 12.5% of all unemployed people cite back pain as the reason for their unemployment, with an estimated 2.5 million people reportedly having back pain every day of the year (9). In the United States, it is estimated that over 140 million days are lost to work because of back pain (10). In a primary-care cohort in the United States, 18% of back pain patients asserted that they were unable to obtain or maintain full-time work over a 3-year period because of their pain (11). Back pain, however, is not the only pain problem having a significant impact on functioning. For example, in the primary-care cohort study, 13% of people with headache also noted excessive disability experienced due to their symptoms (11).

Health Care for Chronic Pain

Another way to view the data on chronic pain is to examine how the symptoms impact health-care utilization. In the United States in 2004, 10.1% of all physician office visits and 13.9% of all emergency-room visits were due to reports of musculoskeletal symptoms and 15.6% of all emergency-room visits were for general symptoms such as pain (12). Furthermore, in the United States, 17% of patients seen in primary care report persistent pain (13) and 5% of all patients treated in primary care receive a prescription for an opioid (14). In the national survey in the United States mentioned previously, 4.2% of adults reported that they had taken an opioid in the past month for pain relief (6).

Based on a national survey of pain specialists conducted in 1995, an estimated 2.9 million Americans (1.1% of the population) are treated annually by health-care professionals specializing in chronic pain (15). This figure does not, of course, include patients treated by primary-care physicians or specialists who do not consider themselves pain specialists, nor does it include visits to practitioners of complementary and alternative medicine modalities, or self-medication using over-the-counter preparations.

In the previously mentioned study conducted in Australia examining health-care utilization, Blyth et al. (3) examined health-care utilization in people with chronic pain. They found that individuals who experienced chronic pain with a high level of impediment in activities of daily living demonstrated a twofold increase in visits to primary-care settings and hospitalizations and a fivefold increase in emergency-room visits during a 12-month period, as compared to individuals who did not report chronic pain. These findings were obtained after adjusting for known predictors: age, gender, general health, comorbidities, psychological distress, and access to health care (3). An Internet-based survey of 2569 people with fibromyalgia syndrome determined that over 50% of this sample reported five or more visits to health-care providers in the previous year. Thirteen percent noted 12 or more visits in this time period and 29% sought treatment at a hospital emergency department at least once, and some as many as four times in the previous year (16).

The figures enumerated attest to the significant numbers of people who report that they experience chronic pain and that pain significantly impacts their lives. Chronic pain, however, not only affects the individual reporting the symptoms but his or her significant others. If we consider spouses, partners, and family members, then the absolute numbers of people in the population affected by pain expand geometrically, leaving only a minority of the population untouched at any one point in time. Few, if any of us, will completely avoid an intimate relationship with persistent pain symptoms at some time during our lives.

DIRECT COSTS OF CHRONIC PAIN

Clinicians have an extensive arsenal available to treat people with chronic pain—pharmacological preparations (e.g., opioids, nonsteroidals, anticonvulsants, antidepressants, NMDA antagonists, topical preparations), operative procedures, physical modalities (e.g., ultrasound, transcutaneous electrical nerve stimulation, diathermy), regional anesthesia (e.g., epidural steroids, neural blockade), neuroaugmentation modalities [e.g., spinal column stimulators (SCSs), implantable drug delivery systems (IDDS), etc.], multidisciplinary pain rehabilitation programs (MPRPs) (e.g., interdisciplinary pain centers, functional restoration programs), and complementary and alternative medicine modalities (e.g., chiropractic, acupuncture, massage, biofeedback).

The direct costs for the totality of these approaches are astronomical and underscore the extremes undertaken to ward off the human suffering associated with chronic pain. In the United Kingdom, back pain alone is estimated to cost society $26–$49 billion each year (17). Direct costs associated with migraine in the United States are estimated to be in excess of $2.4 billion (18). De Lissovy et al. (19) estimated that the cost of treatment, per patient, in the first year following failed back surgery for pain was approximately $34,716 in the United States.

The annual total of both direct and indirect costs for chronic pain is estimated to be as high as $294.5 billion per year (20), with back pain alone estimated to cost in excess of $100 billion per year (21), i.e., approximately 2% of the annual gross domestic product of the United States (22). Cousins (23) suggested that the costs of health care for patients with chronic pain might exceed the combined costs of treating patients with coronary artery disease, cancer, and AIDS.

Pharmacological Costs

The vast majority of symptoms associated with chronic pain are managed with medication. Pain medications are the second most frequently prescribed drugs (after cardiac–renal) during visits to physicians' offices and emergency departments, accounting for 12% of all medications prescribed in ambulatory visits (24). As noted previously, 4.2% of adults in the United States reported taking an opioid for pain management in the preceding month (6). According to pharmaceutical industry data, pain is a $13.2-billion market (A Chappell, Eli Lilly Company, personal communication, October 2004).

Over the past decade, there has been a surge of papers extolling the virtues of opioids to treat chronic pain not associated with cancer. Additionally, there has been recognition that the negative consequences previously feared (e.g., addiction, drug diversion) may not be as common as previously thought in this patient population. The prevalence of abusive behaviors may, however, be substantial. For example, based on urine toxicology screens, procurement of drugs from multiple prescribers, diversion, and prescription forgery, the numbers may exceed 20% (25) and may be as high as 40% (25).

In 1999, over 3 million prescriptions were written for one opioid alone, Oxycontin® (27). The costs of drugs do vary by location; thus, the cost of one 20-mg tablet of Oxycontin® in two locations in Atlanta, GA, in the year 2000 ranged from $3.34 to $3.84 per tablet (28). Straus noted that a typical failed back surgery syndrome patient in two practices in Atlanta, along with NSAIDs and other drugs (e.g., muscle relaxants, antidepressants, anxiolytics, anticonvulsants), might be prescribed five 20-mg tablets a day. Therefore, the annual costs for Oxycontin® alone would exceed $6903 per year, not including related physician visits or laboratory work.

There has been growing support for the use of anticonvulsants, antidepressants, and topical preparations for neuropathic pain syndromes. The cost of these medications also varies by location. Again, in Atlanta in 2000, Straus (28) reported that one frequently prescribed anticonvulsant medication for neuropathic pain, Neurontin®, costs $1.89 for each 300-mg tablet (this was prior to it going off patent, and generic versions are available at lower prices). Based on the data provided by Straus, failed back surgery patients would spend almost $2088 per year for

Neurontin® alone. This is a relatively conservative figure, as patients may be prescribed up to four times the dosage stipulated by Straus.

Surgical

After medication, perhaps the most common treatment for persistent pain is surgery. Approximately 31,000 lumbar surgeries are performed primarily for pain each year at a conservatively estimated cost of $27,577 per operation (29). Using these figures, the cost of lumbar surgery in the United States would exceed $8.6 billion each year. There are, of course, many other frequently used surgical procedures that are performed to alleviate pain other than lumbar surgery. Information on the frequency with which these surgical procedures are performed and their costs are more difficult to obtain than those for back pain. There is, however, no doubt that the cost is substantial. (Please refer to chap. 6 in this book for more detailed information on problems associated with spine surgery for chronic pain.)

Implantable Devices

Over the past quarter century, technological advances have resulted in the development of a number of sophisticated implantable devices (i.e., SCSs, IDDS) that are used to treat patients with chronic pain. Segal and Stacey (30) suggested that by 1996, 10,000 SCSs had been implanted worldwide, with 7000 implanted in the United States. Bell et al. (31) projected that the 5-year cost required for treating and maintaining patients with SCSs in the United States would be $144,255. Thus, in the United States by 1996, over $0.5 billion had been committed to these devices, related services, and treatment for adverse events. In 2006, correcting for inflation, this cost would exceed several billion dollars.

IDDS are being advocated to treat recalcitrant chronic pain (32). The costs for this technology can be quite expensive. The initial costs for screening, hospital, and professional charges can range from $27,577 to $55,134. De Lissovoy et al. (19) suggested that the 5-year costs of IDDS would range from $82,893 to $125,102. However, if the annual costs for medical management range from $13,000 to $19,000, then treatment with IDDS would be expected to "break even" in 4–10 years. Similar calculations for SCSs suggest that the 5-year expected costs would be $76,180 and thus the break-even point would occur in 4–6 years.

Multidisciplinary Pain Rehabilitation Centers

Based on the Marketdata survey (15), only about 176,850 (6% of those treated by pain specialists) of chronic pain patients are treated at MPRPs. Using the average figure of nonsurgical health-care expenditures of $44,990 (33), 7 years as the mean duration of pain, and the mean number of surgeries of 1.7 (34) at an average cost of $15,000–$30,000 (35), we estimate that the cost of health care alone *prior* to treatment of patients at MPRPs in 2006 would be in excess of $67–$135 billion. Involvement of multiple disciplines at an MPRP is labor intensive and costly. This is in part due to the number of clinicians involved in providing treatment, and each of the clinicians involved expects payment for the services he or she provides. Based on the average cost of treatment at MPRPs ($15,339) (15) and the number treated (176,850), the annual cost of treatment at MPRPs would exceed $2.7 billion.

INDIRECT COST ASSOCIATED WITH CHRONIC PAIN

Health-care expenditures comprise only a portion of the costs associated with chronic pain. The majority of the costs are associated with disability compensation, lost productivity, and lost tax revenue, among others. Frymoyer and Durett (35) projected the costs for back pain alone, the most prevalent chronic pain syndrome, to exceed $34 billion for health care, $18.9–$71 billion for disability compensation, $6.9 billion for lost productivity, and $7 billion in legal services. Indirect costs associated with migraine are anticipated to exceed $30 billion each year in the United States (18). Again, using U.S. data, patients with rheumatoid arthritis are projected to incur over $21 billion in medical expenditures and work loss (36). Pain is not just costly in the United States but in other parts of the world as well, for example, in the state of Victoria (Melbourne), Australia, over $151 million was paid out in claims for back pain in 1996–1997 (37). We have not mentioned the costs associated with the multiple medical and mental comorbidities generally experienced by individuals with chronic pain nor have we addressed the costs of utilization of health care for comorbid conditions, which are estimated to be high (38).

What is evident from the figures presented is that chronic pain is both prevalent and is, regardless of how it is treated, exceedingly expensive. Additionally, despite the high cost of treating chronic pain, relief for many individuals with chronic pain remains elusive and total elimination of pain is exceedingly rare, which is why it is called *chronic* pain. As we shall see next, although there have been phenomenal advances in the knowledge of neurophysiology, anatomy, and biochemistry, along with the development of potent analgesic medications and other innovative medical and surgical interventions, we have not eliminated pain and disability as problems for a significant portion of the population.

EFFICACY OF TREATMENT FOR CHRONIC PAIN

As noted, a large and growing number of treatments are available to manage acute and chronic pain. Since the number of people affected and the costs are astronomical, it is legitimate to ask how effective—both clinically and economically—are treatments that are currently available to manage chronic pain. It is impossible to provide a single answer to this deceptively simple question beyond, "it depends." It depends on (1) knowledge of the mechanisms involved as the source or cause of pain, (2) individual variations in patients treated, (3) the criteria used to determine success, (4) the methods used for assessing these criteria, (5) the design of the studies that attempt to establish effectiveness, and (6) the data analytic method selected to evaluate the outcomes. The emphasis on evidence-based medicine (EBM) and the newer concept of "pay for performance" makes these questions of effectiveness, both clinical and cost, particular concerns to society. In the remainder of this chapter, we will consider treatment efficacy.

EVIDENCE-BASED MEDICINE

The prevalence of pain, the diversity of treatment available, the inconsistency in the outcomes of clinical trials, and the inability to compare results between studies directly has led to considerable consternation and repeated calls for "more and better research." The inadequacy of the data and the practice of relying on clinical judgment have resulted in pleas for "evidence-based medicine," a phrase that has progressed from a buzzword to a mantra. In 1996, one of the initial proponents of EBM, David Sackett, referred to EBM as the "conscientious, explicit and judicious use of current best evidence in making decisions about the care of individual patients" (39). After criticism was raised about the apparent failure to include clinical experience in decision making based solely on published research, Sackett et al. (40) attempted to address the concerns by noting that EBM involved "the integration of best research evidence with *clinical expertise* and *patient values* (emphasis added)." The primary goal of EBM is to improve health outcomes through the deployment of the most effective interventions.

Why is EBM needed? There are a number of cogent reasons. There have been rapid advances in health care, but a lag between evidence and practice, with great variability among providers in the use of evidence presented in published studies. Only about 15% of medical interventions currently in practice are supported by solid scientific outcome data.

EBM emphasizes on standardization of methods to appraise data and to promote more efficient use of available health-care resources. Promulgation of EBM may serve to overcome clinical entropy. As a process, EBM provides methods to synthesize multiple published studies that meet established standards and consequently are carefully designed and well controlled. The use of explicit inclusion criteria should assure quality control, in contrast to reviews based on "box scores" of trials regardless of quality, lack of standards for inclusion, and with no guarantee of comprehensiveness. Rather, studies may be "cherry picked" to support the authors' preconceived biases. The promise of EBM is that potential sources of bias will be minimized (or at least transparent), resulting in the validity of the conclusions being maximized.

The steps of EBM consist of (1) formulation of questions to answer and information needs, (2) seeking answers supported by the best evidence, (3) examination of the quality of the evidence, (4) application of evidence to implement best health-care practice, and (5) evaluation of health-care practice. The sources of evidence are derived from published studies, available reviews, abstracts, and unpublished studies and data. They are typically acquired from the following:

- Cochrane Collaboration reviews
- other published systematic reviews
- commissioned reviews
- published studies using MEDLINE, CINAHL, Embase, PubMed, and other databases
- abstracts and unpublished studies and data
- references in published articles and chapters in edited books

There are a number of standards for judging the quality of evidence. A common approach is to weigh the quality of evidence in a hierarchy with meta-analysis of multiple well-designed controlled studies at the top and case studies at the bottom. The latter should be given the least value. These would then be followed by well-designed experimental studies, well-designed quasi-experimental studies and non-randomized controlled, single-group pre–post, cohort, time series, or matched-case controlled studies, well-designed nonexperimental studies such as comparative and

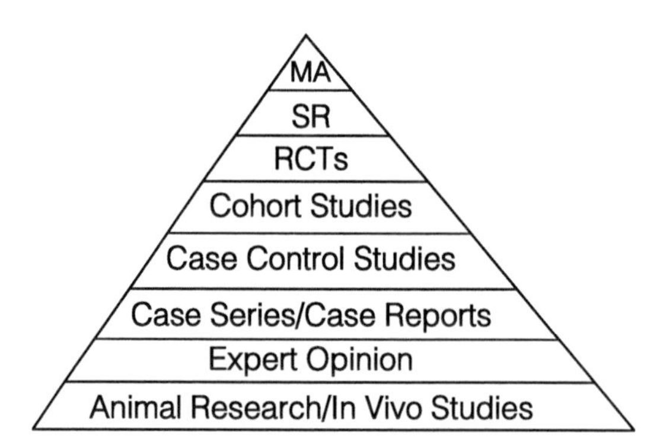

FIGURE 1 Hierarchy of evidence in evidence-based medicine (1). Abbreviations: MA, meta-analysis; SR, systematic reviews; RCTs, randomized controlled trials.

correlational descriptive, and case studies. Figure 1 illustrates that much of medical practice is based on the weakest but largest sources of information—case reports and clinical examples.

Given the advantages of EBM enumerated, one wonders why there is such resistance among practitioners. Among the concerns most commonly raised are practitioners' perceptions of a loss of autonomy. There appears to be a related belief that EBM will diminish clinical experience and expertise, as well as interfering with provider–patient relationship. Other criticisms have been raised that EBM will be used solely for cost containment (i.e., financially motivated). Furthermore, although the methods described may sound good, there are a number of issues that mitigate some of the enthusiasm for EBM (Table 1). EBM has become almost synonymous with double-blind randomized control trials. The assumption by some is that such trials are the only way to determine the validity of the claim of treatment effectiveness. However, there is as much disagreement as to what qualifies as acceptable evidence as this is what qualifies as good clinical practice. Some of the issues that need to be considered when evaluating randomized trials are enumerated in Table 2.

Although inmeta-analyses and systematic reviews of randomized controlled trial (RCT) are given the greatest weight in EBM, we need to be cognizant of the limitations beyond the technical ones noted in Tables 1 and 2. There is inherent subjectivity regardless of the technical sophistication reported, and one should be wary of a false sense of certainty created by EBM. Examination of EBM reviews reveals (1) inconsistency among conclusions of different reviews, even using similar quality ratings, (2) variability of results among outcome criteria, (3) inconsistency in use of inclusion criteria in selecting studies to retain, (4) variability in outcome criteria and measures across studies (ease of measurement vs. relevance), and (5) technical bias favors research investigators' know how to perform.

We can also note some EBM paradoxes: (1) no definitive evidence *whatsoever* has accumulated to show that "medicine by EBM" is superior to "medicine as usual" (43)—there is no evidence for EBM. That is, no studies have reported that the use of EBM to guide practice actually produces better clinical outcomes. (2) Case

TABLE 1 Some Challenges with and Concerns about the EBM Approach

- Oversimplifies the complex and interpersonal nature of clinical care
- Provides information about groups, not individual patients (reverence of group data for individual)
- Generalization from clinical trials to clinical practice ("efficacy" vs. "effectiveness" trials)
- Absence of published studies ("absence of evidence is not evidence of absence") (41)
- Heterogeneity in quality of studies combined
- Combining marginally related studies
- Inconsistency among conclusions of different reviews, even using similar quality ratings
- Variability of results among outcome criteria
- Inconsistency in use of inclusion criteria
- Inclusion criteria are not representative of clinical practice (e.g., exclude those who are medically frail, depressed, history of drug abuse)
- Intensity of monitoring in a clinical trial may be substantially different from what occurs in clinical practice
- Variability in outcome criteria and measures (ease of measurement vs. relevance)
- Time lag from review to publication (EBM is always "old medicine")
- Studies of interventions that are likely to have commercial value are most likely to be supported (e.g., drug trial vs. physical therapy trial)
- Data obtained in commercially supported studies are more likely to be positive
- Feasibility of RCTs for some interventions is limited if not impossible
- Technical bias favors research investigators' know how to do
- Positive results are more likely to be published "file draw problem" (42)
- Exclusive ("evangelical") reliance on RCTs (RCTism) as the sole means to establish "the truth"
- Idolatry of statistical significance, worship of *p* value, statistical significance does not necessarily equate with clinical importance

TABLE 2 Some Problems with Randomized Controlled Trials

- Sample included in clinical trials may not represent clinical practice inclusion and exclusion criteria (e.g., exclude women of child-bearing age, limits on age, presence of depression.)
- Difficulties with blinding (participants and providers may be able to detect treatment received)
- Ethical concerns about use of placebo treatment
- Patient willingness to be randomized in a placebo or experimental trial
- Method of recruitment will influence representativeness of the sample (e.g., referral bias, clinical vs. community sample.)
- "Denominator problem" (i.e., number of participants is known but the number eligible is unknown, except in population-based studies)
- Characteristics of volunteers for RCT (not all eligible will volunteer)
- Studies of interventions likely to have commercial value more likely to be conducted (e.g., pharmacological intervention vs. physical therapy)
- Precision of diagnoses
- Problem of dropouts and how to handle the "missing" data
- Short trial duration (typically $<$3–6 mo)
- Determining appropriate comparators
- Appropriate statistical analyses (multiple end points)
- Provide information about groups, not individuals
- Often only report statistical significance and not clinical meaningfulness or meaningful results to patients
- Bias toward studies that are easy (known methods) to conduct

examples may reveal discrepancies in RCT; yet, case reports are low in hierarchy of evidence deemed acceptable. (3) EBM, which aims to eliminate bias, can be a source of bias itself. (4) If all RCTs yielded the same results, systematic reviews would not be needed.

We do not want to throw the baby out with the bath water nor do we want to worship RCTs and p values. EBM is an important tool that must be balanced with clinical experience. EBM is not a textbook, cookbook, substitute for clinical judgment, a standard of care (legal issues), or a way of cost-cutting medicine (ethical issues). Caveat emptor!

COST-EFFECTIVENESS OF TREATMENTS FOR CHRONIC PAIN PATIENTS

A number of criteria have been used to evaluate the effectiveness of different pain treatment approaches and modalities. Self-reports of pain and adverse events are the most commonly used endpoints. Other criteria examined include functional activities, return-to-work (RTW), health-care utilization, and to a lesser extent reduction in disability compensation. One simple way to think about cost-effectiveness is to consider the cost to achieve a positive outcome for a particular patient. A simplified formula to determine cost-effectiveness is

$$\text{Cost-effectiveness} = \frac{\text{Cost of treatment X}}{\text{\% Who achieve outcome}} \text{ vs. } \frac{\text{Cost of treatment Y}}{\text{\% Who achieve outcome}}$$

When costs are not involved, one refers to the sum as the cost benefit rather than cost-effectiveness. We will examine each of the above-mentioned criteria for both clinical effectiveness and cost-effectiveness where data are available.

Pain Reduction

Medication

As noted previously, the first-line treatment for pain consists of a host of pharmacological agents. As has also been noted, pharmaceutical industry data indicate that over 312 million prescriptions for analgesic medications were written in the year 2000 in the United States, more than one prescription for analgesics for every man, woman, and child (M. Williams, Merck pharmaceuticals, personal communication, November 18, 2001).

Despite their frequent use, currently available medications do not eliminate pain. For example, the average pain reduction for patients placed on "long-term opioids" is approximately 31%, when effects reported in studies are weighted by sample size (44). We placed "long-term" in quotation marks, as the duration of treatment in the majority of the published RCTs ranges from a week to 3 months, although they may be followed by an open-label extension (45). The weighted mean duration of randomized controlled trials of opioids is approximately 5 weeks (44).

At a recent consensus meeting of specialists who treat neuropathic pain, tricyclic antidepressants, anticonvulsant drugs, and topical preparations were viewed as the treatments of choice (46). Seldom, however, do these pharmacological agents reduce pain below a rating of 4 on an 11-point numerical rating scale (e.g., 0–10 with 10 being the highest level of pain), with only 30–40% of patients reporting at least a 50% reduction in pain (47,48). It is noteworthy that the inclusion criterion for many drug trials is a pain intensity rating of 4. Thus, many participants in a "successful" (statistically significant) clinical trial of a drug would be eligible for inclusion in a subsequent clinical trial! This observation is not included to denigrate the reduction of pain by 30–40%, but rather to acknowledge that these treatments are not providing "cures" for chronic pain.

A common outcome criterion used in drug trials is the "number needed to treat" (NNT) to achieve a 50% reduction in pain beyond what would have achieved with a placebo. Several meta-analyses have reported using this criterion for a range of antidepressant and anticonvulsant medications for different pain syndromes, primarily neuropathic pain. Pooling the data from these trials reveals that the NNTs to achieve 50% pain reduction were 2.9 (47). That is to say, for every three people receiving an antidepressant or anticonvulsant for their pain, only one will experience at least 50% pain relief that he or she would not have experienced with a placebo. Conversely, two of the three treated patients will have less than a 50% reduction in pain. We will return to the criteria on which to base conclusions about clinical effectiveness. As is the case for opioids, the duration of trials for anticonvulsants and antidepressants is relatively brief, usually less than 3 months.

Obviously, medications do not eradicate all pain for the majority of patients treated. This does not mean that these drugs are not beneficial, only that we need to be cautious in what outcomes can reasonably be expected. The data also suggest that there is a need to consider treatment combinations that may potentially improve outcomes, since individual drugs do not completely eliminate the problem of pain for the majority of patients. For a more in-depth analysis of the utilization of opioids for the treatment of chronic pain, please refer to chapter 5 in this book.

Surgery

Persistence of back pain, and to a lesser extent other chronic pain syndromes, frequently leads to surgery. However, a number of studies reveal that significant pain may persist following surgery (49). For example, in an early study, Dvorak et al. (49) studied 575 back pain patients who had surgery for herniated disks and noted that 70% continued to report back pain up to 17 years following surgery. Similar results have been reported in more recent studies. Lehmann et al. (50) showed that 75% of patients who underwent spinal fusion for back pain continued to report pain following surgery. North et al. (51) noted that 66% of patients who underwent repeat surgery for back pain continued to experience pain 5 years following surgery, and Fritzell et al. (52) reported that following lumbar surgery, pain improved by an average of 30%, with only 17% "pain free" following spinal fusion.

Spinal Cord Stimulators SCS

Several studies of SCSs have reported impressive results in pain reduction for carefully selected patients with pain of long duration. For example, in a well-designed study, North et al. (53) reported on a long-term follow-up (mean 7 years) for a consecutive series of patients. They noted that 52% of 171 patients receiving permanent implants reported at least 50% relief of pain, and 60% indicated that they would undergo the procedure again even though they still continued to have at least some pain. In a systematic review, Turner et al. (54) reviewed 39 studies of SCS for low back pain and concluded that on average, 59% of patients experienced at least 50% reduction in pain.

More recently, Van Buyten et al. (55) reported that 4 years following implantation of an SCS, 61% of patients continued to report that their pain ranged from "uncomfortable" to "horrible," with fewer than 37% of the patients rating their pain in this category at follow-up than prior to implantation. One caution in interpreting these results is that the follow-up excluded 22 patients who had the stimulators removed, 20 of whom could not be contacted, and another 22 who had died (none attributed to the SCS). Burchiel et al. (56) presented 1-year follow-up data and reported that 40% of implanted patients indicated at least 50% reduction in pain. However, the absolute percent average change in pain severity reported was only 18.6%, decreasing from a mean rating of 7.31 to 5.95 (scale ranges from 0 to 10). Once again, these results indicate that following treatment, patients continue to report that their pain is at least at a moderate level of severity and they would be eligible for participation in another clinical trial with the inclusion criterion of pain severity at a level of 4. These data raise questions regarding the meaning of categorical ratings of percent of pain reduction. For example, a reduction in pain of 18.6% would not reach the somewhat liberal criterion of clinical significance, 30% reduction, as suggested by Farrar et al. (57). Moreover, the data indicate that patients continued to experience substantial pain severity after receiving the implant.

A number of SCS studies consumptions report significant reductions in consumption of analgesics. North and colleagues (53) reported that 58% of patients treated with SCS demonstrated a reduction in or elimination of analgesic medication consumption. In a retrospective study, Kumar et al. (58) reported that 40% of patients no longer used prescription analgesics, and Ohnmeiss et al. (59) reported that 2 years after implantation, 84% of patients decreased or eliminated opioids. In one recent study, SCS has been reported to reduce consumption of opioids by 35% (45), and another study (60) noted a 76.7% decrease in oral pain medication following implantation of an intraspinal infusion system. In contrast, however, in a prospective study, Burchiel et al. (56) found that only 7% of patients reported elimination of opioid use 1 year after the implant. The medication sparing effects for implantable therapies and MPRP can provide significant savings in costs for medication and health care. It is important, however, to acknowledge that none of the available treatments for chronic pain have been demonstrated to eliminate all pain for all patients.

IDDS

Significant reductions of pain have also been reported for IDDS for both chronic pain associated with cancer and other pain syndromes (e.g., back pain). Good to excellent results have been reported in most published studies. For example, Hassenbusch et al. (61) and Paice et al. (62) both reported a mean pain reduction of approximately 60% following epidural infusions in mixed samples of patients with different pain syndromes. In a small study ($n = 16$), Kumar and colleagues (63) reported a mean 57.5% reduction in pain at a follow-up of over 2 years, with 44% ($n = 7$) patients reporting greater than 50% reduction of pain. These results are particularly impressive, since the patients who were included had inadequate pain control following conservative approaches, long-term use of opioids, and implantation of an SCS.

In a systematic review of intrathecal opioids, Turner et al. (in press) (64) reported that the proportion of patients with $\geq$50% pain relief at 6 months ranged from 38% to 56%, with the pain reduction decreasing in longer follow-ups from 30% to 44%. Based on their review, the authors concluded that

> on average ... patients [who] receive permanent IDDS, ... pain seems to improve, but *increases* in opioid dosage and change in medication are often needed to maintain pain improvement. Long-term effects ... remain *unclear*. ... the effectiveness of IDDS in improving pain and function, as compared with a placebo, natural history, or other treatment is unknown. Drug side effects and other complications requiring additional surgeries are *common* [emphasis added].

It is important to be alert to the mixed diagnosis of patients treated across and within studies using the same treatment, as some syndromes may be more or less responsive to the treatment. For example, in contrast to the Hassenbusch et al. (61) and Paice et al. (62) studies, Hassenbusch et al. (65) found that pain reduction was only 39% for a sample of patients with neuropathic pain who were implanted, while in a mixed sample of patients with predominantly neuropathic pain, Anderson and Burchiel (66) found that only one-half (11/22) of patients achieved at least a 25% reduction in pain.

MPRPs

The reduction of pain following treatment at MPRPs has been reported to be statistically significant in several meta-analyses (34,67,68), with two meta-analyses (34,69) reporting that the mean pain reduction for patients treated at MPRPs is 37%. Once again, we note that the majority of patients continue to experience considerable pain. Interestingly, the pain reduction achieved at MPRPs is accompanied with a significant decrease (63%) in prescription pain medication (34). These results may seem somewhat paradoxical given the growing use of medications to treat chronic pain, but may reflect a referral bias to MPRPs.

Regardless of the treatment, it generally appears that pain is reduced by between 30% and 40%, but in fewer than 50% of patients. If the results indicate that disparate treatments produce roughly the same outcome, then the issue of cost becomes especially relevant. How much does it cost to produce comparable outcomes? Consideration of the data reviewed suggests that MPRPs are substantially more cost-effective than the alternatives. For example, using the cost-effectiveness formula presented earlier and the estimated costs of treatment, the cost of one patient achieving the average reduction in pain for MPRPs would be $30,678, compared to spinal surgery that would cost $55,154. Based on these figures, MPRPs would create the same outcomes at 44% of the cost. It should also be noted that these figures do not consider additional costs associated with adverse events.

Iatrogenic Complications and Adverse Events

At least as important as reduction in pain severity are the potentials for iatrogenic complications and adverse events that may result from the treatment. Selection of any intervention must balance the positive outcomes with potential negative consequences. Each of the treatments for chronic pain patients, perhaps with the exception of MPRPs, has the potential for undesirable consequences.

Medications

Long-term use of medication raises concerns about tolerance, tolerability, drug misuse and abuse (i.e., opioids), and side effects including neurotoxicity (47,70). Studies of chronic pain patients taking opioids on a long-term basis suggest that over

45% may be engaging in aberrant drug-taking behaviors (26). There are always contraindications based on the patient's medical condition, age, child-bearing status, co-occurring medical conditions, and other medications prescribed.

Surgery

Studies have reported that a significant percentage of chronic pain patients treated with surgery report that their pain is *worse* following surgery (50,71,72). Malter and colleagues (73) reported complication rates of 18% and 7% for back pain patients having lumbar surgery involving fusion and with laminectomy or discectomy alone, respectively. Reoperation rates were 18% and 15% for fusion and nonfusion patients. Up to 33% of back surgeries are repeated because of problems associated with previous surgery (71). Subsequent operations do not guarantee resolution of pain. Some studies acknowledge the poor results achieved for reoperations (51,72). Bell et al. (31) suggested that there is a 10% probability of a repeat surgery in every succeeding year following lumbar surgery.

SCS

In a systematic review of outcome studies for SCS, Turner and colleagues (54) reported that a review of 13 studies indicated that, on average, 42% of patients experienced complications requiring interventions related to the procedure itself or malfunctions of the device. Although many of the complications are minor, some require substantial medical or surgical intervention and, consequently, cost.

Two recent case series reported complications associated with SCS. In Canada, Kumar and colleagues (74) reviewed their 10-year experience with SCS with 160 patients and noted 51 adverse events in 42 (39 related to hardware and 12 biological) of 160 patients implanted. The mean cost of complication averaged $6241, with some exceeding $20,000. In the United States, Rosenow et al. (75) reported on 289 patients who received 577 procedures between 1998 and 2002, 43.5% of which involved revision or removal of hardware, with poor pain relief being the most common indicator for revision. In this study, 46% of implanted patients required hardware revisions and 22.5% required multiple revisions.

Health-Care Utilization

Many treatments for chronic pain may actually increase rather than decrease health-care utilization. For example, placing patients on long-term opioids requires additional medical monitoring. Similarly, implantation with SCS or IDDS requires routine monitoring, replacements of the devices as needed, and refilling of drug reservoirs for IDDSs. All invasive interventions have the potential for creating additional medical problems that need to be treated as do prescriptions for medications that potentially produce adverse events that require medical attention.

In contrast to the above-mentioned treatments, in a meta-analysis of 42 published studies on the efficacy of MPRPs, Flor et al. (34) reported significant reductions in health-care utilization following treatment at MPRPs. Most of these trials had only short-term follow-ups. A recent long-term follow-up study (76) reported significant reductions of hospital admissions by a factor of 1.5 along with a significant reduction of in-hospital days (10-days fewer) occurring following treatment at a MPRP. Importantly, these reductions were maintained 10 years following treatment.

Physical Functioning

Outcomes regarding changes in pain severity are dependent on patients' self-reports. There are a number of factors that can bias patients' responses. Moreover, the relationship between pain reports and functional behavior is modest. As a consequence, evaluation of the effectiveness of pain treatment approaches should consider functional outcomes such as improvement in physical activity and, when appropriate, RTW, along with reductions in pain severity.

Medications

Inspection of the pharmacological studies for pain reveals a striking lack of attention to functional outcomes. For example, in one systematic review of antidepressants for neuropathic pain (48), only 1 of 20 studies included *any* indication of improvements in physical functioning following initiation of treatment. The emphasis in the pharmacological literature is almost exclusively on pain relief and adverse events. There are no data demonstrating that significant numbers of patients return to work, and minimal data on improvement in functioning following treatment with long-term opioids (77), tricyclic antidepressants (47,78–80), or anticonvulsant medication (78–81). Similarly, outcome studies for regional anesthesia ignore RTW as an outcome. Only 1 of 14 studies examining the efficacy of regional blockage for complex regional pain syndrome included functional measures as an outcome (82).

IDDS

As is the case for pharmacological studies, outcome research for IDDS rarely attends to the impact of treatment on functioning. In the 18 studies described in a recent review of intrathecal morphine (83), only 4 included outcomes related to functional activities. When functional outcomes are reported, the results are not particularly impressive. For example, Paice et al. (62) noted that only 22.8% of a mixed sample of cancer and noncancer patients with pain reported "great" increases in activities of daily living; however, 24.6% reported no change and 3.8% indicated a *decrease* in functional activities.

SCS

In contrast to pharmacological, regional anesthesia, and IDDS studies, investigators evaluating the effectiveness of SCS, surgery, and MPRP have, more frequently, considered changes in functional outcomes along with pain severity. For example, in a retrospective study of SCS, Van Buyten et al. (55) noted a 26.6% improvement in daily activities at follow-up. Kumar et al. (58) found a 37.5% reduction in the number of patients reporting restrictions in their activities following implantation of an IDDS.

Surgery

The evidence regarding the efficacy of surgery for improving function in patients with chronic pain is quite limited. In one of the few studies to examine this outcome, Gallon (84) noted that 58% of back pain patients who had surgery described themselves as *worse* on a measure of physical functioning, compared to 30% of patients who indicated that they were more disabled following standard care. Another study by Fritzell et al. (52) found that only around 30% of patients reported functional improvements following spinal fusions.

MPRPs

Flor and colleagues (34), in their meta-analysis, reported a 43% increase in physical activities following treatment in MPRPs. We can use the cost-effectiveness formula to compare the outcomes of SCS and IDDS compared to those of MPRPs. Once again using the formula presented, it appears that the cost to improve physical functioning would be $35,672 ($15,339/.42) for MPRPS, $112,781 ($30,000/.266) for SCS, and between $73,539 ($27,577/.374) and $147,024 ($55,134/.275) for IDDS. Based on these figures, we can conclude that MPRPs are two to four times more cost-effective than SCS and IDDS for producing improved physical functioning of patients with chronic pain.

Return-to-Work

Many studies reporting on changes in physical activities have relied on patients' self-reports. A more objective measure of function is RTW. There are a number of caveats that need to be taken into consideration, however, when considering rates of RTW. RTW may have little to do with the *readiness* of an individual to resume job-related activities (85). For example, the mean duration of pain for patients treated at MPRPs is 7 years (34), and someone who has been off of work for such a long period may not have a job to which to return. Additionally, their skills may be outdated, making return to their previous job difficult. Economic factors (e.g., the job market) will also influence whether someone returns to gainful employment following treatment. Finally, administrative decisions regarding appropriateness of RTW may be primary, with little consideration given to the presence of the patients' symptoms or physical capacities. Furthermore, research does not report whether individuals are returning to a full-time status or regular work duties versus more limited job functions. These limitations, however, apply equally to all treatments; therefore, even though there are significant limitations, RTW rates can be used to compare different treatments.

RTW rates following lumbar surgery have been reported to be as low as 20% (51). Examination of outcomes of lumbar surgery for worker compensation patients reveal that none of the patients in the sample actually returned to work (86).

One recent study reported 50% RTW following radiofrequency facet joint denervation for the treatment of low back pain (86). At first, this outcome seems quite impressive; however, the group of patients treated with *sham therapy* showed almost the identical rate of RTW. These sobering results underscore the necessity of developing and using appropriate placebo treatments.

Studies of patients who have been implanted with SCSs suggest that from 5% to 40% eventually returned to work (51,53,87,88). One of the few studies of the results of IDDS on RTW indicates that none of the patients ($n = 16$) returned to gainful employment (65). These outcomes can be compared to the RTW rates reported for patients treated at MPRPs, which range from 48% to 65% (34).

The outcomes following treatment at MPRPs are quite impressive given the long pain duration (mean = 7 years) for treated patients (34). Two meta-analyses (34,69) confirmed that the long-term effects on RTW for pain patients treated at MPRPs were very positive and the results were superior to other active treatments.

Once again, using the cost-effectiveness formula mentioned earlier, it becomes apparent that MPRPs are substantially more cost-effective if the criteria is RTW, with MPRPs being 12 times more cost-effective than conventional medical care, 17.5

times more cost-effective than SCS, and 30 times more cost-effective than surgery (89).

Closure of Disability Claims

Disability payments may exceed medical costs for chronic pain sufferers by a factor of five. An important outcome, at least from a societal perspective, is closure of disability claims. Once again, we need to invoke a caution. As in the case for RTW, closure of disability claims may depend on administrative decisions and not on pain per se. Only outcome studies for MPRPs and one for SCS (56) have reported changes in disability claims following treatment. Flor et al. (34) noted an approximate 50% reduction in rates of disability following treatment at MPRPs. This rate can be compared with the study of SCS conducted in the United States (57) that reported a 20% reduction (not statistically significant) in disability status 1 year following implant. Again, using the cost-effectiveness formula, we find that MPRPs would require $30,678 to close one disability claim compared to SCS, which, at a conservative cost of $30,000, would convert into a cost-effectiveness rate of $150,000 ($30,000/.20). This rate is 4.9 times greater than that required to close a single disability claim compared to the cost for this result following treatment at an MPRP.

Thomsen et al. (90) used social records instead of self-reports to evaluate the efficacy of an MPRP. They obtained data on disability and welfare costs for a period of 6 months prior to entry to a 4-month waiting list and at a 9-month follow-up after termination to evaluate the efficacy of an MPRP. The fact that the data were not obtained from self-report is particularly noteworthy. The authors identified significant reductions in social transfers (welfare benefits, sickness benefit, and pensions). These investigators noted a 63% decline in benefits during the follow-up period.

CONCLUSIONS FROM RESEARCH ON COMMON TREATMENT FOR CHRONIC PAIN

It would be impossible to review the voluminous research on clinical trials for chronic pain. However, it is useful to cite some of the conclusions based on meta-analyses and systematic reviews published in the literature. Reviews of the most common treatments for chronic pain draw some sobering conclusions. For example, in reviewing the literature on the long-term use of opioids, Von Korff and Deyo (91) opined that there have not been adequate trials to prove the "*safety and effectiveness of long-term opioid therapy*" in chronic noncancer pain. Please refer to chapter 5 in this book for additional analysis of problems with chronic opioid therapy. De Kleuver et al. (92), after reviewing the 15-year history of total disk replacement for back pain (arthrodesis), concluded that there were *insufficient data* on the safety and efficacy of the procedures and suggested that total disk replacement should be considered as an experimental procedure. Gibson et al. (93) noted that "*There is no acceptable evidence of the efficacy of any form of fusion for degenerative lumbar spondylosis, back pain or instability.*" Deyo et al. (94) concurred but went one step farther and concluded that the results have been "disappointing." These sobering evaluations have not, however, resulted in any decline in the frequency with which these procedures are being performed. In fact the numbers have more than doubled from around 50,000 in 1995 to almost 120,000 in 2001 (95). Based on a recent Cochrane review, van Tulder et al. (96) suggested that cognitive interventions combined with exercise (rehabilitation) is recommended for chronic low back pain, and fusion surgery may be considered only in carefully selected patients *after* active rehabilitation programs during a 2-year period of time have failed.

Koes et al. (97) conducted a systematic review and concluded that the benefits, *if any*, of epidural corticosteroid injections for sciatica due to herniated nucleus pulposas are only short term. Sanders et al. (98) agreed, concluding that "despite growing use, there is currently no demonstration for the utility of using epidural steroid or facet joint injection .... and such therapies are not recommended [for chronic pain patients] ...." Cochrane reviews of randomized trials involving patients with low back pain suggest that there is a lack of convincing evidence supporting injection therapies for low back pain (99). Based on a review of 44 published studies, Merrill (100) similarly concluded that the scientific literature provides little proof of long-term benefit for those patients treated with nerve blocks, epidural steroids, facet injections, or IDET. Van Tulder et al. (96) concurred and noted that "... facet joint, epidural, trigger point and sclerosant injections have not clearly been shown to be effective and can consequently not be ... recommended." Yet, in the United States, epidural steroid injections are the most commonly performed pain management procedures (101).

Turner et al. (64) summarized the data on IDDS and concluded that on average, patients who received permanent IDDS experienced some reductions in pain, although this was accompanied by increases in opioid dosages often needed to maintain pain improvement. However, the long-term effects remain unclear and the effectiveness of IDDS in improving pain and function, as compared with a placebo, natural history, or other treatment, is unknown. These authors also alert us that drug side-effects and other complications requiring additional surgeries are commonly observed.

A multinational study conducted in the United States, Europe, and Israel (102) investigated the benefits of surgery, manipulation, traction, heat and cold, massage, TENS, physical therapy, and back schools, and found that almost none of these frequently practiced medical interventions for low back pain had any positive effects on health measures or work resumption. Similar observations have been made regarding some of the most popular complementary and alternative medicine interventions. For example, there is some recent, limited support for the application of acupuncture on neck and shoulder pain. Nevertheless, the vast majority of studies to date continue to show little to no clinically significant improvement over time for acupuncture applied to chronic pain syndrome patients (98,103).

It is important to reiterate that in our review and analyses, we have had to combine and contrast data from very different studies with diverse populations, varying outcome criteria even for ostensibly the same constructs (e.g., physical functioning, health-care utilization). Moreover, we have relied on studies conducted in different countries. Despite these concerns, we can observe some general trends. There is no question that chronic pain is prevalent and costly. Moreover, there are no cures, and a substantial percentage of patients treated with any of the available interventions will continue to experience significant levels of pain and disability despite the best efforts of health-care providers. Careful examination of outcomes leads to a general conclusion that MPRPs produce clinical outcomes that are at least as good as the alternatives but at significantly lower costs. Paradoxically, there continues to be resistance of third-party payers to approve and reimburse for treatments at MPRPs—so much for the impact of EBM on payers and the growing reliance on "pay for performance."

We might be viewed as being nihilistic in concluding that nothing works, but there continues to be countless patients seeking and being treated with costly interventions with potentially devastating, adverse consequences. There is, of course, a problem of group analyses, as the need turns from the question of what works to the question of what works for whom. Few studies have performed responder analyses. One recent study comparing the effectiveness of two commonly used treatments for chronic pain (cognitive-behavior therapy and operant behavioral therapy) found that pretreatment patient characteristics were predictive of response to treatment. If confirmed, these types of responder results will permit the prescribing of treatment to patients based on psychological as well as physical characteristics as is commonly used in decisions regarding candidates for surgery.

There is a great need for research that goes beyond asking the questions of whether a particular treatment is effective in terms of addressing a set of questions. In particular, it is important to determine which treatments are effective for patients with a given set of physical and psychological characteristics, whether these treatments are most likely to produce desirable outcomes on specific criteria, and how these treatments compare to the available alternatives. Since none of the currently available treatments have proven to be capable of eliminating pain and restoring functioning to a significant proportion of patients, attention also needs to be given to combining various treatments (i.e., combinations of several medications, medications with somatic treatments, invasive procedures, and psychological treatments). Clinicians and investigators need to work more closely together to translate clinical outcomes into clinical practice. We can do better and we must do better in providing appropriate treatment for the large number of people who have chronic pain.

ACKNOWLEDGMENTS

Preparation of this manuscript was supported in part by grants from the National Institute of Health (AR 47298 & 44724).

REFERENCES

1. Verhaak PFM, Kerssens JJ, Dekker J, et al. Prevalence of chronic benign pain disorder among adults: A review of the literature. Pain 1998; 77:231–239.
2. Volinn E. The epidemiology of low back pain in the rest of the world. A review of surveys in low- and middle-income countries. Spine 1997; 22:1747–1754.
3. Blyth FM, March LM, Brnabic AJM, et al. Chronic pain in Australia: A prevalence study. Pain 2001; 89:127–134.
4. National Assembly for Wales. Welsh Health Survey. Cardiff: Government Statistical Service, 1999.
5. Beregman S, Herrstrom P, Hogstrm K, et al. Chronic musculoskeletal pain, prevalence rates and sociodemographic associations in a Swedish population study. J Rheumatol 2001; 28:1369–1377.
6. National Center for Health Statistics. Health, United States, 2006 with Chartbook on Trends in the Health of Americans. Hyattsville, MD: U.S. Government Printing Office, 2006.

7. Nachemson AL. Newest knowledge of low back pain. A critical look. Clinical Orthopedics 1992; 82:8–20.
8. Lousberg R. Chronic pain. Multiaxial Diagnostics and Behavioral Mechanisms. Thesis, University of Maastricht, 1994.
9. Elliott AM, Smith BH, Penny KI, et al. The epidemiology of chronic pain in the community. Lancet 1999; 354:1248–1252.
10. Guo H-R, Tanaka S, Halperin WE, et al. Back pain prevalence in US industry and estimate of lost workdays. Am J Publ Health 1999; 89:1029–1035.
11. Stang P, Von Korff M, Galer BS. Reduced labor force participation among primary care patients with headache. J Gen Intern Med 1998; 13:296–302.
12. Hing E, Cherry DK, Woodwell DA. National Ambulatory Medical Care Survey: 2004 Summary. Vital Health Statistics 2006; (374):1–30.
13. Gureje O. Persistent pain and well-being: A World Health Organization study in primary care. JAMA 1998; 280:147–151.
14. Olsen Y, Daumit GL, Ford DE. Opioid prescriptions by U.S. primary care physicians from 1992 to 2001. J Pain 2006; 7:225–235.
15. Marketdata Enterprises. Chronic Pain Management Programs: A Market Analysis. New York: Valley Stream, 1995.
16. Bennett RM, Jones J, Turk DC, et al. An internet survey of 2,596 people with fibromyalgia. BMC Musculoskeletal Disorders 2007; 8:27.
17. Maniadakis N, Gray A. The economic burden of back pain in the UK. Pain 2000; 84:95–103.
18. Hu XH, Markson LE, Lipton RB, et al. Burden of migraine in the United States: Disability and economic costs. Arch Intern Med 1999; 159:813–818.
19. De Lissovoy G, Brown RE, Halpern M, et al. Cost-effectiveness of long-term intrathecal morphine therapy for pain associated with failed back surgery syndrome. Clin Ther 1997; 19:96–112.
20. National Academies of Sciences and Institute of Medicine. Musculoskeletal disorders and the workplace: Low back pain and upper extremities. Washington, DC: National Academies Press, 2001.
21. Katz JN. Lumbar disc disorders and low-back pain: Socioeconomic factors and consequences. JBJS 2006; 88(Suppl 2):21–24.
22. Luo X, Pietrobon R, Sun SX, et al. Estimates and patterns of direct health care expenditures among individual with back pain in the United States. Spine 2003; 29:79–86.
23. Cousins MJ. Foreword. In: Fordyce WE, ed. Back Pain in the Workplace. Management of Disability in Nonspecific Conditions. Task Force Report. Seattle: IASP Press, 1995: ix.
24. Schappert SM. Ambulatory care visits to physicians' offices, hospital outpatient departments, and emergency departments: United States, 1996. Vital and Health Statistics, Series 13(134):1–80; National Ambulatory Medial Care Survey. National Center for Health Statistics. Washington DC: Dept. Health & Human Services, 1998.
25. Ives TJ, Chelminski PR, Hammett-Stabler CA, et al. Predictors of opioid misuse with chronic pain: A prospective cohort study. BMC Health Serv Res 2006; 6:46.
26. Michna E, Jamison RN, Pham L-D, et al. Urine toxicology screening among chronic pain patients on opioid therapy: Frequency and predictability of abnormal findings. Clin J Pain, 2007; 23:173–179.
27. Red Book. Drug Topics. Top 200 Brand-name Drugs by Prescription. Montvale, NJ: Medical Economics Publishing Co., 2002.
28. Straus BN. Chronic benign pain syndromes—the cost of intervention. Spine 2002; 27:2614–2619.
29. National Center for Health Statistics. 1997 National Hospital Discharge Survey. Series 13(144). Washington, DC: US Dept of Health and Human Services, Center for Disease Control, 1997.
30. Segal R, Stacey BR. Spinal cord stimulation revisited. Neurol Res 1998; 20:391–396.

31. Bell G, Kidd D, North R. Cost-effectiveness analysis of spinal cord stimulation in treatment of failed back surgery syndrome. J Pain Symp Manage 1997; 13:286–295.
32. Krames ES, Olson K. Clinical realities and economic considerations: Patient selection in intrathecal therapy. J Pain Symptom Manage 1997; 14:S3–S13.
33. Simmons J, Avant W, Demski J, et al. Determining successful pain clinic treatment through validation of cost effectiveness. Spine 1988; 13:24–34.
34. Flor H, Fydrich T, Turk DC. Efficacy of multidisciplinary pain treatment centers: A meta-analytic review. Pain 1992; 49:221–230.
35. Frymoyer J, Durett C. The economics of spinal disorders. In: Frymoyer J, ed. The Adult Spine. Philadelphia, PA: Lippincott-Raven, 1997:143–150.
36. Lubeck PA. Review of the direct costs of rheumatoid arthritis. Pharmacoeconomics 2001; 19:811–818.
37. Buchbinder R, Jolley D, Wyatt M. Population based intervention to change back pain beliefs and disability: Three part evaluation. BMJ 2001; 322:1516–1520.
38. Rizwoller DP, Crounse L, Shetterly S, et al. The association of comorbidities, utilization and costs for patients identified with low back pain. BMC Musculoskeletal Disorders, 2006; 7(72).
39. Sackett DL, Rosenberg WMC, Muir Gray JA, et al. Evidenced based medicine: What it is and what it isn't. BMJ 1996; 312:71–72.
40. Sackett DL, Richardson WS, Rosenberg WMC, et al. Evidence-Based Medicine: How to Practice and Teach EBM. London: Churchill-Livingstone, 1996.
41. Altman DG, Bland JM. Absence of evidence is not evidence of absence. BMJ 1995:311–485.
42. Rosenthal R 'The file drawer problem' and tolerance for null results. Psych Bull 1979; 86:638–641.
43. Miles A, Grey JE, Polychronis A, et al. Current thinking in the evidence-based health care debate. J Eval Clin Pract 2003; 9:95–109.
44. Turk DC. Clinical effectiveness and cost effectiveness of treatments for chronic pain patients. Clin J Pain 2002; 18:355–365.
45. Turk DC, Loeser JD, Monarch ES. Chronic pain: Purposes and costs of interdisciplinary pain rehabilitation programs. TEN: Trends Evidence-based Neurpsychiat 2002; 4:64–69.
46. Dworkin RH, Backonja M, Rowbotham MC, et al. Advances in neuropathic pain: Diagnosis, mechanisms, and treatment recommendations. Arch Neurol 2003; 60:1524–1534.
47. Collins SL, Moore A, McQuay HJ, et al. Antidepressants and anticonvulsants for diabetic neuropathy and postherpetic neuralgia: A quantitative systematic review. J Pain Symptom Manage 2000; 20:449–458.
48. McQuay HJ, Tramer M, Nye BA, et al. A systematic review of antidepressants in neuropathic pain. Pain 1996; 68:217–227.
49. Dvorak J, Gauchat M, Valach L. The outcome of surgery for lumbar disc herniation. I. A 4–17 years' follow-up with emphasis on somatic aspects. Spine 1988; 13:1418–1422.
50. Lehmann TR, Spratt KF, Tozzi JE, et al. Long-term follow-up of lower lumbar fusion patients. Spine 1987; 12:97–104.
51. North RG, Ewend MG, Lawton MT, et al. Failed back surgery syndrome: 5-year follow-up after spinal cord stimulator implantation. Neurosurgery 1991; 28:692–699.
52. Fritzell P, Olle H, Wessberg P, et al. Swedish Lumbar Spine Study Group. Lumbar fusion versus nonsurgical treatment for chronic low back pain: A multicenter randomized controlled trial from the Swedish lumbar spine study group. Spine 2001; 26:2521–2522.
53. North RB, Kidd DH, Zahurak M, et al. Spinal cord stimulation for chronic, intractable pain: Experience over two decades. Neurosurgery 1993; 32:384–394.
54. Turner JA, Loeser JD, Bell KG. Spinal cord stimulation for chronic low back pain: A systematic literature synthesis. Neurosurgery 1995; 37:1088–1096.
55. Van Buyten J-P, Van Zundert J, Vueghs P, et al. Efficacy of spinal cord stimulation: 10 years of experience in a pain center in Belgium. Eur J Pain 2001; 5:259–307.

56. Burchiel KJ, Anderson VC, Brown FD, et al. Prospective, multicenter study of spinal cord stimulator for relief of chronic back and extremity pain. Spine 1996; 21:2786–2794.
57. Farrar JT, Portenoy RK, Berlin JA, et al. Defining the clinically important difference in pain outcome measures. Pain 2000; 88:287–294.
58. Kumar K, Nath R, Wyatt GM. Treatment of chronic pain by epidural spinal cord stimulation: A 10-year experience. J Neurosurg 1991; 75:402–407.
59. Ohnmeiss DD, Rashbaum RF, Boddanffy GM. Prospective evaluation of spinal cord stimulation in patients with intractable leg pain. Spine 1996; 21:1344–1351.
60. Doleys D, Coleton M, Tutak U. Use of intraspinal infusion therapy with non-cancer pain patients: Follow-up and comparison of worker's compensation vs. non-worker's compensation patients. Neuromodulation 1998; 1:149–159.
61. Hassenbusch SJ, Stanton-Hicks MD, Soukup J, et al. Sufentanil citrate and morphine/bupivacaine as alternative agents in chronic epidural infusions for intractable noncancer pain. Neurosurgery 1991; 29:76–82.
62. Paice JA, Penn RD, Shott S. Intraspinal morphine for chronic pain: A retrospective, multicenter study. J Pain Symptom Manage 1996; 11:71–80.
63. Kumar K, Kelly M, Pirlot T. Continuous intrathecal morphine treatment for chronic pain of nonmalignant etiology: Long-term benefits and efficacy. Surg Neurol 2001; 55:79–88.
64. Turner JA, Sears JM, Loeser JD. Programmable intrathecal opioid delivery systems for chronic noncancer pain: A systematic review of effectiveness and complications. Clin J Pain 2007; 23:180–195.
65. Hassenbusch SJ, Stanton-Hicks M, Covington EC, et al. Long-term intraspinal infusions of opioids in the treatment of neuropathic pain. J Pain Symptom Manage 1995; 10:527–543.
66. Anderson VC, Burchiel KJ. A prospective study of long-term intrathecal morphine in the management of chronic nonmalignant pain. Neurosurgery 1999; 44:289–301.
67. Guzman J, Esmail R, Karjalainenen K, et al. Multidisciplinary rehabilitation for chronic low back pain: Systematic review. BMJ 2001; 7301:1511–1515.
68. Morley S, Eccleston C, Williams A. Systematic review and meta-analysis of randomized controlled trials of cognitive behaviour therapy and behaviour therapy for chronic pain in adults, excluding headache. Pain 1999; 80:1–13.
69. Hoffman BM, Papas RK, Chatkoff KD, et al. Meta-analysis of psychological interventions for chronic low back pain. Health Psych 2007; 26:1–9.
70. Breivik H. Opioids in cancer and chronic non-cancer pain therapy—indications and controversies. Acta Anesthesiol Scand 2001; 45:1059–1066.
71. Long DM, Filtzer DL, BenDebba M, et al. Clinical features of the failed-back syndrome. J Neurosurg 1988; 69:61–71.
72. Friedlieb O. The impact of managed care of the diagnosis and treatment of low back pain: A preliminary report. Am J Med Qual 1994; 9:24–29.
73. Malter AD, McNeney B, Loeser JD, et al. 5-year reoperation rates after different types of lumbar spine surgery. Spine 1998; 23:814–820.
74. Kumar K, Wilson JR, Taylor RS, et al. Complications of spinal cord stimulation, suggestions to improve outcome, and financial impact. J Neurosurg Spine 2006; 5:191–203.
75. Rosenow JM, Stanton-Hicks M, Rezai AR, et al. Failure modes of spinal cord stimulation hardware. J Neurosurg Spine 2006; 5:183–190.
76. Jensen MK, Thomsen AB, Hojsted J. 10-year follow-up of chronic non-malignant pain patients: Opioid use, health related quality of life and health care utilization. Eur J Pain 2006; 10:423–433.
77. Turk DC. Clinician attitudes about prolonged use of opioids and the issue of patient heterogeneity. J Pain Symptom Manage 1996; 11:218–230.
78. Sindrup S, Jensen TS. Efficacy of pharmacological treatments of Neuropathic pain: An update and effect related to mechanism of drug action. Pain 1999; 83:389–400.

79. Sindrup SH, Jensen TS. Pharmacologic treatment of pain in polyneuropathy. Neurology 2000; 55:915–920.
80. Sindrup SH, Jensen TS. Pharmacotherapy of trigeminal neuralgia. Clin J Pain 2001; 18:22–27.
81. McQuay H, Carrol D, Jadad AR, et al. Anticonvulsant drugs for management of pain: A systematic review. BMJ 1995; 311:1047–1052.
82. Kingery WS. A critical review of controlled clinical trials for peripheral Neuropathic pain and complex regional pain syndromes. Pain 1997; 73:123–139.
83. Prager JP. Neuraxial medication delivery: The development and maturity of a concept for treating pain associated with failed back surgery syndrome. Spine 2002; 27:2593–2605.
84. Gallon R. Perception of disability in chronic back pain patients: A long-term follow-up. Pain 1989; 37:67–75.
85. Turk DC. Transition from acute to chronic pain: Role of demographic and psychosocial factors. In: Jensen TS, Turner JA, Wiesenfeld-Hallin Z, eds. Proceedings of the 8th World Congress on Pain, Progress in Pain Research and Management. Seattle: IASP Press, 1997:185–213.
86. Franklin GM, Haug J, Heyer NJ, et al. Outcome of lumbar fusion in Washington State Workers' Compensation. Spine 1994; 19:1897–1904.
87. Kupers R, Van den Oever R, Van Houdenhove B, et al. Spinal cord stimulation in Belgium: A nation-wide survey on the incidence, indications and therapeutic efficacy by the health insurer. Pain 1996; 56:211–217.
88. Taylor RS, Van Buyten J-P, Buchser E. Spinal cord stimulation for chronic back and leg pain and failed back surgery syndrome: A systematic review and analysis of prognostic factors. Spine 2004; 30:152–160.
89. Turk DC, Okifuji A. Treatment of chronic pain patients: Clinical outcomes, cost-effectiveness, and cost benefits of multidisciplinary pain centers. Crit Rev Phys Med Rehabil 1998; 10:181–208.
90. Thomsen A, Sorensen J, Sjogren P, et al. Chronic non-malignant pain patients and health economic consequences. Eur J Pain 2002; 6: 345–352.
91. Von Korff M, Deyo RA. Potent opioids for chronic musculoskeletal pain: Flying blind? Pain 2004; 109:207–209; Commentary.
92. de Kleuver M, Oner FC, Jacobs WCH. Total disc replacement for chronic low back pain: Background and a systematic review of the literature. Eur Spine J. 2003; 12:108–116.
93. Gibson JNA, Grant I, Waddell G. The Cochrane review of surgery for lumbar disc prolapse and degenerative lumbar spondylosis. Spine 1999; 24:1820–1832.
94. Deyo RA, Nachemson A, Mirza SK. Spinal-fusion surgery—the case for restraint. N Engl J Med 2004; 7:722–727.
95. Deyo RA, Gray DT, Kreuter W, et al. United States trends in lumbar fusion surgery for degenerative conditions. Spine 2005; 30:1441–1445.
96. Van Tulder MW, Koes B, Seitsal S, et al. Outcome of invasive treatment modalities on back pain and sciatica: An evidenced based review. Eur Spine J 2006; 15:S82–S92.
97. Koes BW, Scholten RJPM, Mens JMA, et al. Efficacy of epidural steriod injections for low-back pain and sciatica: A systematic review of randomized clinical trials. Pain 1995; 63:279–288.
98. Sanders SH, Harden N, Vicente PJ. Evidenced-based clinical practice guidelines for interdisciplinary rehabilitation of chronic nonmalignant pain syndrome patients. Pain Practice 2005; 5:303–315.
99. Nelemans PF, de Bie RA, de Vet HCW, et al. Injection therapy for subacute and chronic benign low-back pain. Cochrane Database of Systematic Reviews, 2006:2.
100. Merrill DG. Hoffman's glasses: Evidence-based medicine and the search for quality in the literature of pain medicine. Reg Anesth Pain Med 2003; 28:547–560.
101. Manchikanti L. The growth of interventional pain management in the new millennium: A critical analysis of utilization in the medicare population. Pain Physician 2004; 7:465–482.

102. Hansson TH, Hansson EK. The effects of common medical interventions on pain, back function, and work resumption in patients with chronic low back pain: A prospective 2-year cohort study in six countries. Spine 2001; 25:3055–3064.
103. Van Tulder M. The Cochrane Library, Issue 3. Oxford: Update Software, 2003.
104. Leclaire R, Fortin L, Lambert R, et al. Radiofrequency facet joint denervation in the treatment of low back pain. A placebo-controlled clinical trial to assess efficacy. Spine 2001; 26:1411–1416.

3 "Carving-Out" Services from Multidisciplinary Chronic Pain Management Programs: Negative Impact on Therapeutic Efficacy

Robert J. Gatchel
The University of Texas at Arlington, Arlington, Texas, U.S.A.

Nancy D. Kishino
West Coast Spine Restoration Center, Riverside, California, U.S.A.

Carl Noe
Baylor Medical Center, Dallas, Texas, U.S.A.

Throughout this book, there are a number of chapters addressing the various key "ingredients" of multidisciplinary chronic pain management programs. As a result, only a brief overview of the therapeutic philosophy of such programs will be provided here. As previously delineated (1,2), such programs are based upon the *biopsychosocial model* of pain and disability. This model is now widely accepted as the most heuristic perspective to the understanding and treatment of chronic pain disorders, and it has replaced the traditional but outdated biomedical reductionist approach (1,3). This biopsychosocial approach views pain and disability as a complex and dynamic interaction among biological and psychosocial factors that perpetuates, and may even worsen, the clinical presentation. This interaction accounts for the frequent individual differences in how pain is expressed and its response to treatment.

In marked contrast, the traditional biomedical approach had always assumed that pain symptoms have specific physical causes and attempts were made to eliminate the cause by directly rectifying the pathophysiology or by blocking/cutting the pain pathways pharmacologically or surgically. Unfortunately, over the years, it became increasingly more apparent that this approach did not eliminate a significant amount of pain and it did not produce any definitive cures for the most prevalent chronic pain syndromes, such as low back pain, extremity pain disorders, peripheral neuropathologies, and so on (2). This failure had the unfortunate effect of holding out the promise of an elusive cure that subsequently affected the patients adversely and perpetuated a dualistic view of mind and body. That is to say, if the pain syndrome could not be "cured," then, it must be "in the patient's head." This produced a great deal of unwarranted stigmatization of many patients who were viewed as not having "real pain." Fortunately, the biopsychosocial approach has now debunked this false dualism and has led to a much more compassionate and effective treatment of chronic pain.

Flor et al. (4) conducted one of the first meta-analyses of multidisciplinary pain management programs, involving 65 published studies, with outcomes measured by variables such as return-to-work, reduced pain levels, improved mood, and decreased health-care utilization. This analysis clearly revealed a significant improvement for those who received multidisciplinary care relative to no treatment, wait-list control, and single discipline treatments. Since that time, the clinical efficacy and cost-effectiveness of multidisciplinary programs have been repeatedly demonstrated, relative to traditional approaches (2). There have also been a number of systematic reviews demonstrating the clinical effectiveness of such programs (5). Finally, van Tulder et al. (6) found "strong evidence" for multidisciplinary treatment approaches, using the Cochrane Collaboration's high methodology and analysis standards. It is also noteworthy that such programs are used and shown to be effective not only in the United States but also in other countries around the world, such as Canada (7), Denmark (8), France (9), Germany (10), Switzerland and England (11), and Japan (12). In England, more than 40 multidisciplinary programs had been established by the year 2000 (13). Unfortunately, Schatman (14,15) has noted that the number of these very effective and cost-efficient programs in the United States has decreased dramatically over the past decade.

MAJOR THERAPEUTIC COMPONENTS OF MULTIDISCIPLINARY PAIN MANAGEMENT PROGRAMS

Again, the major essential components of multidisciplinary pain management programs have been delineated in many previous publications (1,16–19). To briefly review, a coordinated treatment team approach is a necessity, with constant, effective communication among all treatment personnel, through which patient progress can be discussed and evaluated on a daily basis. Consistency is extremely important, ensuring that patients will hear the same treatment philosophy and message from each of the treatment team members. Indeed, chronic pain patients are often in conflict about their own future treatment and prognosis and may seek out any conflict between team members and "outside" health-care professionals and use it to compromise treatment goals that they deem unreasonable or difficult to achieve. Within this multidisciplinary context, formal treatment team meetings should occur at least once a week in order to review patient progress and to make any modifications to the treatment plan for each patient. Individually tailored treatment programs for patients are essential!

In terms of the makeup of the multidisciplinary pain management team, the following discipline members, working together on a daily basis, are essential for therapeutic effectiveness. As will be discussed later in this chapter, any missing discipline component will seriously compromise the therapeutic outcomes of such programs.

- The *physician* serves as the medical director of the treatment program. This medical director must have a complete understanding of the, biopsychosocial philosophy of multidisciplinary care and a firm background in providing medical rehabilitation for the various types of pain disorders frequently encountered in such treatment facilities.
- Most comprehensive multidisciplinary pain management programs may provide anesthesiology services, involving injections, nerve blocks, and other medical procedures. Therefore, a *nurse* is often required to assist the physician, follow-up the procedures, and serve as a physician extender and impact to address patient needs.

- The *psychologist* or *psychiatrist* plays the leading role in the day-to-day maintenance of the psychosocial aspects and status of patient care. It is well known that significant psychosocial barriers to successful recovery may develop as a patient progresses from acute to more chronic stages of a pain syndrome (1). Therefore, comprehensive psychological evaluations are required to identify potential barriers to recovery, as well as a patient's psychosocial strengths and weaknesses. A cognitive-behavioral treatment (CBT) approach can then be used to address such important issues, such as pain-related depression, anxiety, substance abuse, and other forms of psychopathology. Such a CBT approach has been found to be the most appropriate and effective modality to use in multidisciplinary programs (2,20). A *biofeedback therapist* is also important to help train patients in relaxation and physiological self-control techniques to reduce the stress of pain.
- A *physical therapist* is required to interact with patients on a daily basis regarding any issues related to physical deconditioning and reconditioning progression toward recovery. This therapist also plays an important role in educating the patient about the physiological bases of pain, and teaching methods of reducing the severity of pain episodes through the use of appropriate body mechanics and exercise pacing. Again, effective communication with other team members is crucial so that patients' fear avoidance of exercise will not interfere with their physical reconditioning.
- An *occupational therapist* is involved in both the physical and vocational aspects of the patient's rehabilitation. Most patients participating in a multidisciplinary pain treatment program are likely not to be working because of their pain. Frequently, they have become pessimistic regarding the prospect of returning to work or other activities of daily living. The occupational therapist addresses such vocational issues, as well as serving as an advocate for the patient with insurance issues, employer contact, and if needed, vocational retraining. Some multidisciplinary treatment teams include a *vocational counselor* in lieu of an occupational therapist.

Again, for a multidisciplinary program to be maximally effective, all of the above treatment-component team members need to be working collaboratively on a daily basis. As will be discussed next, removing one component from the program will seriously jeopardize successful treatment outcomes.

NEGATIVE IMPACT OF "CARVING OUT" BASIC TREATMENT COMPONENTS FROM MULTIDISCIPLINARY PAIN MANAGEMENT PROGRAMS

Even though multidisciplinary pain management programs have been shown to be therapeutically effective and cost-effective, a major obstacle to their greater use is the lack of understanding by third-party payers who refuse to cover such programs in a misguided attempt to "contain costs." This has paradoxically produced the effect of steering patients away from multidisciplinary treatments that demonstrably reduce health-care utilization, and toward more expensive unimodal therapies associated with poorer outcomes (2). Schatman (14,15) has elucidated the ethical issues associated with third-party payers' refusal to cover multidisciplinary chronic pain management programs.

Unfortunately, more and more Americans are being covered by managed care plans, with 85% of working Americans now enrolled in health maintenance organizations (HMOs) or other forms of managed care (21). As of 1998, more than 6 million Medicare beneficiaries were enrolled in 427 managed care plans, with approximately 88% of these covered by full-risk programs (22). During this period, approximately 78.8 million Americans were members of 647 HMOs nationwide (23). Nevertheless, the managed care organization (MCO) industry growth is no longer accompanied by reliable profits ("News and Trends"), and plans are increasingly focused on managing high-cost areas such as chronic diseases. Due to the prevalence of chronic pain conditions in the population now served by managed care plans, it is important for MCOs to actively respond to the health-care needs of patients with such clinical problems. Many plans, in fact, may find that the cost impact of chronic pain problems is greater than that for all other typically diagnosed chronic conditions (24). Unfortunately, instead of authorizing full multidisciplinary pain management programs, MCOs have been "carving out" portions of comprehensive, integrated programs (i.e., sending patients to different providers for their various needs outside of the comprehensive pain management programs), thus diluting the proven successful outcomes of such integrated programs in an effort to cut costs (25–27). While MCOs may be most guilty of compromising the integrity of chronic pain management services, it is important to note that *all* health-insurance carriers manage health care to a certain degree, and accordingly share in the responsibility for the provision of suboptimal care. They lose sight of the fact that, in the long run, multidisciplinary programs that help chronic pain patients resume productive lives produce much greater long-term cost-effectiveness in terms of future health care, tax, legal, and general economic factors.

Compromising the Effectiveness of Comprehensive Pain Management Programs

Gatchel and colleagues have conducted a number of empirical studies that clearly demonstrated how treatment component "carve-outs" significantly compromise the effectiveness of pain management programs (25,28). For example, the study by Robbins et al. (28) revealed that "carving out" physical therapy services had a negative impact on both the short-term and 1-year follow-up outcome measures in a heterogeneous sample of chronic pain patients treated in a multidisciplinary pain management program. This was true for measures of both physical and psychosocial functioning, with outcome measures including the SF-36, the Oswestry Pain Disability Questionnaire, and the Beck Depression Inventory.

Of equal importance, significant differences in vocational status were found between the two groups. The full multidisciplinary treatment group showed a *decrease* in the percentage of patients who were not working because of their original injury, and these gains were maintained at 1-year follow-up. In striking contrast, the "carve out" group did not show significant changes at either immediate post-treatment or 1-year follow-up. Thus, taken as a whole, these data clearly demonstrate that the "carve out" patients did not achieve the same level of therapeutic benefits relative to the multidisciplinary pain management patients who received all of their treatment in the same clinic. With the growing number of insurance carriers contracting treatment "carve-outs," these data again are especially important to consider due to their illustration of significant compromise of patients' long-term improvement and vocational status.

Impact on Quality-Adjusted Life Years

The negative impact of treatment "carve outs" has also been assessed in another way. Hatten et al. (29) recently conducted a study in which three treatment options were evaluated within a pain management center: (1) a complete multidisciplinary pain management program; (2) medication management alone; and (3) medication management and supplemental anesthetic procedures. Results clearly demonstrated the superiority of the full multidisciplinary pain management program on both psychosocial and functional measures. Of greater importance, these investigators conducted a cost–utility analysis [expressed in cost/quality-adjusted life years (QALYs)]. The calculation of QALYs involves the cost of a specific intervention, relative to the desired improvement in health (in this case, increased functioning and decreased pain). Results of this analysis demonstrated that relative to the other two treatment groups, the multidisciplinary treatment group was associated with a better QALY. Such findings indicate that this type of comprehensive treatment is both less costly *and* more effective than the other less comprehensive treatments. Patients treated through multidisciplinary management improved significantly more on measures of physical functioning, pain intensity and health-related quality of life, and in a more cost-effective manner.

OTHER COMPLEXITIES OF THE PROBLEM

In a series of commentaries in response to the Gatchel and Okifuji (2) review, a number of thoughtful points were raised concerning other potential factors that may be contributing to the underutilization/undercoverage by third-party payers for multidisciplinary pain management programs (2). These are reviewed next.

- *Often, such programs are the last resort for chronic pain patients, after medical and interventional therapies fail to adequately manage the condition*—this, unfortunately, creates the perspective from third-party payers that chronic pain treatment has already been much too costly, thereby making them more skeptical regarding paying for any additional services. What is the remedy? We must do a better job of educating third-party payers that the clinical- and cost-effectiveness of our programs need to be judged against the important reality that the patients who enter such programs are already recalcitrant to other treatments. For example, the average chronic pain patient has had 1.7 surgeries before entering a multidisciplinary program (30). We must, therefore, become more active in educating the public and the medical and insurance communities about the benefit of earlier referral to multidisciplinary pain management programs before more chronic problems develop that may require surgery and other costly interventional procedures.
- *Why are patients referred for interventional approaches rather than comprehensive multidisciplinary pain programs*—this question is quite illustrative of the misperception among health-care providers, in the area of pain, that there is a simple *either/or* type of option available—either conservative care or interventional approaches. In keeping with the true essence of a biopsychosocial multidisciplinary approach, multiple therapeutic modalities (conservative as well as interventional) should always be considered and available in order to maximize treatment gains. Again, better education is needed to change this *either/or* misperception among health-care providers and third-party payers. A multidisciplinary

pain management program should be considered for both acute and chronic cases because the entire spectrum of patients can be taken into account. Both conservative and interventional techniques can be applied, as needed. This is discussed in greater detail in chapter 7 in this book.

- *Why do we have difficulty "selling" the multidisciplinary pain management approach*—there is a panoply of intertwined forces in today's health-care environment that cause this challenge and are difficult to navigate. Unfortunately, many chronic pain clinicians were never trained in the requisite skills needed for dealing with the major forces/stakeholders (i.e., MCOs, government, workers' compensation, health-care policy, lobbying, etc.). Even in the area of political advocacy, in which an important impact can be made (such as maximizing Medicare reimbursement, which serves as the benchmark against which managed care companies base their reimbursement rates), the vast majority of chronic pain practitioners have not yet developed the "political savvy" to advocate for their patients and their profession. Many chronic pain professionals believe that a clear mandate exists: DO we have the veracity to fight against all the intertwined fronts/forces, for ourselves as health-care providers and, more importantly, the patients for whom we have the professional responsibility to care? To start this process, as noted by Turk (31), "Greater collaboration is required among professional groups, consumers of healthcare services, governmental agencies and third-party payers to ensure that the most clinically effective and cost-effective treatments are provided to all likely to benefit from them" (p.13).

IS THERE A "MIDDLE-GROUND" SOLUTION?

It has become obvious that the cost of multidisciplinary pain management has become a major barrier to patients trying to access this evidence-based effective intervention. Third-party payers do not behave as though they have any incentive (i.e., the bottom-line quarterly profit report) to pay for preventive care, even for known high-utilizing patients. Unproven cost-effectiveness is a frequently used excuse made by them for this argument. However, one potential way to increase the efficiency of resource utilization is to employ risk stratification at the time of initial assessment. Gatchel and colleagues have described an early intervention treatment program for acute pain patients who are at high risk for chronicity (32,33). The assessment is simple, brief and allows the opportunity for patients to benefit from interdisciplinary treatment when it is most cost-effective for all parties.

Haldorsen and colleagues (34) have also reported results from an assessment system that identifies high-, moderate-, and low-risk patients with chronic pain. Low-risk patients did well with usual treatment and a low-intensity multidisciplinary pain management program. Moderate-risk patients benefited similarly from both low-intensity and high-intensity multidisciplinary treatments, but not as well with usual treatment. High-risk patients responded best to the high-intensity treatment program. Karjalainen et al. (35) also reported benefit in patients with subacute pain who were treated through a low-intensity multidisciplinary program. Thus, the notion of treating the "right patient with the right program at the right time" is empirically supported. Risk stratification should include three time-defined groups: acute, subacute, and chronic. It would also include three severity-defined groups: low risk, moderate risk, and high risk. "Carve outs" would again disrupt the assessment by a multidisciplinary treatment team and would be expected to disrupt any potential gains made by risk assessment and tailoring treatment programs, as well as compromising the efficacy and cost-effectiveness. Ashburn (36) aptly posed the question: "Interdisciplinary Pain Management: Center of Excellence or Home of the Dinosaur?" The dinosaurs became extinct as a result of a meteor the size of San Francisco striking the Yucatan peninsula of Mexico. Hopefully, the decision making by our species with regard to "carve outs" will be more rational than a random event possibly associated with the Nemesis star!

BIOETHICAL ISSUES

It should be noted that Sanders et al. (37) developed evidence-based clinical practice guidelines for the multidisciplinary rehabilitation of chronic nonmalignant pain syndrome patients. There have also been guidelines developed for specific types of pain, such as acute low back pain (38). Thus, we have developed guidelines, as well as generated evidence-based outcomes research, on the therapeutic effectiveness of such programs (2). In spite of this, as Schatman (14,15) recently pointed out, these effective services are not being approved for use by third-party payers. This is resulting in a steadily decreasing number of such programs in the United States. As highlighted by Schatman (14,15), the number of accredited multidisciplinary chronic pain management programs in the United States has decreased from 210 in 1998 to a mere 84 in 2005 because of lack of appropriate authorization by third-party payers, the resultant great loss of revenue, and the ultimate need to "close the doors" because of financial problems.

In turn, the refusal to cover multidisciplinary chronic pain management creates a serious bioethical issue of which such payers may be accused of when grass-root pain-support groups become more politically active. Indeed, as the growing number of insurance carriers contracting treatment "carve outs" seriously compromises the integrity and effectiveness of multidisciplinary pain management programs, it is important to further highlight the significant medicolegal and ethical concerns this policy creates. The attempt to contain costs in the short term is also short sighted, as chronic pain will continue to be a medical problem requiring future long-term treatment costs. Other important issues to consider are delineated next.

- With the new "Pain Care Bill of Rights" issued by the American Pain Foundation, chronic pain patients are now positioning themselves to begin demanding the best standard of care for their chronic pain (i.e., comprehensive multidisciplinary pain management programs). Obviously, health-care industry operates on the basis of a "business ethos" (i.e., maximizing profits) to the detriment of patient care.
- With the "graying" of America, persons 50 years and older are twice as likely to be diagnosed with chronic pain. Epidemiologic projects suggest a chronic pain prevalence of at least 2% of the population (39). By the year 2030, the U.S. Census Bureau projects that about 20% of the population will be 65 years or older. Thus, the survival and continued growth of multidisciplinary pain programs will be an essential investment for the future health care of senior citizens in the United States. For greater details, please refer to chapter 9 on vulnerable populations in this book.

- Paradoxically, however, because of insurance company policies, multidisciplinary pain management programs are not able to remain open (14,15), thus creating a major crisis to be inherited by the next generation due to the greed and lack of a genuine ethical foundation of the current insurance community!

SUMMARY AND CONCLUSIONS

There is no doubt that the best available approach to chronic pain management from both a therapeutic and cost-effective perspective is a comprehensive multidisciplinary program. Dr. Turk's discussion of this issue (chap. 2) in this volume provides more than ample evidence. Such programs are based upon the heuristic biopsychosocial model of pain and disability. This model views pain and disability as a complex and dynamic interaction among biological and psychosocial factors that perpetuates, and may even worsen, the clinical presentation. As such, all of these variables need to be comprehensively addressed in order for treatment to be successful. Multidisciplinary programs include different discipline components that are integrated into a comprehensive whole. Such an approach is consistent with the phenomenological notion of treating *the person with chronic pain* as opposed to merely treating the pain. For such programs to be maximally effective, all of the treatment-component team members need to be working collaboratively on a daily basis. Removing one component from the program will seriously jeopardize successful treatment outcomes.

Unfortunately, even though multidisciplinary pain management programs have been shown to be therapeutically effective and cost-effective, a major obstacle to their greater use is the lack of understanding by third-party payers who refuse to cover such programs in a misguided attempt to "contain costs." A "risk-stratification" approach may also be a cost-effective preventive approach. By simply "carving out" services, the insurance industry mistakenly assumes that it will decrease costs. However, as was reviewed, this policy has significantly compromised the efficacy of these multidisciplinary pain management programs. Such a policy also raises important bioethical concerns because chronic pain patients are being denied the best standard of care available today to decrease their pain and suffering. There are also significant vocational implications associated with patients' long-term improvement and independent financial security. To satisfy basic bioethical concerns, third-party payers need to move away from what appears to be their major motivational drive and develop concern for the provision of the most effective patient care.

Penny saved is a penny got.

Henry Fielding, *The Miser*

ACKNOWLEDGMENTS

The work presented in this chapter was supported in part by grants from the NIH (3R01 MH 454562, 2R01 DE 10713, and 1K05 MH 071892), the U.S. Department of Defense (DAMD 17–03-1–0055), and Baylor Research Institute, Dallas.

REFERENCES

1. Gatchel RJ. Comorbidity of chronic mental and physical health disorders: The biopsychosocial perspective. Am Psychol 2004; 59:792–805.
2. Gatchel RJ, Okifuji A. Evidence-based scientific data documenting the treatment and cost-effectiveness of comprehensive pain programs for chronic nonmalignant pain. J Pain 2006; 7:779–793.
3. Turk DC, Monarch ES. Biopsychosocial perspective on chronic pain. In: Turk DC, Gatchel RJ, eds. Psychological Approaches to Pain Management: A Practitioner's Handbook. 2nd ed. New York, NY: Guilford; 2002.
4. Flor H, Fydrich T, Turk DC. Efficacy of multidisciplinary pain treatment centers: A meta-analytic flow. Pain 1992; 49:221–230.
5. Guzman J, Esmail R, Karjalainen K, et al. Multidisciplinary rehabilitation for chronic low back pain: Systematic review. Br Med J 2001; 322:1511–1516.
6. van Tulder M, Koes B, Bombardier C. Low back pain. Best Pract Res Clin Rheumatol 2002; 16:761–775.
7. Corey DT, Koepfler LE, Etlin D, et al. A limited functional restoration program for injured workers: A randomized trial. J Occup Rehabil 1996; 6:239–249.
8. Bendix AE, Bendix T, Vaegter K, et al. Multidisciplinary intensive treatment for chronic low back pain: A randomized, prospective study. Cleve Clin J Med 1996; 63:62–69.
9. Jousset N, Fanello S, Bontoux L, et al. Effects of functional restoration versus 3 hours per week physical therapy: A randomized controlled study. Spine 2004; 29:487–493.
10. Hildebrandt J, Pfingsten M, Saur P, et al. Prediction of success from a multidisciplinary treatment program for chronic low back pain. Spine. 1997; 22:990–1001.
11. Angst F, Brioschi R, Main CJ, et al. Interdisciplinary rehabilitation in fibromyalgia and chronic back pain: A prospective outcome study. J Pain 2006; 7:807–815.
12. Kitahara M, Kojima KK, Ohmura A. Efficacy of interdisciplinary treatment of chronic nonmalignant pain patients in Japan. Clin J Pain 2006; 22:647–655.
13. Peat GM, Moores L, Goldingay S, et al. Pain management program follow-ups: a National Survey of Current Practice in the United Kingdom. J Pain Symptom Manage 2001; 21:218–226.
14. Schatman ME. The demise of multidisciplinary pain management clinics? Pract Pain Manage 2006; 6:30–41.
15. Schatman ME. The demise of the multidisciplinary chronic pain management clinic: Bioethical perspectives on providing optimal treatment when ethical principles collide. In: Schatman ME, ed. Ethical Issues in Chronic Pain Management. New York, NY: Informa Healthcare; 2007:43–62.
16. Deschner M, Polatin PB. Interdisciplinary programs: Chronic pain management. In: Mayer TG, Gatchel RJ, Polatin PB, eds. Occupational Musculoskeletal Disorders: Function, Outcomes & Evidence. Philadelphia, PA: Lippincott, Williams & Wilkins; 2000:629–637.
17. Mayer TG, Gatchel RJ. Functional Restoration for Spinal Disorders: The Sports Medicine Approach. Philadelphia, PA: Lea & Febiger; 1988.
18. Turk DC, Gatchel RJ. Psychosocial factors and pain: revolution and evolution. In: Gatchel RJ, Turk DC, eds. Psychosocial Factors in Pain: Critical Perspectives. New York, NY: Guilford; 1999.
19. Wright AR, Gatchel RJ. Occupational musculoskeletal pain and disability. In: Turk DC, Gatchel RJ, eds. Psychological Approaches to Pain Management: A Practitioner's Handbook. 2nd ed. New York, NY: Guilford; 2002:349–364.
20. Gatchel RJ, Rollings KH. Evidence-based review of the efficacy of cognitive behavioral therapy for the treatment of chronic low back pain. Spine J in press.
21. Gatchel RJ. Pain assessment and treatment in the managed care environment: a position statement from the American Pain Society. In press.
22. Centers for Medicare and Medicaid Services. Managed care in medicare and medicaid (Fact Sheet). Washington, DC: Department of Health and Human Services, 1998.

23. America's Health Insurance Plans. Available on www.ahib.org.
24. Fishman P, Von Korff M, Lozano P, et al. Chronic care costs in managed care. Health Aff (Millwood) 1997; 16:239–247.
25. Gatchel RJ, Noe C, Gajraj N, et al. The negative impact on an interdisciplinary pain management program of insurance "treatment carve out" practices. J Work Compens 2001; 10:50–63.
26. Keel P, Wittig R, Deutschman R, et al. Effectiveness of in-patient rehabilitation for sub-chronic and chronic low back pain by a integrative group treatment program. Scand J Rehabil Med 1998; 30:211–219.
27. National Center for Health Statistics. 1997 National Hospital Discharge Survey. Washington, DC: U.S. Department of Health and Human Services, Center for Disease Control, 1997; Series 13, No. 144.
28. Robbins H, Gatchel RJ, Noe C, et al. A prospective one-year outcome study of interdisciplinary chronic pain management: compromising its efficacy by managed care policies. Anesth Analg 2003; 97:156–162.
29. Hatten A, Gatchel R, Polatin P, et al. A cost-utility analysis of chronic spinal pain treatment outcomes: converting SF-36 data into quality-adjusted life years. Clin J Pain 2006; 22:700–711.
30. Turk DC. Clinical effectiveness and cost effectiveness of treatment for patients with chronic pain. Clin J Pain 2002; 18:355–365.
31. Turk DC, Gatchel RJ, eds. Psychological Approaches to Pain Management: A Practitioner's Handbook. 2nd ed. New York, NY: Guilford; 2002.
32. Gatchel RJ, Polatin PB, Noe CE, et al. Treatment and cost-effectiveness of early intervention for acute low back pain patients: a one-year prospective study. J Occup Rehabil 2003; 13:1–9.
33. Gatchel RJ, Stowell AW, Wildenstein L, et al. Efficacy of an early intervention for patients with acute TMD-related pain: a one-year outcome study. J Am Dent Assoc 2006; 137:339–347.
34. Haldorsen EM, Grasdal AL, Skouen JS, et al. Is there a right treatment for a particular patient group? Comparison of ordinary treatment, light multidisciplinary treatment, and extensive multidisciplinary treatment for long-term sick-listed employees with musculoskeletal pain. Pain 2002; 95:49–63.
35. Karjalainen K, Malmivaara A, van Tulder M, et al. Multidisciplinary biopsychosocial rehabilitation for subacute low back pain among working age adults (Review): The Cochrane Database of Systematic Reviews, 2003, (www.cochrane.org).
36. Ashburn MA. Interdisciplinary pain management: center of excellence or home of the dinosaur. Clin J Pain 1996; 12:258–259.
37. Sanders SH, Harden RN, Vicente PJ. Evidence-based clinical practice guideline for interdisciplinary rehabilitation of chronic nonmalignant pain syndrome patients. Pain Pract 2005; 5:303–315.
38. McGuirk B, King W, Govind J, et al. Safety, efficacy and cost-effectiveness of evidence-based guidelines for the management of acute low back pain in primary care. Spine 2001; 26:2615–2622.
39. Verhaak PFM, Kerssens JJ, Dekker J, et al. Prevalence of chronic benign pain disorder among adults: a review of the literature. Pain 1998; 77:231–239.

4 Problems with Chronic Opioid Therapy and the Need for a Multidisciplinary Approach

Jane C. Ballantyne
Division of Pain Medicine, Department of Anesthesia and Critical Care, Massachusetts General Hospital and Harvard Medical School, Boston, Massachusetts, U.S.A.

INTRODUCTION

There are several reasons that during the latter part of the twentieth century, opioid treatment was extended to increasing numbers of patients suffering from chronic noncancer pain, whereas previously it had been used rarely and cautiously for noncancer, nonacute pain. As the understanding of pain and opioid mechanisms improved earlier in the century, opioid therapy for acute and cancer pain was used increasingly, at higher doses than had ever been used. The concept that all pain could be overcome with opioid therapy, at high dose if necessary, was born. Addiction seemed to arise only rarely, and it was conjectured that the existence of severe pain counteracts the euphoric effects of opioids so that addiction is unlikely to arise during pain treatment with opioids. At the same time, pain was seen for the first time as a disease rather than a symptom, pain medicine became a specialty, and pain clinics were built. Opioid therapy became a necessary component of pain management and often the only option left if injections, nonopioid medications, and other adjuncts failed. The somewhat idealistic view that all pain could and should be abolished, using opioids if necessary, took hold.

Unfortunately, what was presented as a noble and obtainable goal—to abolish pain using opioids if necessary—has not fulfilled its promise. We have learned that opioid analgesic efficacy is not always sustained over time and even if the treatment is initially beneficial, it can later lose its efficacy. Also, when opioids are used long-term in the outpatient setting, problematic opioid-seeking arises at a frequency that is concerning. Pain clinics are not the only facilities experiencing the burden of failed opioid treatment, and in particular primary-care practices and some surgical practices feel overwhelmed when the number of opioid-seeking patients increases to the point that they cannot cope with the demands these patients place on medical services. Physicians expecting to be able to treat pain simply and successfully may be unable to cope with the complex biopsychosocial problems associated with opioid dependence. Then, instead of being helped, these patients become even more vulnerable to the inadequacies of chronic disease management inherent in a medical system such as that in the United States that supports long-term care approaches less than it does acute interventions.

ADDICTION

While the therapeutic benefits of opioids have been appreciated for millennia, so have their addicting effects. Physicians have long understood that prolonged opioid treatment is accompanied by addiction risk. Fear of addiction is the main reason for "opiophobia," and the main reason that opioid treatment was not commonly extended to patients with chronic pain until late in the twentieth century. History has also taught that opioid addiction becomes a societal problem only when opioids reach a critical point in availability and usage, as was observed when opium cultivation and usage spread from the middle east to the far east and then on to the western world. The clear message is that not all users become addicted, but a certain proportion does, and so the more the usage is there, the more the addiction will become a problem. Why then did twentieth century physicians feel confident that addiction would not be a problem if opioid therapy was extended to chronic pain patients? This perception was largely based on the greater understanding of opioid mechanisms brought about by the discovery of endogenous opioid systems, the confidence that opioids have unique analgesic properties, and the observation that when treating severe pain, euphoria and other side effects seem muted. Yet the actual experience has been that the addiction does indeed arise during opioid treatment of chronic pain, at a rate that is not dissimilar to that seen in the general population (5–30% of those exposed) (1). Should this deter opioid treatment of chronic pain? The question is, should all patients be denied opioids for the treatment of severe chronic pain because there will be a poor outcome in some? Most people would say no. We can do better than this because we are beginning to gain a depth of knowledge about how and why opioids produce addiction and how addiction can be avoided, and we can use this knowledge to structure opioid treatment of pain so that addiction risk is minimized.

Addiction Mechanisms

Addiction is a chronic neurobiological disease produced by repeated exposure to an addictive drug (or process), characterized by loss of control over drug use (or other behaviors). Opioid addiction arises after repeated opioid use in certain, not all, circumstances. The circumstances that combine to produce drug and opioid addiction can be considered in three categories: (1) psychosocial factors, (2) drug-related factors, and (3) genetic factors (Fig. 1) (2,3). The highest risk for addiction arises when risk factors in each category arise together. Pain patients with no genetic predisposition, no psychosocial comorbidity, and who take stable doses of opioid for the treatment of severe pain in a controlled setting are unlikely to develop addiction. On the other hand, patients with a personal or family history of substance abuse, displaying one or several psychosocial comorbidities, are at risk of developing addiction, especially if the treatment is not carefully structured and monitored.

The so-called "reward circuitry" is central to addiction processes. The "reward center" is located within mesocorticolimbic dopamine systems in the brain, where opioids play a critical role (4). Both dopamine and opioids have a central role in addiction processes, although there is still considerable uncertainty about the exact neural circuitry and neurotransmitters involved (5,6). The predominant role in addiction development of the positive reinforcing (rewarding) effects of addictive drugs mediated through the mesocorticolimbic reward systems is firmly established. At the same time, it is recognized that withdrawal phenomena, acting both

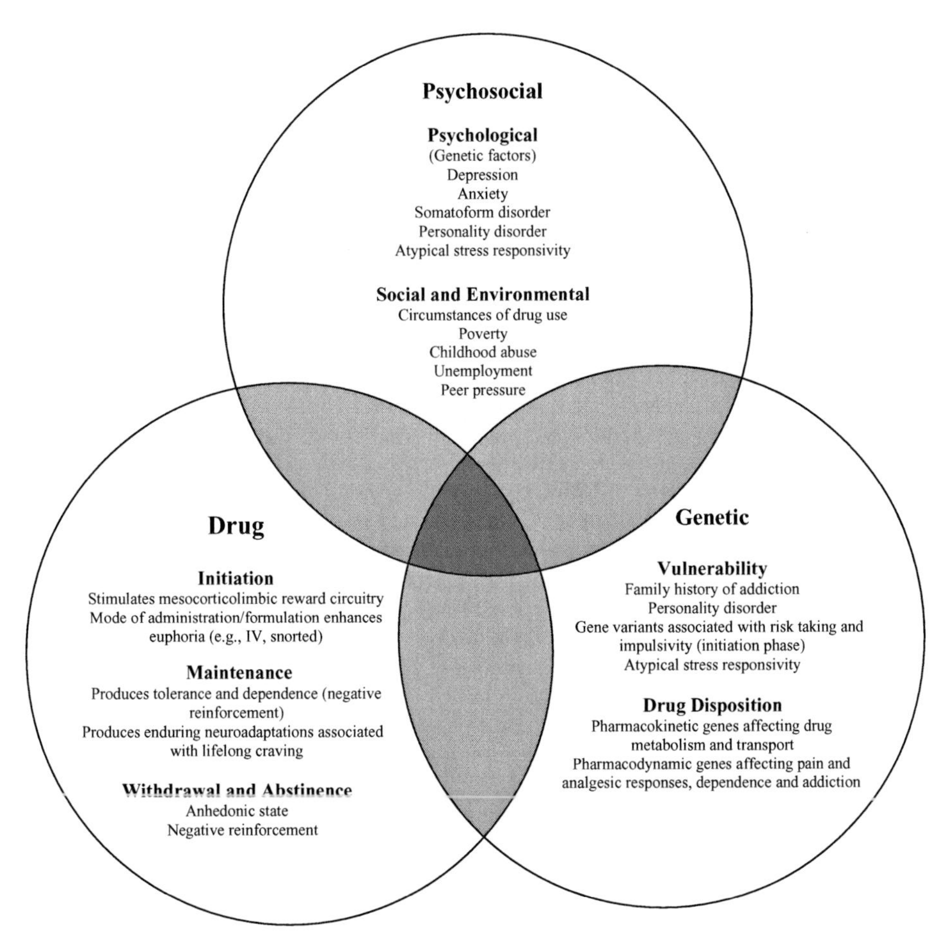

FIGURE 1 The three domains contributing to addiction. Adapted from Ref. 92.

on this reward circuitry, as well as on other systems, contribute to craving and compulsive drug seeking, at least during active use and early abstinence (4,7,8). Withdrawal phenomena are both psychological (withdrawal anhedonia) and physical, and unpleasant feelings and symptoms during withdrawal induce craving. In the case of opioid dependence, upregulation of cAMP pathways in the brain (locus coeruleus) and spinal cord leads to acute physical withdrawal symptoms when administered opioids are reduced or stopped, resulting in excessive central norepinephrine release, and its manifestations (9–11). While withdrawal phenomena are important in early drug-seeking behaviors, it is important to distinguish these from the more enduring effects of addiction, which are learned, reinforced behaviors. As drug addiction develops, drug use combined with behaviors, circumstances, and stressors associated with obtaining and using the drug form a powerful memory imprint through involvement of secondary areas of the brain normally involved in memory, conditioning, and learning (5,6). As with all conditioned responses, this memory is hard to eradicate and is often irreversible, unlike the craving associated with early withdrawal. Continued and uncontrolled drug-seeking behavior is, therefore, probably the most important factor producing the enduring state of addiction (a learned state), whereas craving associated with withdrawal (psychological and physical) may reverse once the patient receiving opioid treatment has been weaned. Perhaps practitioners are most culpable when they abandon opioid-seeking patients to doctor shopping, or worse still, obtaining the drugs they need illicitly, in effect, reinforcing drug-seeking behaviors.

DEFINING AND QUANTIFYING ADDICTION

If we accept that not all problematic opioid-seeking behavior is addiction, our chief difficulty with assessing addiction risk lies in defining exactly what addiction is when it arises in opioid-treated pain patients. Perhaps it is not surprising that we currently have no satisfactory definition or criteria for addiction arising in pain patients, considering that the currently accepted criteria for *substance dependence* [the DSM-IV term for *drug addiction* (12)] were arrived at only after decades of debate, and may still need refining on the basis of new insights derived from scientific discovery. The tolerance and physical dependence that are considered criteria for drug addiction by DSM-IV terminology are inevitable features of therapeutic opioid use, and it is now recognized that they are neither necessary nor sufficient for a person to be addicted (6). This realization came about partly through the experience of treating chronic pain with opioids, which has made it clear that opioid-treated pain patients can become dependent without being addicted. Moreover, in the case of therapeutic opioid use, behaviors that are considered typical of problematic opioid use differ from those listed by DSM-IV and have never formally been accepted as signs of addiction. The types of problematic behaviors associated with opioid treatment of pain are listed in Table 1. A consensus document from American pain and addiction societies attempts to rationalize addiction terminology for use in opioid pain management. It addresses the difficulty of labeling chronic opioid-treated pain patients "addicts" simply because they are opioid tolerant and dependent, and it finds new descriptors for behavioral criteria. It separates out tolerance and physical

TABLE 1 Signs of Prescription Drug Abuse

Self-escalation of dosage
Repeated prescription loss with "classical" excuses
"The pills fell into the toilet bowl"
"I left the prescription in the changing room"
"The airline lost my luggage"
"The dog ate it"
"The vial was stolen from my medicine cabinet"
"The pills were ruined in the laundry"
Multiple prescribers
Frequent telephone calls to the office
Multiple drug intolerances described as "allergies"
Focusing mainly on opioid issues during visits
Visiting office without an appointment

Source: Adapted from Ref. 93.

dependence and lists the following addiction criteria: impaired control over drug use, compulsive use, continued use despite harm, and craving (13). Unfortunately, these definitions have led to further confusion because by separating tolerance and physical dependence from addiction, they imply that there is no psychological component to dependence other than addiction, which is almost certainly not true. The message here is that psychological dependence can be reversible, and therefore patients experiencing this should not be labeled addicts or necessarily treated as such.

At the start of the movement toward broadening opioid therapy to reach those with chronic noncancer and nonterminal pain, addiction rates were considered to be very low. A key paper reporting hospital rates of addiction was taken out of context and widely used to support an extremely low rate of addiction (0.03%) (14). More realistically, Portenoy and Foley, in a seminal paper describing opioid therapy for noncancer pain, reported rates of addiction of 5% (15). Rates of this order were widely accepted, despite the weak level of evidence. Controlled studies made no attempt to evaluate addiction. After a decade or more of acceptance that therapeutic opioid use was unlikely to result in addiction, the medical community began to question the supposed low rates of addiction because of a perceived increase in the number of problematic patients, and because of the documented increase in prescription drug abuse (16). A systematic review published in 1992 reported addiction rates of up to 18.9% (17), yet went largely unnoticed while efforts were made by pain advocates during the 1990s to persuade the medical community that addiction was extremely rare during the treatment of pain. Today, when we are justifiably more concerned, this higher rate has become widely accepted. Whatever figure we believe or accept, whether 5%, 20%, or higher, the true incidence of addiction in opioid-treated chronic pain patients is unknown, and this is partly because we have no accepted definitions or criteria for addiction arising during opioid pain treatment.

ANALGESIC EFFICACY

Short-term Analgesic Efficacy

Randomized controlled trials (RCTs) have been conducted to test the analgesic efficacy of opioids for various chronic pain conditions, including the arthitides and various neuropathic pain conditions (18–20). Measured pain scales from the RCTs show a statistically significant improvement across all the studies, both in cases of painful arthitides and neuropathic pain. The question underlying the trials was whether chronic pain conditions, particularly neuropathic pain conditions, are opioid responsive. (There had been a traditionally held view that neuropathic pain is not opioid responsive.) The randomized studies make it clear that contrary to this traditional belief, neuropathic pain is indeed opioid responsive, although larger doses are required than those needed to treat nociceptive pain (21–28). The RCTs demonstrate clearly that chronic pain conditions respond to opioids at least during the conduct of such trials—up to 8 weeks (20,29). Whether or not analgesic efficacy is sustained over longer periods cannot be determined from these RCTs.

Long-term Analgesic Efficacy

The real question when embarking on a course of opioid treatment for chronic pain is whether analgesic efficacy is maintained over time. Here one must turn to less rigorous forms of evidence, since it is generally not feasible to conduct RCTs over prolonged periods. Current knowledge of long-term analgesic efficacy comes from surveys, case series, and open-label follow-up studies in association with some RCTs (18,19,30,31). Many case series, mainly reporting the use of long-term opioid therapy in pain programs, report satisfactory analgesia for all patients who stay on the treatment (15,18,32). A review of the open-label follow-up studies, however, has shown that 56% of patients abandon the treatment because of lack of efficacy or side effects (19). Moreover, many opioid trials utilize enrichment in their protocols (patients who do not respond are selected out during a pretrial phase), and there is an unusually high dropout rate across opioid trials during enrichment, likely reducing the internal validity of the trials (33). A recent epidemiological study reporting experience with chronic opioid therapy in Denmark in a large mixed cohort of Danish patients showed pain levels [as well as employment records, health-care utilization, activity levels, and quality of life (QOL)] being worse in opioid-treated patients than in a matched cohort of chronic pain patients not receiving opioids (31,34). Overall, the evidence supporting long-term analgesic efficacy is weak.

Treatment in the long-term studies has been based on the traditional premise that dosage should be titrated upward to overcome pharmacological tolerance, this being an inevitable consequence of long-term opioid treatment. In fact, the majority of patients are able to reach a stable, nonescalating effective dose, and analgesic tolerance seems to stabilize over time. Some patients, however, fail dose escalation, reporting no change or a worsening of their pain, despite high doses of opioids (35,36). Some report actual improvement in pain once opioid treatment is discontinued (37,38). The putative mechanisms for failed opioid analgesia may be related to rampant tolerance or opioid-induced hyperalgesia (35,39–43). Advances in basic science help understand these phenomena and their clinical relevance, but it remains unclear exactly what aspects of treatment—drug choice, dose, or timing—cause these phenomena to compromise opioid efficacy. The premise that tolerance can always be overcome by dose escalation must now be questioned (18).

FUNCTION AND QUALITY OF LIFE

Whether long-term opioid treatment can improve patients' function or QOL is clearly a broader issue than whether opioids can reduce a pain score. Surprisingly, only a few of the existing opioid studies have focused on this issue, and there are few available data. RCTs provide mixed results on function—some find improvement, others do not. The focus of the functional testing in RCTs varies with the primary interest of the investigators, for example, physical function, joint tenderness, activity levels and grip strength for arthritis patients, sleep, anxiety, and psychomotor function and disability scores for back pain patients. This variability precludes an overall assessment. Moreover, RCTs have assessed short-term functional achievements only. Several case series report on function, and these consistently report improvement, although the quality of this type of evidence must be questioned (44). Epidemiological studies are less positive and predominantly report failure of opioids to improve QOL in chronic pain patients (31,34,45). Studies specifically assessing cognitive function, including the ability to drive and operate machinery, find that cognitive function, manual dexterity, and reaction times are maintained provided a stable dose of opioid is used (46–50). This is not true when the dosing is irregular or escalates (46,51,52). This becomes an important issue if the goal of treatment is to return to work and full functioning.

PRESENT STATE OF KNOWLEDGE

Despite the existence of several RCTs assessing opioid therapy for chronic noncancer and nonterminal pain, research questions regarding the therapy remain unanswered. The RCTs do not assess the use of high doses (higher than 180 mg morphine per day), or the use of prolonged treatment (extending beyond 32 weeks). Moreover, patients in RCTs are likely to be a biased sample, not reflecting the normal population of patients seeking opioid treatment of pain, many of whom will not accept possible randomization to a placebo. We can claim that opioids provide good short-term efficacy for chronic noncancer pain, including neuropathic pain. Although many physician-reporters describe successful use of opioids over prolonged periods (up to 3 years), we must remain cautious that their good results may be due as much to their careful approach and dedication to their patients as to the drug itself. The secondary improvements in function and QOL (debatably of paramount importance) have not been confirmed by the accumulated evidence to date.

Liabilities pertaining to long-term opioid therapy must also be taken into account, and this evidence comes from focused studies. A few studies suggest that prolonged high-dose therapy has deleterious neuroendocrine effects that could worsen the mood-suppressing effects of opioids and the likely psychosocial comorbidities of chronic pain (18,53–56). More evidence is needed to explain the exact clinical significance of these effects. The problem of iatrogenic addiction remains poorly defined and quantified. Until or unless medical science advances to the point of identifying a marker of addiction, either through advanced imaging or through genetic profiling, addiction can only be regarded as a continuum—a risk that could arise in any patient given the right combination of drug, psychosocial situation, and genetic predisposition. Thus, a cautious approach to both selection and management of opioid-treated chronic pain patients is advisable.

FUTURE DIRECTIONS

During the latter part of the twentieth century, several factors produced a great deal of optimism about the ability of opioids to abolish pain. For the first time, largely because endogenous opioid systems were identified, it was understood just how specific the analgesic effects of opioids are. Not simply soporific or narcotic, like alcohol, anesthetics, and other hypnotics, but specifically pain-relieving, producing analgesia independent of insensibility, especially in the presence of severe pain. Experience with opioid therapy for severe acute and cancer pain taught that pain could be well controlled using opioids without undesired central effects such as somnolence and craving. Why not extend the treatment to patients suffering chronic pain? Would we see the same success, with good analgesic efficacy, controllable side effects, and extremely low addiction liability?

Unfortunately, the hoped-for success of long-term opioid treatment has not been realized, at least not in all settings. While many practitioners have been able to improve the lives of patients with debilitating chronic pain using carefully structured opioid therapy (32), there are others who struggle with issues related to therapeutic opioid use. Practitioners who are not equipped to deal with the demands of complex pain patients, who often become increasingly complex when opioid dependence supervenes, may become overwhelmed when their well-meaning effort to relieve pain turns into a battle to control opioid overuse and worsening pain. Diversion of prescription opioids increases societal drug abuse problems (57). Perhaps most worrying, studies do not support long-term analgesic efficacy, and population studies suggest that when opioids are used liberally for chronic pain in the outpatient setting, the health and well-being of the chronic pain population declines (31,34).

Being Selective

The argument for opioid treatment of pain states that opioids are indispensable for the treatment of pain and suffering (58). This argument is further supported knowing that uncontrolled pain may have deleterious physical (59–61) and psychological sequelae; persistent pain destroys the individual's autonomy and dignity, and compromises the person's decision-making capacity. The "principle of balance" recognizes that opioids are indispensable, that they may also be abused, and that efforts to address abuse should not interfere with legitimate medical practice and patient care (62,63). Yet in the case of chronic pain treatment, on the one hand we may see analgesic efficacy diminishing over time (18,19,37,38), on the other, addressing the potential for dependence, abuse, addiction, and general health deterioration may involve complex and far-reaching considerations that inevitably interfere with treatment success.

Despite the established right of patients to receive opioid treatment for acute, terminal, and chronic pain (64,65), key ethical issues persist. The most intransigent of these during the treatment of chronic pain are centered on whether a patient at risk of deteriorating (most notably, at risk of addiction) should embark on a course of chronic opioid treatment. Could addiction become a greater burden than pain? Who is in a better position to judge whether addiction will arise—the physician or the patient? Does the physician have the tools to identify a likely substance abuser? Does the physician perceive that the patient is incapable of self-determination either because of the pervasive effect of intractable pain, or because of the influence of past or present drug use? Then does the physician's presumption of the patient's incompetence compromise the patient's autonomy? (66)

A substance abuse history may constitute only one component of complex circumstances involving the social situation of both individual patients and their community. Practitioners find themselves deciding whether their patients are likely to abuse or divert on the basis of income, race, social status, criminal record, employment status, being perceived as a malinger or drug-seeker, or being known as a frequent drug offender. They are then either helplessly torn between legal obligation, duty to patients, and duty to the community, or, they may take the more comfortable position of considering only their moral duty to patients. They probably receive little guidance or training that helps them make troubling decisions regarding individual patients, despite the existence of guidelines, mandates, and ethical charters broadly recommending fair distribution and careful selection (62,67). Recognizing that the rapidly changing health-care environment presents physicians with moral–ethical–legal conflicts with which they are ill-equipped to deal, hospitals and

TABLE 2 Screening for Risk

1997	Chabal et al. (70)	Prescription abuse checklist to be used by physicians
1998	Compton et al. (71)	Pilot assessment tool—Prescription Drug Use Questionnaire 42 items for structured interview completed by physicians
2003	Friedman et al. (76)	Screening tool for addiction risk (STAR) 14 true or false questions to be completed by patients
2004	Passik et al. (72)	Pain Assessment and Documentation Tool (PADT) Assesses 41 items related to 4 domains—completed by physicians
2004	Adams et al. (73)	Pain Medication Questionnaire (PMQ) 26-item instrument; self-report, completed by patients and scored by physicians
2004	Butler et al. (74)	Screener and Opioid Assessment for Patients with Pain (SOAPP) 24-item questionnaire; completed by patients
2005	Webster et al. (75)	Opioid risk tool (ORT) 10 yes–no questions to be completed by patients

Source: Adapted from Ref. 93.

specialty bodies have begun developing ethics committees and forums to provide guidance on the specific aspects of individual cases that may not have been captured by the deductive model (62,68,69).

Existing evidence, as described in this chapter, strongly suggests that while long-term opioid therapy might be useful in selected patients, if it is used too broadly, many patients will deteriorate, not only in terms of their pain but also in terms of their general health and well-being. It is easier, of course, to provide opioid treatment for all patients appealing for help with pain. It becomes much more difficult to select suitable patients for opioid treatment. If the treatment is not suitable for all patients in pain, how should patients be selected for treatment? This dilemma presents among the most difficult moral and ethical decisions for physicians facing individuals with uncontrolled and debilitating pain. Since it is known that the risk for individuals predisposed to addiction is increased by giving an addictive drug, does this make the risk of prescribing opioids unacceptable for certain patients, and are there validated methods available to help practitioners identify risk? Physicians need simple tools that can help them stratify risk and identify significant aberrant behaviors should they arise. Several groups have now developed such tools and are in the process of validating them (Table 2) (70–76). These tools, if widely applied, can help physicians provide rational, appropriate opioid therapy, with the secondary benefit that medical charts will contain useful data for outcomes and risk assessment. Thus the first step will be to use measurement tools that provide consistency in reporting, and the second to review and analyze the charts.

NEW GUIDELINES

In advanced countries, it is generally agreed that pain is a disease worthy of treatment with opioids if necessary. Each of these countries, seeing that practitioners need guidance if they are to provide long-term opioid treatment appropriately, has produced guidelines. The principles embodied in these guidelines are remarkably similar, no matter which country they have been developed for. They all suggest careful patient selection and follow-up, careful monitoring (sometimes using drug screening), the use of contracts, consents or agreements, a preference for prescribing by a single practitioner and provision by a single pharmacist, and weaning if treatment goals are not reached (15,18,32,77–85). For guidance on structured opioid pain treatment, the reader may refer to the American guidelines (15,18,78,79).

Certain of the United States, recognizing that the dissemination and proper use of guidelines is limited, have introduced further measures to encourage appropriate prescribing. The State of California has written a new law related to Continuing Medical Education (AB 487: Pain Management and the Appropriate Care and Treatment of the Terminally Ill) that requires Californian physicians to successfully complete 12 units of continuing medical education (CME) on "pain management" and "the appropriate treatment of the terminally ill." This mandated CME provides an opportunity for physicians to learn the principles of ideal pain care, including ideal opioid management. In the state of Washington, a guideline on opioid dosing for chronic noncancer pain is under development by an interagency workgroup on practice guidelines (the Department of Corrections, Department of Health, Department of Labor and Industries, Department of Social and Health Services, and Health Care Authority in collaboration with actively practicing pain management specialists). Interestingly, this guideline suggests dose ranges considered appropriate for different practice settings. For example, it advises that doses above 120 mg morphine equivalent per day should only be provided under guidance from pain specialists. There has been much debate about the concept of dose-determined level of care, especially given the uncertainly about the risk/benefits of high-dose opioid therapy. However, there is certainly very little evidence to support the use of high-dose opioid therapy, and there is reason to believe that high doses may be toxic (notably to neuroendocrine systems) as well as being associated with problematic opioid-seeking behavior (18). This type of restriction seems potentially useful to this author, not least because it could provide a means of identifying problem patients needing more intensive care. The obvious counterargument is that patients needing higher doses will be denied treatment because the higher level of care is not available. This problem will only be solved by making appropriate care (i.e., multidisciplinary pain care) more available.

The Importance of Infrastructure

Countries such as the United States strive to provide the level of health care necessary to produce a population that is robust and functional. People should not have to suffer when treatments are available to reduce suffering. The humane society does not expect people to work through pain. The expectation is that there is a "cure"—be it a tablet, an injection, a course of exercises, or an operation. Unaccountably, health-care payers, and governments alike, ignore the evidence that chronic diseases, including pain, may be best approached through lifestyle changes, often needing intensive help through counseling and training, while the majority of patients are little changed by the quick fixes that governments and third-party payers seem intent on favoring. With regard to the present topic, the combined effect of the demise of multidisciplinary pain programs (38) along with aggressive marketing of "designer" opioids and the accompanying message that all pain must be abolished using opioids, if necessary, has resulted in opioid therapy being overused (86). For the busy practitioner who is only given a few minutes to see patients in follow-up, the easiest way to quickly fix the distressed patient is to prescribe an opioid.

There is strong evidence, discussed in-depth elsewhere in this book, that multidisciplinary pain management and the rehabilitative approach is effective in terms of pain reduction, functional restoration, return to work, and QOL (87–90). The cost-effectiveness of this approach is also well documented, especially considering that many of the alternatives (surgical, interventional, medical) carry significant risk of treatment-associated morbidity, which is costly in its turn (87). Simply recognizing and treating depression and anxiety as part of the multifaceted approach to pain management improves treatment results and long-term outcomes (91). Multidisciplinary and rehabilitation programs also incorporate critical aspects of pain and life quality improvement such as biopsychosocial function, functional restoration, and vocational guidance (88,90). Most important in the context of the present chapter, there is compelling evidence that medication usage is reduced when a multidisciplinary approach is used (87). Thus, within multidisciplinary programs, opioids and other medications are used as adjuncts to other approaches, often being used maximally during periods of intensive rehabilitation, and sparingly or not at all once stability is reached.

For nonpain specialists trying to fulfill their responsibility to manage pain, opioid treatment seems an attractive and feasible option because of its immediate effectiveness and ability to satisfy patients' demands for relief. Physicians have been persuaded that the treatment is effective and safe, yet evidence overwhelmingly suggests that simply providing opioids is not enough, and without support most single practitioners cannot cope with the complexity of patients suffering chronic pain, who are made more complex by opioid treatment with its inherent risk of dependence. Physicians must either dedicate their own time to the proper counseling and monitoring of opioid-treated patients or have additional help from psychologists, physician extenders, and others. Moreover, for optimum results, adjunctive treatment options must be available either within the practice settings where opioids are provided or by arrangement with other facilities. Part of the answer to the problems practitioners face with regard to the lack of availability of resources for helping them manage pain must be to create practice models more appropriate for the management of chronic disease, or to rebuild the multidisciplinary programs that have already proven their efficacy.

CONCLUSIONS

Opioid therapy may seem a simple solution to the problem of intractable pain, but in fact, neither the patients requiring opioids nor the treatment itself are simple. Since no treatment (or treatment combination) currently available does more than partially reduce pain, society must adapt to the idea that pain cannot be completely eliminated. Pain that is severe and prolonged enough to warrant long-term treatment with opioids has a devastating effect on patients' lives. Entering a long-term commitment to opioid treatment must, then, involve much soul searching as to the suitability of the treatment—its likely benefits and likely pitfalls. Opioid treatment can diminish in efficacy over time and is seen to result in deterioration in pain relief, function, and QOL in many patients, despite there being clear benefits in others. Although rates of addiction during opioid treatment of pain are unclear, experience has shown that many patients exhibit problematic opioid-seeking behavior that interferes with treatment success, whether this is actually addiction or not. Most importantly, it is necessary to understand that although opioids can provide short-term relief, such relief may not be sustained, yet the adverse effects of withdrawal (which can include anhedonia, physical withdrawal symptoms, and immediate worsening of pain) often make patients reluctant to discontinue the treatment despite poor analgesic efficacy. Thus the "try and see" approach may seem logical, but in the case of opioids, the approach is fraught with difficulty when patients become dependent and difficult to wean. All in all, the role of opioids in the treatment of chronic pain must be seen as adjunctive, and the medical community must accept that treating chronic pain is never as simple as prescribing an opioid.

REFERENCES

1. Kreek MJ, Nielsen DA, Butelman ER, et al. Genetic influences on impulsivity, risk taking, stress responsivity and vulnerability to drug abuse and addiction. Nat Neurosci 2005; 8(11):1450–1457.
2. Hyman S. Dispelling the myths about addiction. Institute of Medicine. Washington, DC: National Academy of Sciences Press 1997:44–46.
3. Kreek MJ. Drug addictions: molecular and cellular endpoints. Ann NY Acad Sci 2001; 937:27–49.
4. Cami J, Farre M. Drug addiction. N Engl J Med 2003; 349:975–986.
5. Hyman S, Malenka R. Addiction and the brain: the neurobiology of compulsion and its persistence. Nat Rev Neurosci 2001; 2:695–703.
6. Hyman SE, Malenka RC, Nestler EJ. Neural mechanisms of addiction: the role of reward-related learning and memory. Annu Rev Neurosci 2006; 29:565–598.
7. Koob G, Le Moal M. Drug addiction, dysregulation of reward, and allostasis. Neuropharm 2001; 24:97–129.
8. Koob G, Le Moal M. Drug abuse: hedonic homeostatic dysregulation. Science 1997; 278:52–58.
9. Koob G, Maldonado R, Stinus L. Neural substrates of opiate withdrawal. Trends Neurosci 1992; 15(5):186–191.
10. Nestler EJ, Aghajanian GK. Molecular and cellular basis of addiction. Science 1997; 278(5335):58–63.
11. Nestler EJ. Historical review: molecular and cellular mechanisms of opiate and cocaine addiction. Trends Pharmacol Sci 2004; 25(4):210–218.
12. American Psychiatric Association. Diagnostic and Statistical Manual of Mental Disorders, 4th edn (DSM-IV). Washington, DC: American Psychiatric Association; 1994.
13. Savage S, Covington E, Ehit H, et al. Definitions related to the use of opioids for the treatment of pain. A consensus document from the American Academy of Pain Medicine, the American Pain Society and the American Society of Addiction Medicine, 2001.
14. Porter J, Jick H. Addiction rare in patients treated with narcotics (Letter). N Engl J Med 1980; 302(2):123.
15. Portenoy RK, Foley KM. Chronic use of opioid analgesics in non-malignant pain: report of 38 cases. Pain 1986; 25:171–186.
16. Office of Applied Studies. National Survey on Drug Use and Health. Substance Abuse and Mental Services Administration (SAMHSA), 2004.
17. Fishbain D, Rosomoff H, Rosomoff R. Drug abuse, dependence and addiction in chronic pain patients. Clin J Pain 1992; 8:77–85.
18. Ballantyne J, Mao J. Opioid therapy for chronic pain. N Engl J Med 2003; 349:1943–1953.

19. Kalso E, Edwards J, Moore R, et al. Opioids in chronic non-cancer pain: systematic review of efficacy and safety. Pain 2004; 112:372–380.
20. Furlan AD, Sandoval JA, Mailis-Gagnon A, et al. Opioid for chronic non cancer pain: A meta-analysis of effectiveness and side effects. Can Med Assoc J 2006; 174(11):589–594.
21. Watson CPN, Babul N. Efficacy of oxycodone in neuropathic pain. A randomized trial in postherpetic neuralgia. Neurology 1998; 50:1837–1841.
22. Huse E, Larbig W, Flor H, et al. The effect of opioids on phantom limb pain and cortical reorganization. Pain 2001; 90:47–55.
23. Harke H, Gretenkort P, Ladleif HU, et al. The response of neuropathic pain and pain in complex regional pain syndrome I to carbamazepine and sustained-release morphine in patients pretreated with spinal cord stimulation: a double-blinded randomized study. Anesth Analg 2001; 92:488–495.
24. Raja SN, Haythornthwaite JA, Pappagallo M, et al. A placebo-controlled trial comparing the analgesic and cognitive effects of opioids and tricyclic antidepressants in postherpetic neuralgia. Neurology 2002; 59:1015–1021.
25. Gimbel JS, Richards P, Portenoy RK. Controlled-release oxycodone for pain in diabetic neuropathy: a randomized controlled trial [see comment]. Neurology 2003; 60(6):927–934.
26. Watson CPN, Moulin D, Watt-Watson J, et al. Controlled-release oxycodone relieves neuropathic pain: a randomized controlled trial in painful diabetic neuropathy. Pain 2003; 105:71–78.
27. Morley JS, Bridson J, Nash TP, et al. Low-dose methadone has an analgesic effect in neuropathic pain: a double-blind randomized controlled crossover trial. Palliat Med 2003; 17(7):576–587.
28. Rowbotham MD, Twilling L, Davies PS, et al. Oral opioid therapy for chronic peripheral and central neuropathic pain. N Engl J Med 2003; 348:1223–1232.
29. Kalso E. Opioids for persistent non-cancer pain. BMJ 2005; 330:156–157.
30. Moore RA, McQuay HJ. Prevalence of opioid adverse events in chronic nonmalignant pain: systematic review of randomised trials of oral opioids. Arthritis Res Ther 2005; 7(5):R1046–1051.
31. Eriksen J, Sjogren P, Bruera E, et al. Critical issues on opioids in chronic non-cancer pain. An epidemiological study. Pain 2006; 125:172–179.
32. Portenoy RK. Opioid therapy for chronic nonmalignant pain: a review of the critical issues. J Pain Symptom Manage 1996; 11:203–217.
33. Katz N. Methodological issues in clinical trials of opioids for chronic pain. Neurology 2005; 65(12, Suppl 4):S32–S49.
34. Ballantyne JC. Opioids for chronic pain: taking stock. Pain 2006; 125:3–4.
35. Mao J. Opioid induced abnormal pain sensitivity: implications in clinical opioid therapy. Pain 2002; 100:213–217.
36. Mercadante S. Opioid rotation for cancer pain: rationale and clinical aspects. Cancer 1999; 86:1856–1866.
37. Schofferman J. Long-term use of opioid analgesics for the treatment of chronic pain of nonmalignant origin. J Pain Symptom Manage 1993; 8:279–288.
38. Harden RN. Chronic opioid therapy: another reappraisal. Aust Prosthodont Soc Bull 2002; 12(1). Available at http://www.ampainsoc.org/pub/bulletin/jan02/poli1.htm. Accessed on 5/11/07.
39. Mao J, Price D, Mayer D. Thermal hyperalgesia in association with the development of morphine tolerance in rats: roles of excitatory amino acid receptors and protein kinase C. J Neurosci 1994; 14:2301–2312.
40. Mao J, Price DD, Mayer DJ. Mechanisms of hyperalgesia and opiate tolerance: a current view of their possible interactions. Pain 1995; 62:259–274.
41. Chu LF, Clark D, Angst M. Opioid tolerance and hyperalgesia in chronic pain patients after one month of oral morphine therapy: a preliminary prospective study. J Pain 2006; 7(1):43–48.

42. Angst MS, Clark JD. Opioid-induced hyperalgesia: a qualitative systematic review. Anesthesiology 2006; 104(3):570–587.
43. Wilder-Smith O, Arendt-Nielsen L. Postoperative hyperalgesia: its clinical importance and relevance. Anesthesiology 2006; 104(3):601–607.
44. Devulder J, Richarz U, Nataraja SH. Impact of long-term use of opioids on quality of life in patients with chronic, non-malignant pain. Curr Med Res Opin 2005; 21(10):1555–1568.
45. Becker N, Sjogren P, Bech P, et al. Treatment outcome of chronic non-malignant pain patients managed in a danish multidisciplinary pain centre compared to general practice: a randomised controlled trial. Pain 2000; 84(2–3):203–211.
46. Bruera E, Macmillan K, Hanson J, et al. The cognitive effects of the administration of narcotic analgesic in patients with cancer pain. Pain 1989; 39:13–16.
47. Vainio A, Ollila J, Matikainen E, et al. Driving ability in cancer patients receiving long-term morphine analgesia. Lancet 1995; 346:667–670.
48. Galski T, Willimas B, Ehle HT. Effects of opioids on driving ability. J Pain Symptom Manage 2000; 19:200–208.
49. Haythornthwaite JA, Menefee LA, Quatrano-Piacentini AL, et al. Outcome of chronic opioid therapy for non-cancer pain. J Pain Symptom Manage 1998; 15:185–194.
50. Tassain V, Attal N, Fletcher D, et al. Long term effects of oral sustained release morphine on neuropsychological performance in patients with chronic non-cancer pain. Pain 2003; 104(1–2):389–400.
51. Kamboj SK, Tookman A, Jones L, et al. The effects of immediate-release morphine on cognitive functioning in patients receiving chronic opioid therapy in palliative care. Pain 2005; 117(3):388–395.
52. Sjogren P, Christrup LL, Petersen MA, et al. Neuropsychological assessment of chronic non-malignant pain patients treated in a multidisciplinary pain centre. Eur J Pain 2005; 9(4):453–462.
53. Mendelson JH, Mendelson JE, Patch VD. Plasma testosterone levels in heroin addiction and during methadone maintenance. J Pharmacol Exp Ther 1975; 192:211–217.
54. Daniell HW. The association of endogenous hormone levels and exogenously administered opiates in males. Am J Pain Manage 2001; 11(1):8–10.
55. Daniell HW. Hypogonadism in men consuming sustained-action oral opioids. J Pain 2002; 3(5):377–384.
56. Finch PM, Roberts LJ, Price L, et al. Hypogonadism in patients treated with intrathecal morphine. Clin J Pain 2000; 3:251–254.
57. DHHS, SAMHSA: National Household Survey on Drug Abuse Main Findings. Series H-11, 1998.
58. AAPM Council on Ethics. American Academy of Pain Medicine. Ethics Charter. Available at www.painmed.org/productpub/pdfs/EthicsCharter.pdf. 2005.
59. Carr DB, Goudas LC. Acute pain. Lancet 1999; 353(9169):2051–2058.
60. Kehlet H, Dahl JB. Anaesthesia, surgery, and challenges in postoperative recovery. Lancet 2003; 362(9399):1921–1928.
61. Brennan TJ, Kehlet H. Preventive analgesia to reduce wound hyperalgesia and persistent postsurgical pain. Not an easy path. Anesthesiolgy 2005; 103:681–683.
62. Dubois MY. The birth of an ethics charter for pain medicine. Pain Med 2005; 6(3):201–202.
63. Joranson DE, Gilson AM, Dahl JL, et al. Pain medicine, controlled substances, and state medical board policy: a decade of change. J Pain Symptom Manage 2002; 23:138–147.
64. Joranson D, Gilson A. State intractable pain policy: current status. Aust Prosthodont Soc Bull 1997; 7(2):7–9.
65. Drug Enforcement Administration. Physician's Manual: An Informational Outline of the Controlled Substances Act of 1970. Washington DC: U.S. Department of Justice, 1990.

66. Opinions on Practice Matters, sec 8.081:222,223. Code of Medical Ethics, Current Opinions With Annotations, 2004–2005 Ed. Chicago: American Medical Association; 2004.
67. Fields HL. Ethical standards in pain management and research. In: Fields HL, ed. Core Curriculum for Professional Education in Pain. Seattle: IASP Press; 1995:117–123.
68. Dubois MY. Why an "ethics" forum in Pain Medicine. Pain Med 2000; 1(2):105–106.
69. Sullivan M. Ethical principles in pain management. Pain Med 2001; 2:106–111.
70. Chabal C, Erjavec M, Jacobson L, et al. Prescription opiate abuse in chronic pain patinets: clinical criteria, incidence and predictors. Clin J Pain 1997; 13:150–155.
71. Compton P, Darakjian J, Miotto K. Screening for addiction in patients with chronic pain with "problematic" substance use: evaluation of a pilot assessment tool. J Pain Symptom Manage 1998; 16:355–363.
72. Passik SD, Kirsh KL, Whitcomb L, et al. A new tool to assess and document pain outcomes in chronic pain patients receiving opioid therapy. Clin Ther 2004; 26(4):552–561.
73. Adams L, Gatchel R, Robinson RC, et al. Development of a self-report screening instrument for assessing potential opioid medication misuse in chronic pain patients. J Pain Sympt Manage 2004; 27(5):440–459.
74. Butler S, Budman S, Fernandez K, et al. Validation of a screener and opioid assessment measure for patients with chronic pain. Pain 2004; 112:65–75.
75. Webster L, Webster R. Predicting aberrant behaviors in opioid-treated patients: preliminary validation of the Opioid Risk Tool. Pain Med 2005; 6(6):432–442.
76. Friedman R, Li V, Mehrotra D. Treating pain patients at risk: evaluation of a screening tool in opioid-treated pain patients with and without addiction. Pain Med 2003; 4(2):182–185.
77. Collett BJ. Chronic opioid therapy for non-cancer pain. Br J Anaesth 2001; 87:133–144.
78. West J, Aronoff G, Dahl J, et al. Model guidelines for the use of controlled substances for the treatment of pain. A policy document of the Federation of State Medical Boards of the United States, Inc. Federation of State Medical Boards of the United States, Inc, Euless, TX; 1998.
79. Haddox JD, Joranson D, Angarola RT, et al. The use of opioids for the treatment of chronic pain. A consensus statement from the American Academy of Pain Medicine and the American Pain Society. American Academy of Pain Medicine and American Pain Society, 1997.
80. Evidence-based recommendations for medical management of chronic non-malignant pain. Reference Guide for Clinicians. Ontario: The College of Physicians and Surgeons of Ontario; 2000.
81. Jovey R, Ennis J, Gardner-Nix J, et al. Use of opioid analgesics for the treatment of chronic noncancer pain—a consensus statement and guidelines from the Canadian Pain Society, 2002. Pain Res Manage 2003; 8(Suppl A):3A–28A.
82. VA/DoD clinical practice guideline for the management of opioid therapy for chronic pain. Available at www.Oqp.Med.Va.Gov?Cpg/Cpg.Htm. 2006. Accessed on 10/24/2006.
83. Atluri S, Boswell MV, Hansen HC, et al. Guidelines for the use of controlled substances in the management of chronic pain. Pain Physician 2003; 6(3):233–257.
84. Kalso E, Allan L, Dellemijn P, et al. Recommendations for using opioids in chronic non-cancer pain. Eur J Pain 2003; 7(5):381–386.
85. Recommendations for the appropriate use of opioids for persistent non-cancer pain. A Consensus Statement Prepared on Behalf of the British Pain Society, the Royal College of Anaesthetists, the Royal College of General Practitioners, and the Royal College of Psychiatrists. London: The British Pain Society; 2005.
86. Red Book. Drug Topics. Top 200 Brand-Name Drugs by Prescription. Montvale, NJ: Medical Economics; March 6, 2002.
87. Turk DC. Clinical effectiveness and cost-effectiveness of treatments for patients with chronic pain. Clin J Pain 2002; 18:355–365.

88. Flor H, Fydrich T, Turk DC. Efficacy of multidisciplinary pain treatment centers: a meta-analytic review. Pain 1992; 49:221–230.
89. Patrick LE, Altmaier EM, Found EM. Long-term outcomes in multidisciplinary treatment of chronic low back pain: results of a 13-year follow-up. Spine 2004; 29:850–855.
90. Guzman J, Esmail R, Karjalainen K, et al. Multidisciplinary rehabilitation for chronic low back pain: systematic review. BMJ 2001; 322:1511–1516.
91. Lin EH, Katon W, Von Korff M, et al. Effect of improving depression care on pain and functional outcomes among older adults with arthritis: a randomized controlled trial. JAMA 2003; 290:2428–2429.
92. Ballantyne J. Pharmacology and practice of opioid drugs for visceral pain. In: Pasricha P, Willis W, Gebhart G, eds. Chronic Abdominal and Visceral Pain: Theory and Practice; 2006.
93. Fishman SM, Mao J. Opioid therapy in chronic nonmalignant pain. In: Ballantyne JC, ed. The Massachusetts General Hospital Handbook of Pain Management, 3rd edn. Philadelphia, PA: Lippincott Williams & Wilkins; 2005.
94. Ballantyne J. Opioid therapy: is it appropriate in patients with noncancer pain? An evidence-based look at the issue. ASA Refresher Courses in Anesthesiology, vol. 34, Chapter 3, American Society of Anesthesiologists, Philadelphia, PA: Lippincott Williams & Wilkins; 2006.

5 Chronic Pain Management as an Alternative to Spine Surgery

Andrew R. Block and Richard D. Guyer
Texas Back Institute, Plano, Texas, U.S.A.

INTRODUCTION: SPINE SURGERY SUCCESSES AND FAILURES

The life of a patient with chronic back pain (CBP) is marked by uncertainty, stress, and even desperation. CBP patients often suffer major disruption of their lives, loss of employment, high divorce rates, frequent emotional disturbance, and dependency on narcotic pain medication. It is not surprising, then, that many look for the magic bullet, a quick fix to set their lives back on track. For many, spine surgery seems to hold out the possibility of such a solution. After all, most patients trust physicians to be able to "cure" their physical ills. If there is ever an individual considered worthy of trust and respect, it is a highly trained spine surgeon.

A number of well-conducted studies point to the effectiveness of spine surgery for CBP. For example, Atlas et al. (1) compared the 4-year outcomes of surgery with unstructured conservative care for lumbar stenosis. They found that the patients treated surgically had significantly greater relief of pain and higher levels of satisfaction than those treated conservatively. Similarly, in a study by Malter et al. (2), patients who underwent discectomy for lumbar disk herniation had significantly better quality of life, for up to 5 years, than patients who were treated conservatively. Additionally, this study found that the cost-effectiveness of discectomy was quite high, even higher than that for coronary artery bypass grafting for single-artery coronary disease. Finally, Fritzell et al. (3) found that patients treated with spinal fusion had significantly greater pain reduction, improvement in function, and reduction in depression than did patients with similar diagnoses who were treated conservatively, primarily through physical therapy.

Unfortunately, despite such findings of the salutary effects of spine surgery, the CBP patient does not have to look far to obtain evidence of surgery's limited effectiveness. A visit to the waiting room of a busy spine surgeon will reveal a number of patients who continue to experience pain after their initial surgery, and many who go on to multiple surgeries. Often friends, colleagues, and even TV ads by trial attorneys urge caution in undergoing spine surgery. Additionally, much research points to the limitations in effectiveness of spine surgery. For example, Hoffman et al. (4) reviewed the results of all studies examining the outcome of lumbar discectomies. They found a mean success rate of 67%, with about a 10% reoperation rate. Lumbar fusion outcome is similar, as revealed in a study by Turner et al (5). Examining all the then extant studies on fusion, an average success rate of 65–75% was found, lower success being associated with greater numbers of levels fused and with the use of instrumentation. Thus, to the confused, despondent back pain patient, spine surgery may deliver much less than it seems to promise.

WHY DOES SPINE SURGERY FAIL?

There are many potential explanations for the frequent failure of spine surgery, most of which are either inaccessible to, or uncontrollable by, the CBP patient. First, as noted by Birkmeyer and Weinstein, there is a lack of general consensus among spine surgeons about indications for these procedures (6). Perhaps, this explains why the rate of spine surgery in different areas of the country varies by as much as eightfold (6). Second, there are wide variations in the skill and experience of spine surgeons such that in some hands, surgery may be a technical failure. Problems such as persistence of unrecognized lateral recess stenosis, a missed sequestered disk fragment, or spinal instability after fusion can lead to failure of the surgery to relieve pain (7). However, most often even when spine surgery is a clinical failure, it is, simultaneously, a technical success: the patient continues to experience disability and pain despite correction of the underlying pathophysiology. In such cases, the explanation for the limitation of spine surgery effectiveness most often rests on patient selection, particularly in choosing to operate on patients who have a high level of psychosocial "risk" factors.

A growing body of research indicates that aspects of patients' emotional, interpersonal, and vocational presentation can strongly influence the outcome of spine surgery [see (8) for an extensive review]. For example, Spengler et al. gave the widely utilized Minnesota Multiphasic Personality Inventory (MMPI) to patients who were to undergo discectomy and found that patients who scored high on the characteristics of *hypochondriasis* and *hysteria* had much poorer clinical outcome than those who scored low on these dimensions (9). Many other psychosocial factors have been found to be associated with continued pain and disability after technical correction of underlying pathology, including history of substance abuse (10), history of physical abuse and abandonment (11), and depression (12), to name a few. In our own prospective study (13), we created a scorecard listing a wide variety of psychosocial risk factors that had been identified from a literature search to be associated with reduced spine surgery outcome. We found that 44/53 patients who had a high level of psychosocial risk obtained poor clinical outcome from spine surgery (both laminectomy/discectomy and spinal fusion), compared to a clinical failure rate of 3/31 in the group of patients having low levels of psychosocial risk and 23/120 in the moderate level of risk category.

Summarizing, there are a number of reasons to urge caution in considering spine surgery. First, there exists no universally accepted standard for the treatment of spine injuries. Second, spine surgeries, while often effective at correcting underlying pathology, fail to achieve pain relief and recovery of function for 25–35% of patients. Finally, psychosocial factors exert a large influence on the outcome of spine surgery.

CHRONIC PAIN MANAGEMENT PROGRAM AS AN ALTERNATIVE TO SPINE SURGERY

Fortunately, several recent studies demonstrate that there exists a viable, effective alternative to spine surgery—the interdisciplinary chronic pain management program (CPMP). Such programs, as many chapters in this book note, teach patients to manage and cope with pain and its impacts, through a combination of physical conditioning, education, psychological treatment, relaxation training, and vocational counseling. Several recent studies have shown that the CPMP approach can be as effective in treating spine pain patients as is spine surgery. Brox et al. studied 64 Swedish patients with evidence of severe disk degeneration lasting more than 1 year (14). These patients were randomly assigned to undergo either (1) lumbar fusion with posterior transpedicular screws and postoperative physical therapy; or (2) a modified CPMP involving cognitive-behavioral intervention with three daily physical exercise sessions for 3 weeks. At 1-year follow-up, both groups had significant improvements in function, as measured by the Oswestry Disability Index (ODI), but there was no significant difference in functional improvement between those treated surgically and those treated nonsurgically. In addition, there were no significant differences in pain, use of analgesics, emotional distress, and return to work. Fear–avoidance beliefs were reduced significantly more in the nonsurgically treated group [see (15) for similar results]. The early complication rate for the surgically treated group was 18%.

Additional support for the use of CPMP has been obtained by Fairbank et al. (16), who examined 349 patients who were uncertain if they should undergo spine surgery. These patients were randomly assigned to spinal fusion or to "intensive rehabilitation"—a CPMP. The surgical group underwent spine stabilization procedures. Subjects were followed for 24 months. The patients treated with spine surgery showed a slightly greater improvement in function as measured by the ODI, but no other comparisons between the two groups reached significance. Intraoperative complications occurred in 19 patients who underwent surgery. An additional study of these patients (17) found that the cost of CPMP was far less than that for surgery (£ 4256 vs. £7830), while the percentage of patients returning to work at 2 years is equivalent. Thus, CPMP was much more cost-effective than spinal fusion. Turk and Burwinkle (18) in a separate review of the literature confirm and extend such findings. They found that the CPMP approach is approximately 26 times more cost-effective in returning patients to work than is spine surgery.

It appears, then, that CPMP is a viable alternative for both patients who have a high level of identified psychosocial risk, or those who are uncertain about whether to undergo spine surgery. However, there are many other potential candidates for spine surgery who could be benefited by considering CPMP (Table 1). For example, many patients may have expectations of poor outcome, or may be overly optimistic in their hopes. Iverson et al. (19) found that expectations of great pain relief by patients who underwent surgery for spinal stenosis were associated with more pain and less satisfaction at 6 months than were lower expectations of pain relief. (However, in this study higher expectations of improvement in functioning as a result of the surgery were associated with greater improvement in functioning and greater satisfaction.) Thus, for patients expecting to have "no pain" as a result of spine surgery, CPMP may be a valuable alternative. This is also the case for patients who have failed previous spine surgeries, since, as noted by a number of authors including North et al. (20), the success rate for repeat spine surgery is quite low [see also (21)]. Similarly, since substance abuse or overuse is associated with reduced spine surgery outcome (10), patients with such problems would likely be better served by participation in a CPMP than by spine surgery. In cases where a potential surgical patient has any of the characteristics listed in Table 1, CPMP ought to be at least considered as an alternative to surgery.

TABLE 1 Patients for whom CPMP Should be Considered as an Alternative to Spine Surgery

- Patients with moderate or high level of identified psychosocial risk factors
- Patients who are uncertain about whether to have spine surgery
- Patients with unrealistic outcome expectations
- Patients who have comorbid physical problems, such as diabetes, obesity, etc.
- Patients with insufficient findings, who might be considered for exploratory surgery
- Patients who have failed previous spine surgery
- Young patients, especially if being considered for spinal fusion
- Patients who have exhibited noncompliance or drug-seeking behavior

SPECIAL CONSIDERATIONS FOR CPMP TREATMENT OF SURGICAL CANDIDATES

In many ways, the CPMP for a potential spine surgery candidate is similar to that for any other pain condition. The program is multidisciplinary in nature, aimed at improving function, reducing or eliminating narcotic medication use, emotional stabilization, and learning cognitive-behavioral techniques for coping with pain as well as reducing "maladaptive thinking." However, patients with identified spinal pathology have particular concerns that need to be recognized and addressed if treatment is to be effective.

Shifting from Medical Model to Rehabilitation Model

While it may be apparent that potential spine surgery candidates can be effectively treated and surgery avoided through participation in a CPMP, it may be difficult to convince this fact to many patients. As noted earlier, many patients feel as though spine surgery is the quickest and most effective solution to their pain. One of the foundations of the CPMP approach, however, is that the patients come to view pain outside of the traditional medical model, i.e., the pain can be eliminated by a physician removing or ameliorating the underlying physical pathology. Rather, the patient needs to accept that a rehabilitation model is more appropriate. This alternative model posits that the "cure" for the pain is not possible, but it is up to each patient to gradually improve functional ability and pain control in order to recover maximally from the injury. Treatment, then, becomes a matter of learning pain "management" techniques, rather than pain "cure," through guidance by the staff and even by other patients.

It is possible for the CBP patients to accept a rehabilitation model. One way is by actively involving patients in the decision to avoid surgery. A recent research by Deyo et al. (22) demonstrates that carefully providing patients with information about surgery can lead them to be more realistic about the potential benefits and risks of spine surgery. In this study, 393 patients with either herniated disks, spinal stenosis, or other diagnoses were given either an interactive video with a booklet about their surgery or the booklet alone. The percentage of patients with herniated disks who elected to undergo surgery was lower in the videodisk group ($p < 0.08$) compared to the booklet group. Patients in the videodisc group felt better informed than those who received the booklet only.

The results of the Deyo et al. (22) study suggest that if patients are accurately informed about the likely benefits and risks of spine surgery given their particular situation, they are much more likely to opt out of surgery and accept a rehabilitation model. As an example, patients can be informed that they are more likely to obtain poor surgery results if they have high levels of psychosocial distress, if they are undergoing a second or third spine surgery, or if they are dependent on pain medication. Such knowledge can go a long way toward convincing patients of the value of the rehabilitation model.

Of course, the approach taken by the referring physician is critical. Moving to a rehabilitation model requires that the patient makes behavioral changes rather than simply, passively having improvements foisted upon him or her through surgery. In order for the patient to embrace the necessary behavior changes, he or she must see the referring physician, as well as the CPMP approach, as truly the best interest option. Research on "social control" by Tucker et al. (23) demonstrates that individuals' health-related behavior can be strongly influenced by others. When individuals feel "positive" and supported by the other, they are likely to engage in the health behaviors suggested. On the other hand, if the individual feels negatively about the other's attempt to change health-related behaviors (e.g., feels the other is nagging or attempting to induce guilt), then the individual is likely to either ignore the suggestions for behavior change or even hide unhealthy behaviors. Such research implies that the patient must see the referring physician as a supportive advocate, who encourages functional improvements and reduction in medication through an active rehabilitation process, rather than advocating for a surgical procedure, the outcome of which is highly uncertain.

Fear of Worsening Injury

One of the most common beliefs of CBP sufferers is that increasing activity can lead to worsening of the underlying physical condition or increasing pain. There is little empirical justification for such fear, except in cases of spinal instability. However, it is clear that such fears can severely limit the progress made by spine surgery candidates, whether they are treated conservatively or with surgery. For example, den Boer et al. (25) preoperatively assessed patient fears of activity, pain-coping strategies, and outcome expectation in 336 patients who underwent surgery for lumbar radicular syndrome related to prolapsed or sequestered disk compromising the L4, L5, or S1 nerve root. A stepwise regression analysis at 6 months postoperatively found that, after controlling for all other factors, fear of movement/reinjury, negative surgery outcome expectations, and passive pain coping were all associated with poorer surgical outcome. Even more relevant to CPMP, a companion study (25) found that these same factors were associated with poorer work capacity at 6 months postoperatively.

The recent study by Brox et al. (15) demonstrates that CPMP can be effective in reducing fear–avoidance beliefs in spine surgery candidates. In this study, patients with indications for instrumented spinal fusions were randomly assigned to either have a posterior lumbar interbody fusion or to a CPMP consisting of lectures on cognitive coping with pain combined with aggressive rehabilitation. Both groups showed significant improvements in pain, general functioning, and medication use at 1-year follow-up. Further, only the CPMP-treated group displayed a significant reduction in fear–avoidance of physical activity. This group also showed greater improvement in fingertip-to-floor distance than did the surgery group.

These results, taken together with those of den Boer et al. (2006), would imply that CPMP-treated spine surgery candidates may be able to maintain their treatment-related gains better, because their fears of reinjury/movement are directly targeted.

Medication

Historically, one of the main goals of CPMPs is the reduction or elimination of narcotic medications. CPMPs are quite successful at this, as approximately 60–70% of patients are able to eliminate use of narcotics, and a large proportion do not return to narcotic use over the long-term (18). The use of opioids and narcotics in benign chronic pain syndromes is controversial, with some advocating their use in selected cases (24). Often patients with spinal pathology that is potentially correctable with surgery are given large doses of pain medication as an interim measure, to see them through until they undergo the surgery. While such medication certainly provides pain relief, use of narcotics has a number of downsides. First, patients going into surgery are often on such high doses of narcotic medications that achieving postoperative pain control becomes problematic. Second, as surgery is delayed, there is increased likelihood of dependency or addiction, and the patient can also become increasingly lethargic or inactive. Perhaps the most significant aspect of using narcotic medication in the spine surgery candidate is the message that such an approach conveys, i.e., the patient has minimal ability and/or responsibility for pain control. Instead, the idea that pain control can only be ultimately achieved through surgery is reinforced.

As noted throughout this text, the goal of the CPMP approach is to teach patients to take responsibility for their own management and control of pain. This is difficult to do in the best of cases, but in the case of a patient who is automatically given narcotic pain medication to control pain associated with a potential surgical lesion, it is often extremely difficult to help the patient recognize the ability to self-manage pain. Again, education seems to be the key. The randomized studies reported earlier indicate that for patients having indications for laminectomy/discectomy or spinal fusion, treatment with CPMP leads to reductions in pain medication that are equivalent to surgical treatment. This implies that the patient education, physical improvement, and cognitive change can be as effective in managing pain as is spine surgery. If the patient can learn to achieve pain control without surgery or medication, the risk of dependency and physical and cognitive complications are eliminated, with the bonus that the patient can feel a great sense of accomplishment for having overcome the use of these medications.

Authorization

There is one very practical concern in considering CPMP as an alternative to spine surgery—insurance authorization. While insurers certainly recognize the limitations of spine surgery, the idea of paying for a CPMP on a patient with a surgical lesion may certainly give rise to pause. After all, some patients who attempt CPMP as a surgical alternative will go on to have spine surgery. For example, in the study of Rivero-Arias et al. (17), 38 of the 176 patients randomized to CPMP approach subsequently went on to have spine surgery, leading to an additional average of £2128 in additional medical treatment costs. However, insurers should take note that even with the costs of these additional spine surgeries added in, the overall cost for patients treated with the CPMP approach was still only 54% of that for the patients treated conservatively. Thus, the attempt at CPMP, for at least those patients with characteristics listed in Table 1, appears to be quite cost-effective.

Patients may, reasonably, be concerned that if they attempt CPMP as an alternative approach, then the insurer may not authorize subsequent surgery. This is a particular concern in managed care environments and for patients covered by worker's compensation, where holding down treatment costs is an explicit goal of the insurer. In such cases, it is critical to obtain the assurance of the carrier that surgery will be authorized if ordered after CPMP. Without such an assurance, many patients may refuse a CPMP, fearing that they may be left with untreatable surgical lesions.

CONCLUSIONS

A universally accepted approach to the treatment of many spine injuries does not exist. The indications for spine surgery, the types of surgeries undertaken and the rate of spine surgery, vary widely as a function of physician training, physician discipline, and even geography. While only about 2% of patients with spinal pain ever undergo spine surgery, it is clear that surgery, even when indicated and correctly performed, is not always effective in relieving pain and improving functional ability. Research reviewed in this chapter demonstrates that, for selected groups of patients, CPMP can be an effective treatment approach. This approach has the advantages of (1) clinical outcomes that are overall equivalent to those of spine surgery; (2) significant reduction in treatment costs compared to surgery; and (3) limited iatrogenic problems, such as development of scar tissue, infection, or in the case of spinal fusion, development of pseudoarthrosis or transition syndrome (degeneration of disks adjacent to the fused level). Further, the CPMP approach explicitly teaches patients the importance of self-responsibility for health, increasing the likelihood that CPMP-treated patients will maintain gains long after the program has ended. On the other hand, treating the potential spine surgery candidate in a CPMP has potential downfalls also: (1) a number of such patients go on to have surgery after CPMP treatment, adding to total treatment cost and duration; (2) insurers may balk at paying for surgery, if needed, after the patient has participated in a CPMP.

While Table 1 gives suggestions for those patients who should be considered for CPMP as an alternative to spine surgery, this table is speculative. It will be critical in the future to identify not only those patients who are most likely to benefit from spine surgery, but also those who are most likely to benefit from CPMP. In considering CPMP, one does well to keep in mind the patient's desperate search for relief. Reduction of pain is the most central concern of the patient. For the surgeon, pain relief is often an epiphenomenon—a by-product of correcting an identified anatomic problem which may (or may not) be the source of the pain. To the extent that the surgeon is unable to clearly circumscribe a specific "pain generator," the surgery is unlikely to achieve the pain relief so desired by the patient. Further, if excessive pain sensitivity, heavy medication use, depression, or other psychosocial factors alter the patient's ability to perceive pain, then surgery is unlikely to be effective. As spine surgery develops increasingly sophisticated hardware, diagnostic, and surgical techniques, patient selection will become even more important. In this way, we should be able to offer alternatives to patients for whom surgery is unlikely to be effective.

REFERENCES

1. Atlas SJ, Keller RB, Robson D, et al. Surgical and nonsurgical management of lumbar spinal stenosis: four-year outcomes from the Maine lumbar spine study. Spine 2000; 25(5):556–562.
2. Malter AD, Larson EB, Urban N, et al. Cost-effectiveness of lumbar discectomy for the treatment of herniated intervertebral disc. Spine 1996; 21(9):1048–1054.
3. Fritzell P, Hagg O, Wessberg P, et al. 2001 Volvo Award Winner in Clinical Studies: lumbar fusion versus nonsurgical treatment for chronic low back pain: a multicenter randomized controlled trial from the Swedish Lumbar Spine Study Group. Spine 2001; 26(23):2521–2532.
4. Hoffman RM, Wheeler KJ, Deyo RA. Surgery for herniated lumbar discs: a literature synthesis. J Gen Intern Med 1993; 8(9):487–496.
5. Turner JA, Ersek M, Herron L, et al. Patient outcomes after lumbar spinal fusions. JAMA 1992; 268(7):907–911.
6. Birkmeyer NJ, Weinstein JN. Medical versus surgical treatment for low back pain: evidence and clinical practice. Eff Clin Pract 1999; 2(5):218–227.
7. Oaklander AL, North RB. In: Loeser JD, Chapman CR, Turk DC, eds. Bonica's Management of Pain, 3rd edn. Philadelphia, PA: Lippincott, Williams and Wilkins; 2001.
8. Block AR, Gatchel RJ, Deardorff WW, et al. The Psychology of Spine Surgery. Washington, DC: American Psychological Association; 2003.
9. Spengler DM, Ouellette EA, Battie M, et al. Elective discectomy for herniation of a lumbar disc. Additional experience with an objective method. J Bone Joint Surg Am 1990; 72(2):230–237.
10. Spengler DM, Freeman C, Westbrook R, et al. Low-back pain following multiple lumbar spine procedures. Failure of initial selection? Spine 1980; 5(4):356–360.
11. Schofferman J, Anderson D, Hines R, et al. Childhood psychological trauma correlates with unsuccessful lumbar spine surgery. Spine 1992; 17(6 Suppl):S138–S144.
12. Kjellby-Wendt G, Styf JR, Carlsson SG. The predictive value of psychometric analysis in patients treated by extirpation of lumbar intervertebral disc herniation. J Spinal Disord 1999; 12(5):375–379.
13. Block AR, Ohnmeiss DD, Guyer RD, et al. The use of presurgical psychological screening to predict the outcome of spine surgery. Spine J 2001; 1(4):274–282.
14. Brox JI, Sorensen R, Friis A, et al. Randomized clinical trial of lumbar instrumented fusion and cognitive intervention and exercises in patients with chronic low back pain and disc degeneration. Spine 2003; 28(17): 1913–1921.
15. Brox JI, Reikeras O, Nygaard O, et al. Lumbar instrumented fusion compared with cognitive intervention and exercises in patients with chronic back pain after previous surgery for disc herniation: a prospective randomized controlled study. Pain 2006; 122(1–2):145–155.
16. Fairbank J, Frost H, Wilson-MacDonald J, et al. Randomised controlled trial to compare surgical stabilisation of the lumbar spine with an intensive rehabilitation programme for patients with chronic low back pain: the MRC spine stabilisation trial. BMJ 2005; 330(7502):1233.
17. Rivero-Arias O, Campbell H, Gray A, et al. Surgical stabilisation of the spine compared with a programme of intensive rehabilitation for the management of patients with chronic low back pain: cost utility analysis based on a randomised controlled trial. BMJ 2005; 330(7502):1239.
18. Turk DC, Burwinkle TM. Assessment of chronic pain in rehabilitation: Outcomes measures in clinical trials and clinical practice. Rehab Psych 2005; 50:56–64.

19. Iversen MD, Daltroy LH, Fossel AH, et al. The prognostic importance of patient preoperative expectations of surgery for lumbar spinal stenosis. Patient Educ Couns 1998; 34(2):169–178.
20. North RB, Campbell JN, James CS, et al. Failed back surgery syndrome: 5-year follow-up in 102 patients undergoing repeated operation. Neurosurgery 1991; 28(5):685–690.
21. Franklin GM, Haug J, Heyer NJ, et al. Outcome of lumbar fusion in Washington State workers' compensation. Spine 1994; 19(17):1897–1903.
22. Deyo RA, Cherkin DC, Weinstein J, et al. Involving patients in clinical decisions: impact of an interactive video program on use of back surgery. Med Care 2000; 38(9):959–969.
23. Tucker JS, Orlando M, Elliott MN, et al. Affective and behavioral responses to health-related social control. Health Psychol 2006; 25(6):715–722.
24. Portenoy R. Chronic opioid therapy in nonmalignant pain. J Pain Symptom Manage 1990(5):S46–S61.
25. den Boer JJ, Oostendorp RAB, Beems T, et al. Continued disability and pain after lumbar disc surgery: the role of cognitive-behavioral factors. Pain 2006; 123:45–52.

6 Integrating Complementary and Alternative Medicine into Multidisciplinary Chronic Pain Treatment

Gabriel Tan
Michael E. DeBakey VA Medical Center, and Departments of Anesthesiology, and Physical Medicine and Rehabilitation, Baylor College of Medicine, Houston, Texas, U.S.A.

Mark P. Jensen
Department of Rehabilitation Medicine, University of Washington, Seattle, Washington, U.S.A.

In the practice of Western medicine, individuals suffering from chronic pain usually seek medical care with the hope of obtaining a specific diagnosis and curative treatment. When a curative treatment is not available, patients then often expect and are given prescriptions for analgesic medications ("pain killers") for pain relief. Unfortunately, however, specific diagnoses for most chronic pain problems are difficult to make, and treatments are rarely curative. Moreover, although analgesic medications can be effective in relieving acute pain in the short-term, their utility for treating chronic pain is controversial and efficacy is, at best, marginal (1). For example, in a recent review of the efficacy of various treatments for patients with chronic pain, it was noted that the average pain reduction for patients placed on long-term opioids is only 32% (2). In addition, anticonvulsants, tricyclic antidepressants, and topical preparations (considered the treatment of choice for neuropathic pain) seldom result in pain reductions to below a rating of 4 on 0 to 10 numerical scales. Turk (3) concluded that "... none of the currently available treatments eliminates pain for the majority of patients." Thus, despite the availability of multiple biomedical treatments for chronic pain, there remains ample room for additional, and perhaps for some patients, even more efficacious treatments.

PSYCHOLOGICAL INTERVENTIONS FOR PAIN MANAGEMENT

Cognitive-behavioral therapy (CBT) and other psychological interventions provide a viable alternative to traditional Western biomedical pain treatments. A growing body of research supports their efficacy for helping patients better manage chronic pain (4,5). However, like more traditional biomedical-focused pain treatments, psychological interventions are not universally effective (6).

Furthermore, psychological interventions are not without their limitations. First, in order to be successful, they require significant effort and motivation on the part of the patient (7). These treatments also tend to be time-intensive (10 or more 1-hour individual or group sessions is not unusual), and they usually require significant practice of the cognitive and behavioral management skills outside of treatment sessions. In addition, some patients with chronic pain are so wedded to the traditional medical model, where treatments are done "to" them and not by them, that they may have little interest in treatments which require their own efforts. Many such patients who desire a biomedical-focused treatment approach will not participate or follow through with psychologically based therapies such as CBT.

Along these lines, there may be a subset of patients who are particularly skeptical, rational, analytic, and hyposensitive to the emotional/somatic component of psychosocial threats (8). Such patients tend to be reluctant to examine the etiology of negative emotional/somatic information and instead tend to search for physical explanations of and physical solutions for their distress. When these patients are referred for psychological treatment (for a pain problem), they may not show up for the sessions and may not follow through with homework assignments or practice recommendations that are often a part of these psychological approaches. One reason for this apparent resistance may be the belief that seeing a psychologist for pain problems amounts to an admission that their pain is "in the head" and not real.

COMPLEMENTARY AND ALTERNATIVE MEDICINE

Complementary and alternative medicine (CAM) has been defined as "diagnosis, treatment and/or prevention which complements mainstream medicine by contributing to a common whole, satisfying a demand not met by orthodoxy, or diversifying the conceptual frameworks of medicine" (9). According to the National Center for Complementary and Alternative Medicine, CAM includes "treatments and healthcare practices not taught widely in medical schools, not generally used in hospitals, and not usually reimbursed by medical insurance companies" (10). CAM encompasses both nontraditional treatments used in association with conventional Western medical practices as well as alternative medical interventions intended to replace traditional Western medical practices (11).

CAM interventions have been increasing in popularity over the past two decades due to dissatisfaction with traditional Western medicine, the availability of information on the Internet, the influence of marketing forces, and the desire of patients to be more actively involved in their own medical decision making (12). Eisenberg and colleagues (13) estimated that the U.S. public spent between $36 billion and $47 billion on CAM treatments in 1997. A recent U.S. national health survey of 31,044 adults found that 36% of the population surveyed used CAM therapies during the prior 12 months (14). This percentage increased to 62% if prayer for health reasons was included in the definition of CAM. Back pain, neck pain, and joint pain are among the problems for which CAM therapies are most commonly sought (14).

EFFICACY OF CAM THERAPIES

The National Institute of Health Office of Alternative Medicine (OAM) and the National Center for Complementary and Alternative Medicine (NCCAM) have grouped CAM therapies into four domains: biologically based medicine, energy medicine, manipulative and body-based medicine, and mind–body medicine. In addition, the NCCAM also defines a separate domain, "whole or professionalized CAM practices" (e.g., acupuncture and homeopathy).

Using the guidelines of the Clinical Psychology Division of the American Psychological Association for quantifying treatment efficacy (15). Tan and colleagues have examined the efficacy of various CAM therapies for chronic pain (16). Their findings indicate that the efficacy of CAM therapies varies considerably from modality to modality, with efficacy ranging from 2 (possibly efficacious) to 5 (highly efficacious). Hypnosis is rated at levels 4–5; biofeedback, acupuncture, and massage therapies at levels 2–4. Chiropractics, meditation, yoga, and glucosamine/chondroitin for arthritis have been assigned level 3 (probably efficacious).

USE OF CAM MODALITIES TO ENHANCE OUTCOMES AT THE MEDVAMC

This chapter will select three CAM modalities, used at the Michael E DeBakey VA Medical Center (MEDVAMC), to illustrate how their inclusion can enhance the outcomes of a pain management program. Two therapies, hypnosis and biofeedback, were selected because they have been shown to be among the most robust in terms of evidence for efficacy in the literature (16). A third modality to be discussed is cranial electrotherapy stimulation (CES), given the authors' experience that CES and hypnosis can be successfully incorporated into an existing pain practice (63,78).

Hypnosis

The use of hypnosis for pain relief in the West dates back to the 1770s when Anton Mesmer used hypnosis to treat a large number of problems, although he attributed treatment successes to his ability to direct the "magnetic fluid" that existed in all material (17). Before the availability of chemical anesthesia, hypnotic anesthesia had been used to successfully perform surgical procedures causing minimal pain (18,19). A meta-analysis of 18 studies by Montgomery et al. (20) found strong support for hypnotic analgesia as a valid and reliable phenomenon with 75% of clinical and experimental subjects reporting significant pain relief. Patterson and Jensen (21) supported this conclusion for both acute and chronic pain conditions. Hilgard and Hilgard (22) proposed three general classes of pain management approaches using hypnosis: direct suggestion for pain reduction (e.g., an area becoming numb, or "you will feel no pain"), alteration of the experience of pain (e.g., letting the pain fade away as the drop of water ripples and spreads outward in the lake, or the pain sensation going from hot to cool), and redirection of attention (e.g., hypnotic suggestion to become absorbed and intrigued by an internally generated event or scene). Overall, research indicates that hypnotic analgesic interventions have a significantly greater impact on pain reduction as compared to no treatment, medication management, physical therapy, and education/advice (23).

The efficacy and mechanism of action of hypnosis on irritable bowel syndrome (IBS) has recently been reviewed (24). A special issue of the *International Journal of Clinical and Experimental Hypnosis* (volume 54:1, 2006) has been devoted exclusively to this topic. The findings are unequivocal in showing that the hypnosis is highly efficacious for the treatment of IBS.

Biofeedback

Biofeedback is the process of providing real-time information from psychophysiological recordings about the levels at which physiological systems are functioning.

Electronic biofeedback devices are designed to objectively record tiny changes in physiological functions noninvasively which could not be readily detected by other means. Most devices record physiological responses from the surface of the skin. The information recorded by surface sensors is sent to a computer for processing and then displayed on a monitor and/or through speakers. The patient and therapist can attend to the display of information and incorporate it into the processes they are attempting to modify. The physiological parameters most often recorded for biofeedback include muscle tension [the surface electromyogram (SEMG)], near surface blood flow (done by recording skin temperature), heart rate, sweating or galvanic skin response (GSR), brain waves (EEG), and respiration rate. Recently clinicians have been exploring the efficacy of neurofeedback for pain management (25–28).

A number of reviews of the efficacy literature on biofeedback for pain have been published (29–31); we present a very brief summary of this literature below. Perhaps the strongest evidence for the efficacy of biofeedback comes from research examining its efficacy for migraine and tension headache (32,33). Rains et al. (34) reviewed the relevant meta-analyses and concluded that biofeedback is highly efficacious for tension-type headaches. Comparative studies have shown that biofeedback is at least as, or more, effective than standard interventions such as medication and relaxation training for both tension and migraine types of headache (35). Regarding muscle-related orofacial pain, a comprehensive review concluded that biofeedback treatment of orofacial pain is effective when the pain is due to muscle rather than originating in the temporomandibular joint (36). Several studies have shown that biofeedback was as effective or better than splint therapy for orofacial pain and gains (in terms of pain reduction) were maintained for longer periods with biofeedback than with other treatments (37,38). A recent review (39) of 12 randomized controlled trials (RCTs) concluded that SEMG training with adjunctive CBT is an efficacious treatment for temporomandibular disorders and both SEMG training as the sole intervention and biofeedback-assisted relaxation training are probably efficacious treatments. For musculoskeletal back pain, reviews on efficacy of mixed behavioral interventions including biofeedback indicate that these can be very successful with chronic LBP (40–43). Reviews of studies of the efficacy of biofeedback on LBP have generally concluded that biofeedback is likely to help some patients with muscle-related back pain, and at an overall improvement rate of about 65% relative to 33% for placebo and no improvement for no-treatment controls (44).

Additional studies have investigated phantom limb pain, of which two types have been found to be amenable to biofeedback: burning and cramping pain. Studies have shown that nearly all amputees with cramping limb pain are helped by SEMG (45). The success rate for cramping limb pain (relative to burning pain) has been encouraging, as about half of the patients with burning limb pain have not been able to benefit from biofeedback (45). Many authors do not differentiate types of phantom pain when applying biofeedback but still report success (46,47). Regarding fibromyalgia, a series of studies has confirmed that psychophysiological intervention combining SEMG biofeedback and EEG-driven stimulation (a type of EEG biofeedback where a dominant frequency is selected and moved up and down as the situation demands) is effective in the treatment of fibromyalgia (48–50). These investigators identified diffuse muscular coactivation as a potential source of pain in fibromyalgia syndrome, and SEMG biofeedback has been successfully used to reduce the pain in these paired tender points (48,49).

Biofeedback as a Diagnostic and Self-monitoring Tool

Although biofeedback is often thought of as a treatment tool and its usual definition does not include psychophysiological assessment, it has been our experience (shared by other clinicians) that biofeedback equipment can be used for diagnostic and/or self-monitoring purposes. We are thinking, for example, of a patient recently referred to us with a chronic history of headaches that interfered with his employment as a manager of a store. He had been seen by neurology who placed him on Imitrex, which gave inconsistent relief. He was hooked up to a biofeedback machine with bilateral placement of SEMG electrodes on the upper trapezes. While obtaining baseline measures, he exhibited a slight increase in muscle tension that corresponded with each inhaling breadth and then subsided when he exhaled. This pattern was indicative of a braced breathing posture, which contributed to cumulative tension and muscle spasm, and was determined to be a likely contributor to his headache via the phenomenon of referred pain. He reported being totally unaware of this bracing posture. He was instructed to continue breathing but to do so without the muscle tension when inhaling. He learned this with the help of the visual feedback of his EMG muscle activity. After six training sessions, he reported significant decrease in the episodes and intensity of the headaches, and was able to eventually taper off his Imitrex.

Observing one's real-time psychophysiological recordings on a screen while one is performing a task or simply sitting still often creates an increased self-awareness and impetus for change. It is one thing to tell a patient that his or her standing posture is putting excessive stress and tension on the back. It is another to hook up the patient with SEMG electrodes in selected sites on the back so that he or she can directly observe real-time changes in SEMG recordings during different activities. The simple observation of how a corrected posture can reduce muscle tension may provide sufficient motivation and feedback information for some patients to self-correct the posture. In practice, however, several training sessions are usually needed to make the appropriate adjustments. Although the example given here refers to the use of SEMG electrodes to measure muscle tension, the same principles would apply to other biofeedback modalities as well.

Physiological Stress Profiling

Another common application of biofeedback training is to perform physiological stress profiling (PSP) while the patient is hooked up to several biofeedback modalities simultaneously and is subjected to a variety of stressful stimuli such as a sudden loud noise (with little or no warning) in order to produce a startle response, or is asked to perform increasingly difficult mental arithmetic tasks. Observing which physiological measures respond to the stressor, and in particular which ones remain reactive even after the stressor is removed, can provide useful feedback to both the patient and the therapist concerning how the patient responds to stress. For instance, some patients may display increased heart rate and shallow breathing in response to and following a stressor, others may show decreased finger temperature, and still others may display significant bracing of the neck muscles. More important for patients with chronic pain is the ability to rebound, that is, for the reactive physiological response systems to return to normal, prestress levels after the stressful stimuli are removed. Inability to rebound is often a contributing factor to many pain conditions such as back and neck pain, and headaches.

Biofeedback as an Adjunctive Therapy for Pain Relief

Biofeedback can be used as the sole treatment for pain or as an adjunctive treatment in combination with other interventions. One method is to combine it with pain medication with the goal of tapering off the medications as the patient acquires better pain management skills through biofeedback. Biofeedback is also often combined with psychotherapy as a part of behavioral intervention, or is used as one modality in a multidisciplinary treatment approach.

Some patients may be so distracted by pain that achieving some degree of relief with medication may be necessary before he or she can focus on the biofeedback training. As progress is made, the medication can be gradually reduced and even eventually tapered off. Also, there is some evidence that when combined with microcurrent electrical stimulation, the combined therapies are more effective than either one alone (51).

Biofeedback to Treat Pain-related Symptoms and Interference on Functioning

In addition to reducing pain, biofeedback therapies can be used to treat pain-related symptoms such as depression, excessive fatigue, chronic anger, sleep problems, and excessive anxiety. Biofeedback may be used to address other issues that can affect the outcome of pain management such as addiction to alcohol and pain medication (51,52).

As indicated above, biofeedback for pain often works by first identifying the patient's individual physiological dysfunctions that may be contributing to the pain, helping the patient recognize when those dysfunctions are occurring, and then helping the patient correct them by watching the display and attempting to implement a variety of corrective strategies. For example, most people with chronic muscle-related pain are often not as able as people without pain to be aware of muscle tension (53). They then tend to keep the muscles very tense over long periods of time, which can cause or contribute to chronic pain. Biofeedback can be used to calibrate sensations coming from the muscles with actual levels of tension so that people do not remain more tense than necessary for longer than necessary.

Adverse events or negative side effects of biofeedback therapy for pain are rarely an issue. However, there are potentially serious side effects of other behavioral therapies commonly used conjointly with biofeedback, such as progressive muscle relaxation (PMR) training. Side effects may occur when biofeedback is used to treat conditions other than pain. For example, precipitation of panic attacks or hyperventilation may occur when respiratory alterations are induced among some individuals with significant anxiety or asthma, and there is a potential to trigger cardiac events when PMR is used with individuals with known (or unknown) cardiac problems (51).

The mechanism of action for biofeedback in pain management has not been fully established. However, there is increasing evidence that for chronic muscle or myofascial pain syndromes, pain modulation with biofeedback can occur in part because of increased perceptions of control and decreases in pain-related catastrophizing, as well as by learning lowered arousal techniques that keep sympathetic pathways to trigger points from being maintained (51,54). For pain conditions such as fibromyalgia, phantom limb pain, and other centrally mediated pain, biofeedback may counter the effects of central sensitization through decreasing sympathetic overload, parasympathetic withdrawal, and stress hormones (54,55). There is also some evidence that changing improper muscle contraction and blood flow patterns has a direct effect on pain caused by these problems (56).

To conclude, biofeedback is a nonpharmacological intervention that can work directly or indirectly to help patients deal with pain. The direct approach, which teaches patients to correct the physiological problem causing the pain, is highly efficacious for several pain problems. The indirect approach involves helping patients modulate their pain experience as well as modulate how pain affects functioning. Biofeedback used for pain treatment has no known toxic effects and minimal side effects; it can be used as the sole treatment for pain or as an adjunctive treatment in combination with other interventions. Sufficient meta-analyses, detailed reviews, assessments by U.S. government–sponsored panels, and high-quality studies with long-term follow-ups of significant numbers of patients have concluded that biofeedback can be highly efficacious for assessing and treating a variety of disorders whose main symptom of interest is pain (e.g., 29–31).

Cranial Electrotherapy Stimulation (CES)

It involves "the application of a small amount of current, usually less than one milliampere, through the head via ear clip electrodes" (57). The CES device we use is called "Alpha-Stim," which has been approved by the U.S. Food and Drug Administration (FDA) as a treatment for depression, anxiety, and insomnia (58). Based on the finding that patients with chronic pain frequently have comorbid affective disorders, CES began to gain popularity as an adjunctive intervention for pain management in the 1990s.

A small, but growing, body of controlled studies has reported on the efficacy of CES in reducing pain in patients with fibromyalgia, tension headaches, spinal pain, dental pain, and unspecified chronic pain (56,58). For example, in a double-blind, placebo-controlled study, 60 patients with fibromyalgia were randomly assigned to 3 weeks of 1-hour daily CES treatments, sham CES treatments, or a wait-list control condition. In this study, treated patients showed significant improvements in pain, sleep, well-being, and quality of life and no placebo effect was found among the sham-treated controls (58). In another double-blind study in which 50 dental patients were randomly assigned to receive real ($N = 30$) versus sham ($N = 20$) CES, 24 of the 30 patients (80%) who received CES were able to undergo dental procedures without other anesthesia, while 15 of the 20 (75%) sham CES patients requested anesthesia (59). Our own double-blind, placebo-controlled pilot study on central neuropathic pain (below the level of injury) associated with spinal cord injury indicated significant reduction in pain intensity postsession that was greater for the active CES treatment than the sham CES treatment (60). A multisite study is currently in its second year of implementation which will hopefully further elucidate the efficacy, effectiveness, and long-term effects of this treatment.

Although the mechanism(s) of action of CES on pain is (are) still unclear, it is generally believed that the effects are mediated through a direct action on brain activity in the limbic system, hypothalamus, and/or reticular activating system (61). It also has been suggested that CES reduces anxiety and depression, thereby indirectly elevating the pain threshold (62). In addition, CES (and self-hypnosis training) can serve a useful "Trojan horse" function to persuade patients to become involved in psychologically based interventions. A practical feature of CES is that a clinician simultaneously can carry out psychotherapy while the patient is "hooked up" to the device. Once patients learn that they can modify pain with changes in brain activity using CES, they may become more willing to consider other treatments that alter brain activity, such as CBT.

THE MICHAEL E DEBAKEY VETERANS AFFAIRS MEDICAL CENTER PAIN MANAGEMENT PROGRAM

The experience of the primary author will be described to illustrate how three CAM modalities (hypnosis, CES, and biofeedback) have been successfully integrated into an existing (anesthesiology-based) multidisciplinary pain management program. As with many pain management programs, this one includes a psychological component which offers CBTs in group and individual settings, along with other psychological services in the assessment and treatment of patients suffering from chronic pain.

Past experience had revealed a number of limitations to the services we traditionally offered, the most notable one being a consistently high rate of no-shows for initial appointments and/or limited follow through after the initial appointment. This pattern led us to consider providing CAM interventions for pain, which we thought would be of interest to at least a subset of our patients. A second limitation of the services we initially offered was related to the nature and characteristics of our pain population. Many of our patients travel long distances (60–150 miles) to reach the MEDVAMC and they have limited means to get to the center. To serve their needs, our interventions need to be brief and provide relatively quick results. A third factor that led us to consider CAM approaches was the severity of the pain conditions in our veteran population, which made pain relief a primary goal for many of our patients—a goal that is not entirely consistent with CBT, which tends to focus on improvement in function rather than pain relief, per se. Veterans who receive care from a VA medical center also differ from the population at large in several significant ways. They are more likely to be older, have poorer health status, be smokers, be heavy drinkers, have psychiatric problems, be socioeconomically disadvantaged, be homeless, and have more severe pain intensity, pain interference, depression, and disability when compared to nonveterans (63).

We have found that VA patients with chronic pain referred to our services are often not prepared for psychotherapy because they do not view their primary (pain) problem as affective or psychological in nature. Rather, like many patients with chronic pain, these patients consider pain as primarily a physical problem, and they want a "real" physically focused treatment. Our experience also has been that patients referred to our service are not likely to continue with an intervention that does not provide symptom relief in a short period of time. Therefore, we have developed a case-management approach where we aim at "connecting" quickly with the patient and focusing at first on providing quick symptomatic relief. Here is a typical sequence of service provision:

(a) All patients referred to the pain program complete and return a clinical questionnaire by mail, which is scored for risk factors and need for psychosocial interventions.
(b) Patients, thus identified, are scheduled to attend an education/orientation meeting followed by a brief 30-minute screening, before or concurrent to seeing a pain anesthesiologist. The meeting is structured to educate patients

about chronic pain by questioning and (hopefully) debunking a purely biomedical focus and introducing the notion that decreasing pain interference and mind and body reconditioning also might be important. By conceptualizing pain management as "brain" management, alternative interventions such as CES and self-hypnosis training, as well as CBT, are introduced. The expected impact is that patients will begin to adopt a different, more biopsychosocial conceptualization for the management of their pain.

(c) CAM interventions, designed specifically to achieve initial pain relief (and indirectly to initiate the process of teaching patients self-management skills), are explained and made available to those who are interested. On average, 70–80% of patients attending this initial orientation/education class and screening have indicated a desire to pursue CAM interventions.

(d) When the patients are seen in subsequent individual sessions, the focus is to utilize CAM interventions such as CES to provide a "physical" treatment that typically results in immediate relief in pain or decrease in other symptoms. A preliminary analysis of 97 individual sessions where CES has been used since the beginning of this program indicates an average postsession pain reduction of 2.02 points on a 0 to 10 Likert scale or a 33.3% average reduction. Psychological interventions are not the main focus of treatment at first but are woven into the sessions for those who are interested. Patients are encouraged to participate concurrently in our education, support, and skills training groups.

This case management focus has been implemented with very positive and encouraging results. Preliminary data indicate that as many as 80% of veterans suffering from chronic pain chose to participate in the CAM therapies either as the sole treatments or in combination with more traditional therapies. Of the first 97 patients where CES was used alone or in combination with psychotherapy, an average pain reduction of 33.3% was achieved within 10 sessions, most of which occurred in the first 3 sessions (63). The veterans were found to be quite receptive to CAM interventions. We concluded that although no formal data were available for comparison, this model of service delivery appears to have substantially decreased the no-show rate since its introduction (63).

We would now like to describe two cases involving the use of CES and self-hypnosis. Since these cases are described in detail elsewhere in another publication (64), the presentation here is brief, and interested readers are referred to the previous publication for more detail.

Case Illustration 1: JS

JS is a 60-year-old married African-American male who was referred to the pain clinic by his primary-care physician (PCP), presenting with the complaint of worsening pain in his lower back and hip secondary to an injury in Vietnam. When asked to rate how much pain interfered with his daily life using the Brief Pain Inventory (BPI) Pain Interference scale, he rated the amount of interference as 9/10 for general activity, 9/10 for mood, 8/10 for walking ability, 8/10 for normal work, 8/10 for relations with people, 9/10 for sleep, and 9/10 for enjoyment of life. In addition, on a categorical scale of distress, he rated his current level of distress as "high." Previous treatments for his pain conditions included (a) chiropractor ("caused a lot more pain"), (b) massage ("made me feel really good but cost money"), (c) physical therapy ("made me feel good but did not do anything with the pain"), and (d) medications (on various pain medications in the past—currently has good relief from Tramadol and Naproxen as prescribed by his PCP).

In addition to chronic pain, JS also suffered from combat-related posttraumatic stress disorder (PTSD). JS has been enrolled in the Mental Health Trauma Recovery Program for veterans suffering from PTSD since 2001. He was first seen by mental health due to sleep problems and nightmares. He endorsed symptoms of intrusive thoughts from his Vietnam experiences, hypervigilance, heightened startle reflex, and isolation. He denied having used alcohol or illicit drugs due to his religious beliefs.

JS has been married for 33 years to his second wife and describes their relationship as "very good" and his wife as being "very supportive." He stays at home most of the time doing household chores and helping out the neighbors with chores. Although generally isolated from others, he maintains frequent contact with his brother and neighbor.

JS developed a back injury and PTSD while serving in combat in Vietnam. As with many Vietnam veterans who suppressed their emotional trauma without full resolution, he "went on with life as usual." As he got older and retired from employment, he had more unoccupied time to himself and some of the unresolved conflicts began to surface. The reexperiencing of his trauma in the form of nightmares likely led to increased muscle tension and bracing postures which, in turn, triggered, escalated, and exacerbated his previous chronic back pain condition.

The initial treatment goals were to reduce pain, stabilize and improve sleep, and help him regain a sense of control over his daily activities. The treatment plan consisted of CES to reduce anxiety and improve sleep, develop and practice skills for monitoring stress levels and responses to stress, and hypnosis to help modulate his pain while making a long-distance trip and to begin the resolution of his trauma. Following an initial screening, JS was seen for a total of nine individual sessions. A typical session commenced with his completing a Likert scale where he was asked to rate his pain intensity from 0 to 10. The CES device and how it works was briefly explained together with the common sensation of "tingling" or "pins and needles" on his ear lobes as the current was increased. He was also made aware that some individuals might feel slightly light-headed initially as the body adjusted to the introduction of microcurrent delivered to the brain, but that this sensation typically disappeared after a few minutes. Next, JS was connected to the CES device with two ear clip electrodes, followed by a fine tuning of the level of current intensity from 0 to 6 on the device (the larger the number, the higher the ampere) by the therapist in order to determine the highest level the patient can tolerate without the feeling of discomfort. After the unit was turned on, JS was asked to report when he first noticed any sensation. The current was then increased to the point of causing discomfort and then the current was reduced until the discomfort disappeared. Finally, his progress and the previous session were discussed. The content of the discussion varied depending on JS's needs and desired treatment goals. Each session ended with a post–pain-intensity rating and a homework assignment if appropriate.

In addition to the patient's self-reported improvement in his pain and related symptoms, comparison of pre- and postpsychometric testing using the BPI and the abbreviated form of the Center for Epidemiological Scale-Depression (CESD) indicated a number of improvements including significant reductions in pain intensity, pain interference, and depressive symptomatology. The findings indicated that JS benefited from the interventions, which included CES and self-hypnosis training. In addition to decreased pain intensity, he reported meaningful reductions on pain interference in all aspects of his daily functioning. Although he was only mildly depressed before treatment, some improvement in depression was also noted. Perhaps equally significant was the substantial reduction in pain medication use and the ability to function with minimal assistance from health-care providers.

Case Illustration 2: EC

Unlike the case of JS where hypnosis was employed as an "adjunct" to CES and psychotherapy, this case illustrates the use of hypnosis as the primary CAM modality. Although EC terminated his therapy prematurely due to transportation difficulties, his case was selected because it represents a classic example of how hypnosis can be used to treat pain in a person who appears to have moderately high hypnotic ability.

EC is a 63-year-old white male who also presented with chronic LBP. He sustained an injury in 1980 while working on an oil rig and spent 8 days in traction. He previously was examined by the anesthesiologist–pain specialist and given the diagnoses of lumbar spondylosis and facet disease. EC also reported severe intractable headaches that significantly interfered with his ability to focus and concentrate. Prior to treatment, EC reported on the BPI that his worst pain was 9/10, least pain was 6/10, average pain was 6/10, and current pain was 9/10. Pain interference was reported as 8/10 for general activity, 5/10 for mood, 5/10 for walking ability, 7/10 for normal work, 7/10 for relations with other people, 8/10 for sleep, and 8/10 for enjoyment of life. Satisfaction with life was rated as 6 to 7 out of 10.

EC had been responding partially to Percoset as prescribed by his PCP. He found a chiropractor helpful for a while, and he had been treated with traction and nonsteroidal anti-inflammatory drugs (NSAIDs). He denied having any history of mental-health problems or treatment, but he did acknowledge some symptoms of depression (fatigue, depressed mood, irritability). He consumed two to four beers a day and one pack of cigarettes per day pretreatment, but he denied using any illicit drugs. He reported a history of heavy alcohol use and previously smoked two to three packs of cigarettes per day. He previously had tried to quit smoking by using the nicotine patch and Zyban, which did not help. However, he reported that he subsequently was able to cut down on his smoking with the help of hypnosis (provided by other clinicians prior to being seen by us for pain).

EC had been separated for 7 years from his wife after many years of marriage. He was residing at his daughter's house because his house had been destroyed in a fire and was being rebuilt with help from his son. He reported that he was not active in the community; however, he maintained contact with his family and a few friends.

EC worked as a welder and pipe fitter for most of his life. He was unemployed and receiving social security disability due to "asbestosis" when he started treatment. He stated that he could not find a job due to back pain and his age.

It was clear from his presentation that EC was a "no nonsense" type of person whose primary expectation from treatment was to achieve pain reduction so that he could "move on" with his life. Although he acknowledged some depression, he denied having any mental-health problem or treatment in the past. The fact that he was able to obtain some help from hypnosis to reduce his cigarette smoking was a clue that he might be able to follow through and benefit from this intervention for pain as well. Treatment goals were pain reduction in order to be able to enjoy activities, such as offshore fishing and golf, and improved physical condition. Treatment focused on training in self-hypnosis, but a stretching exercise program was also initiated as a means of increasing his ability to engage in daily activities.

After the initial screening, EC was seen for a total of five sessions with hypnosis as the primary intervention. Far-eye-fixation induction procedure was used, followed by several deepening procedures. Following the induction, the verbal suggestion was given that EC would be able to use his mind to decrease his pain intensity and that, as he gained mastery of hypnosis, his pain would interfere less with his life activities. He was given the further suggestion that he would be able to transfer his pain from one location to another if he desired so. He reported pre- to postsession pain reduction from 7/10 to 4/10 at the first session, suggesting a moderate degree of responsivity to hypnotic analgesia suggestions.

At the beginning of the second session, EC reported that he was able to transfer his pain from his head to his hand and to make his pain go away at times, which allowed him to focus on accomplishing more tasks involved in the rebuilding of his house. He also reported that his pain had been less "bothersome" and he had been practicing "relaxation" like he did in the last therapy session. During this session, hypnotic induction and deepening procedures were repeated along with the posthypnotic suggestion of being able to increase behavioral activities without being bothered by pain. EC reported a pre- to postsession pain reduction from 6/10 to 0/10. In addition to hypnotherapy, he was taught several slow-motion reconditioning stretches from Chinese Qigong and the need for reconditioning was emphasized.

During the third session, EC continued to report his ability to transfer pain from his head to his hand. He stated that his back pain had decreased and he had been feeling more comfortable in general. In addition, he reported being able to mow his lawn for the first time in over a year. Finally, he reported reducing the use of his pain medication from four to two pills a day. He said that he practiced the slow-motion stretching taught in the previous session. The hypnotic training was repeated as before along with the suggestion that he would be able to substitute the sensation of "drifting and floating" for "rocking and jerking." EC was seen again for hypnosis with further focus on transforming the sensation of "rocking and jerking" to "floating and drifting" to prepare him for a future deep-sea fishing trip. He reported a pain reduction from 8/10 to 5/10 during the fourth session. At the beginning of the fifth and final hypnotherapy session, EC reported continued progress. He also reported being "stressed" by having to baby sit several children belonging to friends and relatives who had unexpectedly dropped them off at his daughter's house where he was residing. Despite the higher level of stress, he reported pre- to postsession pain reduction from 8/10 to 0/10.

At the end of the fifth and final session, EC stated that he would have to take a break from the treatment due to lack of transportation. He noted that he was much more comfortable now than he was prior to treatment, and he expressed confidence in his ability to apply his hypnotic skills on his own.

The cases presented here illustrate the potential for CES, self-hypnosis training, and their combination to help individuals with chronic pain experience less pain, gain control over pain symptoms, and minimize the effects of pain on their lives. The focus of both CES and the self-hypnosis training provided to these patients was on pain relief. In the second case, the hypnosis also included suggestions for increased activity and ability to function despite pain; hypnotic suggestions that may be underutilized in the treatment of chronic pain conditions (65). Many, but not all, patients are able to achieve meaningful reductions in the severity of pain with these interventions. For some of these patients, the pain relief can last for weeks, months, and even years (65).

Many patients with chronic pain begin treatment with a bias toward wanting treatments that are biomedical-focused and directly impact their experience of pain. For these patients who subsequently respond well to CES and/or self-hypnosis training, CAM interventions can be an effective means of engaging them and helping them achieve some reduction in their experience of pain. When effective for reducing pain and also improving other symptoms, such as global distress and sleep interference, these interventions can also be used as a way of helping patients learn that a direct "cause" of their pain need not necessarily be diagnosed and "fixed" in order for them to achieve relief (66).

Improvements that occur in some patients following CES and hypnosis may be enough for many patients. However, for patients seeking additional pain relief or reduced interference with functioning, the benefits obtained from CAM treatments such as CES or self-hypnosis training can be used as evidence for the potential efficacy of other psychological treatments that alter how the brain processes pain information, such as CBT. As more is learned about the specific effects of these and other CAM treatments for pain, they can be incorporated into and used in conjunction with other more traditional pain treatments, as a way to maximize the overall efficacy of pain treatment. In this way, we can seek to ensure that the greatest number of patients receive the most appropriate care.

Case Examples Using Biofeedback

The previous two cases demonstrated the use of CES and self-hypnosis involving veterans previously seen in the VA. Next, we will present two biofeedback cases provided by colleagues in the private practice settings in order to provide a balance between descriptions of patients seen in a government-based tertiary teaching hospital and those seen in the private sector.

Case Illustration 3: JJ[a]

Presenting Problem: JJ is a 42-year-old married, Caucasian female who has two children. She was referred by her general practitioner with the diagnosis of tension headache, which did not seem to respond to treatment. The tension-type headache

[a] Courtesy of Richard Gervitz, Private Practice, San Diego, California.

was of at least 10 years duration. Patient had "tried everything" including a variety of NSAIDs. She obtained temporary relief from chiropractic manipulation and acupuncture, but her symptoms typically returned within 24 hours. JS has good health habits (exercise, nutrition, etc.), and there were no notable stressors reported at intake. The patient was a medical receptionist at a large medical clinic. On assessment, her pain pattern matched the Travell and Simons Trigger Point (TP) manual for suboccipital and upper shoulder muscles (67). Her pain referred forward to forehead and temples. Trigger points were present and showed local tenderness, referral, and a twitch response.

Case Conceptualization: The case was conceptualized using the sympathetic (TP) model described by Gervitz et al. (54). It was hypothesized that ongoing subtle stressors created internalizing cognitions and thus prolonged sympathetic drive to the TPs. The goal of therapy was to break the vicious cycle setup by stress leading to muscle tension, tension leading to pain, and the pain leading to more stress.

Assessment and Treatment: Biofeedback assessment revealed moderate sympathetic arousal [skin conductance, temperature, heart rate variability (HRV) parameters, etc.] at baseline and at recovery from a stressor. This information was used in an extensive educational module which encompassed charts, videos of needle TP studies, and slides of muscle spindles to effect a change in attribution of pain etiology. Two sessions were used to educate the patient including conducting a PSP (as described earlier), a standard biofeedback procedure whereby the patient was hooked up to several biofeedback modalities and subjected to a number of stressful stimuli in order to determine how she responded physiologically to these stressful stimuli and how fast/slow she recovered from the stress reaction. Once the patient showed an understanding of the model, biofeedback was begun. The rationale for the treatment was presented as restoring balance to the autonomic nervous system thereby reducing excessive sympathetic flow to the TPs. Two biofeedback modalities were used in JJ's treatment protocol: SEMG and HRV biofeedback. The EMG was a frontalis threshold training program where the patient was instructed to decrease her frontalis muscle tension down to below one μV. In each session, the EMG biofeedback preceded the HRV biofeedback. JJ was able to reach less than one μV at the frontalis muscle after five training sessions (indicated markedly low levels of muscle activity). HRV biofeedback training began with breathing training using capnometer readings as benchmarks. Increasing abdominal breathing was observed over the course of the training sessions. Once resonant frequency was found (6.5 breaths per minute), she was given access to home-pacing devices (EZ-Air and an audio disk) and instructed to spend two 10-minute sessions a day practicing the breathing exercise. The patient quickly developed good self-regulatory skills and henceforth therapy began to focus on the underlying environmental conditions related to her pain and her reaction to them. Several workplace situations were identified as likely to interact negatively with her personality style so as to produce prolonged periods of increased stress and tension at work. Acceptance and commitment concepts (ACT) were introduced to promote better coping (68). At this point, her pain was 80% reduced and the remaining sessions concentrated on maintaining self-regulation skills and on generalization of the ACT concepts. At the 3-month mark, the patient was 90% pain free. The total number of treatment sessions was eight.

Case Illustration 4: BK ("Beth")[b]

This case involves a patient seen at the Productive Rehabilitation Institute of Dallas for Ergonomics (PRIDE) program. The PRIDE is a tertiary-level, chronic pain management facility in Dallas, TX. The clientele are almost exclusively injured workers who have been unsuccessful with previous treatments and have become significantly disabled. Most of the patients have been unable to work or function normally with daily activities for at least 6 months and some for up to several years. The general goals of the program are to increase each patient's physical conditioning, flexibility, and ability to function; to address psychosocial obstacles that might interfere with increased functioning; to provide extensive biopsychosocial education; and to facilitate a return to productive employment and normal daily activity.

The main phase of the program is 15 days of physically and educationally intensive treatment. This is preceded by 10 to 15 less-intensive preprogram visits. All program patients receive 5–10 "biofeedback classes" (psychophysiologically oriented classes) and 5–8 individual biofeedback sessions. The classes take place in the preprogram phase, and the majority of individual biofeedback sessions take place in the intensive phase.

There are three primary biofeedback treatment goals. First, education and rationale for mind–body interventions are provided to help patients "buy into" the treatment, follow through with homework, and utilize the skills on a daily basis. This education is provided primarily in the class. Second, training in specific relaxation techniques is provided, including a guided relaxation induction which is performed daily in the class, and periodically, as needed, in individual biofeedback sessions. Each patient is provided with two relaxation tapes, a tape player, and batteries. Patients are exposed to a variety of relaxation strategies (including breathing focus, body scanning, mental imagery, open focus, and self-coaching with autogenic-type phrases) so that they can choose the specific techniques that work best for them. Patients are encouraged to practice with their tapes daily until they can perform the techniques independently.

Third, in order to maximize success with relaxation and biofeedback training, patients are taught ways to generalize their self-regulation skills outside of treatment. Emphasis is placed on the use of slow, diaphragmatic breathing, along with "scanning" the body and releasing tension, periodically throughout the day. This goal also involves identifying specific muscle bracing and postural habits with SEMG, teaching patients increased awareness and control over these habits, and encouraging patients to monitor and correct these habits independently as part of their normal daily routine.

Biofeedback session protocol

Some traditional biofeedback protocols involve gradual shaping of a desired response toward a goal with minimal therapist instruction (31). Because of time

[b] This case example first appeared in Biofeedback 2004; (69). It is reprinted with the permission of the Biofeedback Magazine and the Association of Applied Psychophysiology and Biofeedback.

limitations in our program, individual biofeedback training tends to be very directive (similar to traditional golf lessons). When a training goal is identified, patients are actively shown how to reach the goal with verbal and tactile cuing, visual demonstration, and visual (and sometimes auditory) feedback. Patients are encouraged to develop both a somatosensory recognition of goal success and a specific behavioral strategy for achieving the goal. A heavy emphasis is placed on independent practice of skills outside of treatment sessions (64,70).

A typical biofeedback session is structured in the following way:

1. Discuss the follow through and success with homework.
2. Briefly review previous sessions and decide on a training focus for the current session.
3. Hook up an appropriate electrode placement and obtain a baseline measure of the particular physiological response being monitored. (If the baseline looks appropriate, then review what it revealed with the patient, hook up another electrode placement, and obtain another response baseline.)
4. Establish a specific training goal.
5. Show the patient how to reach the goal.
6. Reduce feedback as the patient becomes proficient at reaching the goal.
7. Assign homework to practice the newly learned skills.

CASE EXAMPLE

Beth was a 35-year-old female who was working as a recovery analyst for an insurance company at the time of her injury. She was injured in 2002, about 14 months prior to beginning treatment, when pulling out a 300-pound file drawer that had not been locked in properly. The drawer came out and fell on top of her. Beth reported a history of work injuries, including a neck injury in 1991, resulting in a two-level fusion; shoulder and back strain in 1993; and torn left and right rotator cuffs in 1999, resulted in surgeries to both shoulders. Her medical diagnosis at the time of her PRIDE treatment included chronic right lumbar radiculopathy, chronic old postoperative right cervical radicular syndrome; chronic old postoperative right shoulder impingement, chronic right hip dysfunction, chronic right elbow dysfunction, right wrist dysfunction, deconditioning syndrome, and chronic pain syndrome. She presented with major depressive disorder with anxious features, agitation, sleep disturbance, and family stressors, and she demonstrated some medication dependence on Lortab. At the time of her first doctor's visit, she reported a 10 out of 10 pain level.

Beth participated in five classes and six individual biofeedback sessions. Biofeedback therapy was begun several weeks into her rehabilitation program. By this time, Beth had tapered off of her Lortab and begun taking Paxil. Beth reported some improvement in her pain level and sleep success, which she attributed to her stretching exercises and to her Paxil. She had begun her "biofeedback classes," and received her first relaxation tape a few days before her initial individual biofeedback session. Though she reported pain in a number of body parts, her right shoulder and neck were her primary complaints. A synopsis of each session is provided below (71).

Session 1

Placements (reclining)	Two 5-min baselines	Best with training
Wrist-to-wrist SEMG (μV)	18.0–15.0	2.0
Ankle-to-ankle SEMG (μV)	6.5–5.0	3.5
Left hand temperature (°F)	93.7–95.0	N/A
Respiration	6 BPM, thoracic, forced	6 BPM, abdominal, smoother

Self-report: Patient had begun using her relaxation tape with moderate relaxation success, though she reported some difficulty in becoming comfortable and staying focused.

Session notes: During this baseline, Beth tried to perform the breathing technique that had been described in her classes. Pace was good, but breathing style was primarily thoracic and overly effortful. She was surprised at her muscle tension levels at the baseline and thought that she was more relaxed than she was. During training, Beth had a tendency to be impatient and to force relaxation. It required moderate to maximal cuing to achieve SEMG relaxation. She made some improvement in allowing her breathing to flow more abdominally and effortlessly with visual and verbal cues.

Session 2

Placements (reclining)	5-Min baseline	Best with training	Average during induction
Wrist-to-wrist SEMG (μv)	33.0–23.0	2.0	<3
Ankle-to-ankle SEMG (μv)	23.0–15.0	3.5	<3
Left hand temperature (°F)	93.0–94.8	N/A	>94
Respiration	6–8 BPM, thoracic, strained	6–8 BPM, abdominal, smoother, less strained	6–8 BPM, abdominal, smooth, less strained

Self-report: Patient reported daily use of relaxation tape, generally good success with relaxation, and inconsistent success with decreased pain.

Session notes: The physical therapist requested biofeedback intervention today to address a pain "flare-up" in her neck and shoulder. Beth was initially very tense. She seemed fearful and pain-focused. She was trying to use her breathing and relaxation skills during the baseline, but she appeared to be forcing and struggling. Education about the "pain>>>>fear>>>>tension cycle" was provided. Beth was successful in reducing muscle tension, smoothing her breathing pattern, and reducing her fearful "struggling" approach to pain, with visual feedback and verbal cuing. An autogenic-type relaxation induction was performed. She maintained good relaxation during the exercise. She reported good success with focusing away from pain during the induction, and a reduced pain level at the end of the session.

Session 3

	20-Sec baselines			After training		
First SEMG placements	Sitting	Standing	Recovery	Sitting	Standing	Recovery
Left cervical to upper trapezius (μv)	2.7	3.9	5.0	1.5	3.0	3.0
Right cervical to upper trapezius (μv)	3.3	4.5	9.0	1.8	3.0	3.6

Second SEMG placements	20-Sec baselines		After training	
	Sitting	Neck flexion	Sitting	Neck flexion
Left cervical to mid trapezius (μv)	8.0–6.0	5.0	2.5	3.5
Right cervical to mid trapezius (μv)	8.8–6.0	5.5	2.5	3.5

Self-report: Patient reported daily practice with her relaxation tapes, good success with relaxation, good success with focusing away from pain, and success with decreased pain most of the time.

Session notes: Beth continued to report pain and stiffness in her neck and right shoulder. Recovery problems were noted in her right neck and shoulder following a contraction (with first EMG placements). We worked on contract/recovery trials with visual feedback, verbal cues, and an emphasis on somatosensory awareness of muscle activity. Beth demonstrated increased awareness of muscle bracing versus relaxation and good progress with recovery following contractions. Specific strategies such as "head floating" and "shoulders dropping heavy" seemed to help her relaxation success. Postural imbalance was noted while sitting in a chair, including head forward and rounded shoulders. With verbal cuing and visual feedback (with second SEMG placements), she was able to correct her posture and reduce excessive muscle bracing in her neck and upper back. Patient's physical therapist had previously requested that biofeedback be utilized to help her increase inhibited neck movement (72). We worked on relaxation while stretching her neck into forward flexion (with second SEMG placements). She demonstrated improved relaxation and improved range-of-motion during neck flexion with breathing cues and auditory feedback. Beth was encouraged to monitor posture and muscle bracing, and to practice relaxed neck stretches, at every opportunity during the day.

Session 4

Placements (reclining)	5-Min baseline	Practice
Wrist-to-wrist SEMG (μv)	<3	<3.0
Ankle-to-ankle SEMG (μv)	<3	<3.0
Respiration	5–6 BPM, abdominal, smooth	6–8 BPM, abdominal, smooth

Self-report: Patient reported daily practice with relaxation tape, good success with subjective relaxation, good success with decreased pain, and improved success with sleep at night. She reported frequent focus on scanning and self-regulating muscle tension in her neck and shoulders and good follow-through with relaxed stretches. She verbalized, "When my body is more tense, my pain is more irritating. When I'm relaxed, I don't notice it as much."

Session notes: Beth demonstrated good carry-over with general relaxation training from previous sessions. She spent some time practicing breathing maintenance with mental focus on a meditative phrase. We discussed her progress to this point.

Session 5

First SEMG placements	20-Sec baselines			After training		
	Sitting	Standing	Recovery	Sitting	Standing	Recovery
Left cervical to upper trapezius (μv)	1.5	2.8	2.8	N/A	N/A	N/A
Right cervical to upper trapezius (μv)	1.9	3.0	3.0	N/A	N/A	N/A

	20-Sec baselines		After training	
2nd SEMG placements	Sitting	Neck flexion	Sitting	Neck flexion
Left cervical to mid trapezius (μv)	4.0–3.0	2.0	1.5	N/A
Right cervical to mid trapezius (μv)	4.0–3.0	2.1	1.5	N/A

Self-report: Patient reported daily relaxation practice, both with the relaxation tapes and independently, without the tapes. She reported frequent focus on scanning and self-regulating muscle tension in her neck and shoulders and good follow-through with relaxed stretches. She reported consistent success with relaxation, pain control, and sleep at night. She verbalized "I feel so much better since you taught me how to relax my neck. It doesn't get as stiff and painful now."

Session notes: Good carry-over with neck and shoulder relaxation. Beth needed some additional practice to establish consistency with postural balance. Developing and using a specific postural strategy, rather that just relying on somatosensory cues, helped to improve her consistency. I had her verbalize her postural strategy several times as she practiced.

Session 6

SEMG placement (walking)	30-Sec baseline	Best with training
Left to right upper trapezius (μV)	9.0	<5.0

Self-report: Continued success in all areas. Also, feeling stronger and more confident in general.

Session notes: I placed a portable SEMG unit on patient's shoulders, and let her walk around the facility with auditory feedback in order to facilitate generalization of muscular relaxation skills. Her walking SEMG levels were only moderately elevated compared with many other patients with similar symptoms who often show SEMG levels above 20 μv. We worked on relaxed and balanced posture during standing and walking, and did some contract/recovery practice.

CONCLUSIONS

It can be challenging to provide effective biofeedback and psychophysiological interventions within the time restrictions of a brief, intensive, rehabilitation program. To optimize success, one should "sell" mind–body and self-regulation concepts, in order to encourage independent practice with the techniques. Individual biofeedback therapy sessions must be efficient and goal-directed in order to maximize treatment time. Treatment must be individualized to meet the specific needs of each patient. One must prioritize the treatment focus and recognize that there isn't time to "fix" everything. Support from other treatment team members in reinforcing self-regulation principles is extremely helpful.

Beth was an especially adept patient. It generally takes more treatment time for the average patient to develop and carry-over the skills that she learned. She made strong gains in all areas of her treatment program. I attribute Beth's success to her determination and willingness to follow-though independently with homework. At the completion of the treatment program, she reported confidence in her ability to return to employment and get on with life. She reported a decreased pain level and only minimal functional limitations due to pain. In Beth's words, "I'm tired of sitting around. This is my body, and I'm going to take control of it."

INCORPORATING CAM THERAPIES INTO MULTIDISCIPLINARY PAIN PRACTICES

Interest in incorporating CAM therapies into multidisciplinary pain treatment is not new. For example, in 2001, the NCCAM and the Royal College of Physicians cosponsored a conference in London where experts in the field met to discuss the question, "Can alternative medicine be integrated into main stream care?" Subsequent to this conference, another was held in Edmonton entitled "North American Research Conference on Complementary and Integrative Medicine."

Developing an integrative health care program within the Veterans Administration Hospitals (VHA) is the focus of a recent article (73). The authors outlined a systematic way of incorporating CAM modalities into a conventional medical facility by following these steps: identifying scientifically supported therapies for inclusion, education of providers and patients on the modalities; development of a clinical research protocol, exploration, development, and evaluation of new models of integrative health care; and reintegration of physical, emotional, mental, and spiritual life values into health care and health education.

In incorporating CAM modalities into a multidisciplinary pain management program, several issues should be considered. First, not all CAM modalities are equally efficacious. For example, although not everyone responds to these treatments, and their immediate efficacy is not always maintained, hypnosis, biofeedback, and massage therapies for LBP and shoulder pain all have a degree of support for their efficacy over and above a number of control conditions and in some cases, other treatments (16). Pulsed electromagnetic fields (PEMFs) have demonstrated support for its efficacy for migraine and osteoarthritis only and no other pain condition (16). CES, massage therapies for neck and other pain conditions, spinal manipulation therapy, meditation, and yoga appear to be promising treatments, but more research is needed to replicate preliminary findings. The CAM treatments that show more mixed results include herbal and dietary interventions (perhaps due to the fact that this CAM treatment really represents hundreds of different interventions, so mixed results would certainly be expected), therapeutic touch, craniosacral therapy, Reiki, qigong therapy, and homeopathy (16). However, even these interventions might be helpful for a subgroup of patients.

Acupuncture appears to belong to a category of its own. While there are multiple meta-analyses and clinical trials attesting to the efficacy of this modality as analgesia and for the treatment of a wide variety of medical conditions, relatively few have focused on the treatment of chronic pain conditions (16). As was noted by Tan et al. (16), this may be partially due to the fact that acupuncture was originally developed as an integral part of Traditional Chinese Medicine (TCM) which has a very different paradigm for conceptualizing health and illness (16). Using Western scientific methods such as RCTs to assess the efficacy of a treatment modality based on a completely different paradigm to treat non-TCM chronic pain conditions as defined by Western diagnosis may be like comparing apples and oranges. In short, the efficacy of acupuncture for analgesia is not in dispute, but research on its efficacy in treating chronic pain has mixed results.

In addition to efficacy, there are other issues relevant to practitioners when making decisions to use or incorporate CAM modalities into their pain practice. These include additional requirements for training and equipment, known side effects or potential toxic effects, safety in combining CAM and other modalities, likely acceptance by clients and the public (which raises the issue of long-term compliance), and ease of incorporation into traditional pain management practices (16).

Additional Requirements

The use of biofeedback requires specialized equipment and training, and the use of hypnosis requires special training. A number of treatments, including acupuncture, homeopathy, massage, and chiropractic care, require that a practitioner be licensed. Also, some modalities can be expected to produce concrete results in just a few sessions for some patients (e.g., CES, hypnosis, biofeedback), while others may require longer commitment of time and effort (e.g., yoga, meditation). In general, even when they are effective, CAM modalities as a group tend to require more time than traditional medical pain interventions to achieve results.

Side and Toxic Effects

Another important issue is that, as compared to traditional pain interventions, CAM modalities as a group have fewer known and documented side effects or toxic effects. For example, the "side effects" of training in self-hypnosis for chronic pain are overwhelmingly positive (66). This may explain, at least in part, their popularity relative to traditional medical interventions, which tend to be invasive and tend to undermine patient self-efficacy and control.

Combining CAM and Other Modalities

Another issue that should be considered by clinicians is the fact that some CAM modalities can be combined safely with each other and traditional pain interventions to produce additive or synergistic effects. For example, CES can easily be administered along with self-hypnosis or biofeedback training or with psychotherapy. In this way, any potential benefits of the individual treatments could potentially be combined to provide maximum pain relief for the patient.

There is an increasing interest in combining traditional medical treatments to maximize pain relief, but there is no reason that more established CAM modalities should not be at least considered when developing multimodal treatment plans (74,75). Additional research is needed to examine the use of individual CAM therapies with other CAM approaches and CAM with traditional interventions both in terms of safety and synergistic effects. Recently, there have been some concerns about the combined use of medication with herbal preparations (76,77). Some herbal preparations should be avoided completely due to their rapid, negative, and irreversible actions (76,77).

Acceptance, Compliance, and Ease of Incorporation

The popularity of CAM therapies for chronic pain has been partially fueled by the current lack of efficacious traditional medical treatments for certain conditions. However, after a patient's initial desperation for relief and the curiosity about and novelty of new treatments have worn off, the issue of long-term compliance may quickly emerge as a potential road block to successful positive outcomes. There are few data that would indicate which CAM therapies are more likely be accepted and adhered to, and which are not. In the absence of such data, one might assume that those CAM modalities that most resemble currently accepted medical treatments might have an advantage. Thus, the use of herbal and dietary supplements may result in greater compliance, since the public has been acculturated to the idea of taking medication to get well and stay well. Treatments that utilize sophisticated equipment such as biofeedback, CES, PEMF, and perhaps, acupuncture may also be more easily accepted by the chronic pain patient population. The idea of "massaging" away tension and pain has been ingrained in the human psyche, as has chiropractic care to reduce pain. Hypnosis has been presented in the popular media and by entertainers as a powerful "mind control" intervention so that some members of the public are anxious about losing control with hypnosis treatments, and others have unrealistic beliefs about the effects of hypnosis. Yoga, meditation, healing touch, and qigong may have a foreign connotation, and may appeal only to a subset of the general public. The ease of incorporation of CAM modalities into pain practices and adherence to the techniques is likely to be influenced by the level of public acceptance.

Other Advantages of CAM Use

There may also be instances in which the use of CAM leads to a greater acceptance of traditional interventions. A case in point is the use of CES to increase acceptance of psychological interventions such as CBT. Tan et al. (78) have shown that the use of CES helps veterans become more willing to engage in psychologically based or mind–body therapies because CES was perceived by veterans to be a "real" physical treatment that could produce rapid pain reduction and was credible in treating "real" pain. Once engaged, the veterans became more amenable to participating in and benefited from other mind–body or psychological therapies.

In conclusion, some CAM modalities can provide chronic pain sufferers with significant relief and for some individuals; this relief is maintained over time. While more research is needed to specify the mechanisms of different CAM treatments, enough evidence exists to support offering at least a subset of these (in particular, biofeedback, self-hypnosis training, and CES) to those patients who express an interest in these interventions. As more is learned about the efficacy of these approaches, and as the modalities with established efficacy are more consistently provided to individuals with chronic pain, we can anticipate a corresponding reduction in the disability and suffering associated with chronic pain conditions.

REFERENCES

1. Eriksen J, Sjøgren P, Bruera E, et al. Critical issues on opioids in chronic non-cancer pain: An epidemiologic study. Pain 2006; 125:172–179.
2. Turk DC, Loeser JD, Monarch ES. Chronic pain: purposes and costs of interdisciplinary rehabilitation programs. TENS 2002; 4:64–69.
3. Turk DC. Clinical effectiveness and cost-effectiveness of treatments for patients with chronic pain. Clin J Pain 2002; 18:355–365.
4. Keefe FJ, Abernathy AP, Campbell LC. Psychological approaches to understanding and treating disease-related pain. Annu Rev Psychol 2005; 56:601–630.
5. Morley S, Eccleston C, Williams A. Systematic review and meta-analysis of randomized controlled trials of cognitive behavior therapy and behavior therapy for chronic pain in adults, excluding headache. Pain 1999; 80:1–13.
6. McCracken LM, Turk DC. Behavioral and cognitive-behavioral treatment for chronic pain: Outcome, predictors of outcome, and treatment process. Spine 2002; 27:2564–2573.
7. Jensen MP, Nielson WR, Kerns RD. Toward the development of a motivational model of self-pain management. J Pain 2003; 4:477–492.

8. Wickramasekera I. Secrets kept from the mind but not the body or behavior: the unsolved problems of identifying and treating somatization and psychophysiological disease. Adv Mind Body Med 1998; 14:81–132.
9. Ernst E. Prevalence of use of complementary/alternative medicine: a systematic review. Bull World Health Organ 2000; 78:252–257.
10. Arnold K. Alternative medicines gain in popularity, merit closer scrutiny. J Natl Cancer Inst 1999; 91:1104–1105.
11. Chiappeli F, Prolo P, Cajulis OS. Evidence-based research in complementary and alternative medicine I: history. Evid Based Complement Alternat Med 2005; 2:453–458.
12. Engel LW, Straus SE. Development of therapeutics: opportunities within complementary and alternative medicine. Nat Rev Drug Discov 2002; 1:229–237.
13. Eisenberg DM, Davis RB, Ettner SL, et al. Trends in alternative medicine use in the United States, 1990–1997: results of a follow-up national survey. JAMA 1998; 280:1569–1575.
14. Barnes PM, Powell-Griner E, McFann K, et al. Complementary and alternative medicine use among adults: United States, 2002. Adv Data 2004; 343:1–19.
15. Chambless DL, Hollon SD. Defining empirically supported therapies. J Consult Clin Psyhol 1998; 66:7–18.
16. Tan G, Craine MH, Bair MJ, et al. Efficacy of selected complementary and alternative medicine (CAM) interventions for chronic pain. J Rehabil Res Dev 2007; 44(2):195–222.
17. Barabasz A, Watkins JG. Hypnotherapeutic Techniques, 2nd edn. Oxford, UK: Routledge; 2004.
18. Kroger WS. Clinical and Experimental Hypnosis. Philadelphia, PA: Lippincott; 1963.
19. Esdaile J. Mesmerism in India and its Practical Application in Surgery and Medicine. Hartford, CT: Silas Andrus and Son; 1957.
20. Montgomery GH, DuHamel KN, Redd WH. A meta-analysis of hypnotically induced analgesia; how effective is hypnosis? Int J Clin Exp Hypn 2000; 48:138–153.
21. Patterson D, Jensen MP. Hypnosis and clinical pain. Psychol Bull 2003; 129:495–521.
22. Hilgard ER, Hilgard JR. Hypnosis in the Relief of Pain. New York: Brunner/Mazel; 1994.
23. Jensen MP, Patterson DR. Hypnotic treatment of chronic pain. J Behav Med 2006; 29:95–124.
24. Tan G, Hammond DC, Gurrala J. Hypnosis and irritable bowel syndrome: a review of efficacy and mechanism of action. Am J Clin Hypn 2005; 47:161–178.
25. Kropp P, Siniatchkin M, Gerber WD. On the pathophysiology of Migraine-Links for "empirically based treatment" with neurofeedback. Appl Psychophysiol Biofeedback 2002; 27:203–213.
26. Flor H. The modification of cortical reorganization and chronic pain by sensory feedback. Appl Psychophysiol Biofeedback 2002; 27:215–227.
27. Sime A. Case study of trigeminal neuralgia using neurofeedback and peripheral biofeedback. J Neurother 2004; 8:59–71.
28. deCharms RC, Maeda F, Glover GH, et al. Control over brain activity and pain learned by using real-time functional MRI. Proc Natl Acad Sci 2005; 102:18626–18631.
29. Sherman R, Hermann C. Clinical efficacy of psychophysiological assessments and biofeedback interventions for chronic pain disorders other than head area pain. Manuscript under review.
30. Sherman RA. Biofeedback. In: Lebowitz E, ed. Complementary and Alternative Medicine in Rehabilitation. New York: Churchill Langston 2006:125–138.
31. Tan G, Sherman R, Shanti B. Biofeedback pain interventions. Pract Pain Manage 2003; 3:12–18.
32. Blanchard EB, Andrasik F. Management of Chronic Headaches. New York: Pergamon Press; 1985.
33. Blanchard EB, Greene B, Scharff L, et al. Relaxation training as a treatment for irritable bowel syndrome. Biofeedback Self Regul 1993; 18:125–132.

34. Rains JC, Penzien DB, McCrory DC, et al. Behavioral headache treatment: history, review of the empirical literature, and methodological critique. Headache 2005; 45:S92–S109.
35. Blanchard EB, Hillhouse J, Appelbaum KA, et al. What is an adequate length of baseline in research and clinical practice with chronic headache? Biofeedback Self Regul 1987; 12:323–329.
36. Gevirtz R, Glaros A, Hopper D, et al. Temporomandibular disorders. In: Schwartz M, ed. Biofeedback. New York: Guilford Press; 1995:411–428.
37. Dahlstrom L, Carlsson SG. Treatment of mandibular dysfunction: the clinical usefulness of biofeedback in relation to splint therapy. J Oral Rehabil 1984; 11:277–284.
38. Hijzen TH, Slangen JL, van Houweligen HC. Subjective, clinical and EMG effects of biofeedback and splint treatment. J Oral Rehabil 1986; 13:529–539.
39. Crider A, Glaros A, Gevirtz R. Efficacy of biofeedback-based treatments for temporomandibular disorders. Appl Psychophysiol Biofeedback. In press.
40. Neblett R, Gatchel RJ, Mayer TG. A clinical guide to surface-EMG-assisted stretching as an adjunct to chronic musculoskeletal pain rehabilitation. Appl Psychophysiol Biofeedback 2003; 28:147–160.
41. Newton-John TR, Spence SH, Schotte D. Cognitive-behavioral therapy versus EMG biofeedback in the treatment of chronic low back pain. Behav Res Ther 1995; 33:691–697.
42. van Tulder MW, Koes B, Malmivaara A. Outcome of non-invasive treatment modalities on back pain: an evidence-based review. Eur Spine J 2006; 15(Suppl 1):S64–S81.
43. van Tulder MW, Ostelo R, Vlaeyen JW, et al. Behavioral treatment for chronic low back pain: a systematic review within the framework of the Cochrane Back Review Group. Spine 2001; 26:270–281.
44. Flor H, Birbaumer N. Comparison of the efficacy of electromyographic biofeedback, cognitive-behavioral therapy, and conservative medical interventions in the treatment of chronic musculoskeletal pain. J Consult Clin Psychol 1993; 61:653–658.
45. Sherman RA, Devor M, Jones D, et al. Phantom Pain. New York: Plenum; 1996.
46. Belleggia G, Birbaumer N. Treatment of phantom limb pain with combined EMG and thermal biofeedback: a case report. Appl Psychophysiol Biofeedback 2001; 26:141–146.
47. Harden RN, Houle TT, Green S, et al. Biofeedback in the treatment of phantom limb pain: a time-series analysis. Appl Psychophysiol Biofeedback 2005; 30:83–93.
48. Donaldson CC, MacInnis AL, Snelling LS, et al. Characteristics of diffuse muscular coactivation (DMC) in persons with fibromyalgia—part 2. NeuroRehabilitation 2002; 17:41–48.
49. Donaldson CC, Snelling LS, MacInnis AL, et al. Diffuse muscular coactivation (DMC) as a potential source of pain in fibromyalgia—part 1. NeuroRehabilitation 2002; 17:33–39
50. Mueller HH, Donaldson CC, Nelson DV, et al. Treatment of fibromyalgia incorporating EEG-Driven stimulation: a clinical outcomes study. J Clin Psychol 2001; 57:933–952.
51. Swartz MS. Biofeedback: A Practioner's Guide, 2nd edn. New York: The Guilford Press; 1995.
52. Peniston EG, Kulskosky PJ. Alpha-theta brainwave training and beta endorphin levels in alcoholics. Alcohol Clin Exp Res 1989; 13:271–279.
53. Sherman RA. Pain Assessment and Intervention from a Psychological Perspective. Wheat ridge, Colorado: Association of Applied Psychophysiology and Biofeedback; 2003.
54. Gervitz R, Hubbard D, Harpin E. Pscyhophysiologic treatment of chronic low back pain. Prof Psychol Res Pr 1996; 27:561–566.
55. McNulty WH, Gervirtz RN, Hubbard DR, et al. Needle electromyographic evaluation of trigger point response to a psychological stressor. Psychophysiology 1994; 31:313–316.

56. Sherman RA. Biofeedback. In: Lebowitz E, ed. Complementary and Alternative Medicine in rehabilitation. New York: Churchill Livingston; 2003:125–138.
57. Kirsch DL, Smith RB. The use of cranial electrotherapy stimulation in the management of chronic pain: a review. NeuroRehabilitation 2000; 14:85–94.
58. Lichtbroun AS, Raicer MC, Smith RB. The Treatment of fibromyalagia with cranial electrotherapy stimulation. J Clin Rheumatol 2001; 7:72–78.
59. Clark MS, Silverstone LM, Lindenmuth J, et al. An evaluation of the clinical anagelsia/anesthesia efficacy on acute pain using the high frequency neural modulator in various dental settings. Oral Surg Oral Med Oral Pathol 1987; 63:501–505.
60. Tan G, Rintala DA, Thornby JI, et al. Using cranial electrotherapy stimulation to treat pain associated with spinal cord injury. JRRD 2006; 43:461–474.
61. Giordano J. How Alpha-Stim Cranial Electrotherapy Stimulation Works. Mineral Wells, TX: Electromedical Products Inc; 2006.
62. Tan G, Jensen MP, Robinson-Whelen S, et al. Coping with chronic pain: a comparison of two measures. Pain 2001; 90:127–133.
63. Tan G, Colon-Garcia F, Jensen MP. A model for expanding psychological services to veterans suffering from chronic pain. Poster presented at the Association of VA Psychology Leaders Annual Conference, Dallas, 2006.
64. Neblett R. Active SEMG training strategies for chronic musculoskeletal pain—part 1. Biofeedback 2002; 30:28–31.
65. Patterson DR, Jensen MP. Hypnosis and clinical pain. Psychol Bull 2003; 129:495–521.
66. Jensen MP, McArthur KD, Barber J, et al. Satisfaction with, and the beneficial side effects of hypnosis analgesia. Int J Clin Exp Hypn 2006; 54:432–447.
67. Travell J, Simons R. Myofascial pain syndrome: The Trigger Point Manual. Baltimore, MD: Williams and Wilkins; 1983.
68. Gevirtz RN. The muscle spindle trigger point model of chronic muscle pain. Biofeedback 2006; 34:53–56.
69. Neblett R. Biofeedback therapy within an interdisciplinary chronic pain management program. Biofeedback 2004; 32:13–19.
70. Neblett R. Active SEMG training strategies for chronic musculoskeletal pain—part 2. Biofeedback 2002; 30:39–42.
71. Cram JR. Kasman G. Holtz J. Introduction to Surface Electromyography. Gaithersburg, MD: Aspen Publication; 1998.
72. Neblett R, Mayer TG, Gatchel RJ. Theory and rationale for surface EMG-assisted stretching as an adjunct to chronic musculoskeletal pain rehabilitation. Appl Biofeedback Self Regul 2003; 28:147–160.
73. Overall JC, Smeeding S, Osguthorpe SG. Developing an Integrative health care program. Fed Pract 2006; 23:16–31.
74. Gilron I, Bailey JM, Tu D, et al. Morphine, gabapentin, or their combination for neuropathic pain. N Engl J Med 2005; 352:1324–1334.
75. Gilron I, Orr E, Tu D, et al. A placebo-controlled randomized clinical trial of perioperative administration of gabapentin, rofecoxib and their combination for spontaneous and movement-evoked pain after abdominal hysterectomy. Pain 2005; 113:191–200.
76. Fugh-Berman A. Herb-drug interactions. Lancet 2000; 355:134–138.
77. Hu Z, Yang X, Ho PC, et al. Herb-drug interactions: a literature review. Drugs 2005; 65:1239–1282.
78. Tan G, Alvarez J, Jensen MP. Complementary and alternative medicine (CAM) approaches to pain management. J Clin Psych 2006; 62:1419–1431.

7 The Impact of Interventional Approaches when used Within the Context of Multidisciplinary Chronic Pain Management

Michael Hatzakis, Jr.
Bellevue Rehabilitation Associates, Bellevue, Washington, U.S.A.

Michael E. Schatman
Consulting Clinical Psychologist, Bellevue, Washington, U.S.A.

INTRODUCTION

There are numerous interventions currently employed to treat individuals with chronic pain, many at great cost to the health-care system (1–4). Turk and Swanson (chap. 2 in this book) review a long list of these interventions, including medications, surgery, and implantable stimulators, for their effectiveness in treating pain. Most provide modest decreases in pain in the short-term, and some have a long-term impact (2). Turk and Swanson observe, however, that the majority of studies on these interventions are limited by the short-term and highly focused nature of the outcomes used to assess the impact of such interventions rather than measuring impact upon overall functioning and well-being. A formidable body of literature appears to support the assertion that multidisciplinary pain rehabilitation centers (MPRCs) may be at least as effective as other treatments to reduce actual pain levels (5,6). Additionally, the literature suggests that MPRCs represent a more cost-effective approach to the management of chronically painful conditions and are associated with other clinically relevant outcomes, such as reductions in health-care utilization (6,7), lowered opioid use (6,8), increased physical functioning (5,9), and higher rates of return to work compared to interventions such as surgery or spinal procedures alone (6,7,10). The study of MPRCs involves more holistic end points that address the overall needs of the individual, such as improved rates of return to work and decreased overall levels of disability. Accordingly, the study of MPRCs enjoys methodological advantages over the arguably narrower outcomes often measured, such as Likert scale pain intensity changes or opioid usage. Despite their strong empirical support, only 6% of those with chronic pain treated by pain specialists are treated within the context of the MPRC (11).

Interventional approaches to the management of chronic pain are commonly used, despite the extremely weak empirical support for their long-term efficacy (12–17). It has been noted that the health-insurance establishment has continued to provide remuneration for the seemingly endless numbers of invasive procedures that are performed on patients with chronic pain, despite their lack of efficacy (18). Ethical problems associated with interventionalists' persistent use of injection therapy in isolation for the treatment of chronic pain, despite the lack of empirical support for such practice, have been aggressively noted (18,19). Chapter 2 in this volume notes the paradox of the insurance industry's willingness to continue to fund numerous injections, while the empirically supported MPRCs are increasingly struggling to obtain third-party reimbursement for their patients. Schatman (20,21) has attributed this phenomenon to the health-insurance industry's lack of a sound ethical foundation, while chapter 2 in this volume also notes that this all-too-common practice is clearly not fiscally sound.

INTERVENTIONS THAT HAVE THE POTENTIAL TO MODULATE THE EFFECTIVENESS OF THE MPRC APPROACH

In addition to lacking empirical support for their clinical efficacy and cost-efficiency, the potential adverse effects of some of the commonly used interventional approaches to chronic pain are substantial and often irreversible. Such interventions include spinal surgery, intrathecal and intradural drug delivery systems, spinal cord stimulators, and intradisk electrotherapy, all of which are associated with potentially serious iatrogenic complications as well as being associated with equivocal long-term clinical efficacy and cost-efficiency. Other interventional techniques have a significantly lower rate of associated adverse events and a sufficiently high rate of *short-term* efficacy. These interventions include, but are not limited to, zygapophysial joint injections, selective nerve root blocks, trigger point injections, and acupuncture. Although they should not be considered panaceas, the short-term relief that these procedures provide may be valuable in modulating the patient's *degree of engagement* in a comprehensive multidisciplinary rehabilitation program. Each of these interventions has been associated with a reported degree of short-term relief of pain such that when used in the context of a pain rehabilitation program, they may provide a powerful impact on the patient's ability to tolerate and benefit from other aspects of a multidisciplinary approach. For example, short-term pain relief may enhance concentration (22–26), thereby improving the chronic pain patient's ability to participate in and benefit from program components such as psychological and vocational counseling, biofeedback, and educational presentations. Most important, however, is the effect of short-term relief on the chronic pain patient's ability to tolerate therapeutic exercise.

The use of procedures for the short-term reduction of pain and increasing mobility has been supported empirically on the premise that their use fosters great activation and/or participation in a therapeutic program. For example, the theories developed by Simons and Travell (27–30) suggest that myofascial pain often presents in the form of taut bands or trigger points. These trigger points are observed as exquisite local tenderness that is explained by sensitization of the nerve endings of group III and group IV fibers. Clearly, if muscles contain points of heighten sensitivity with increased pain upon activation, it follows that the individual, who naturally wants to reduce pain, will become increasingly kinesophobic. The development of kinesophobia will hamper the chronic pain patient's ability to fully engage in therapy. Often, he or she will require high doses of analgesics (including opioids) to remain active. The theory that muscles with active trigger points fatigue easily has also been supported (31). If, however, one were able to anesthetize these highly sensitized nerve endings for a period of days or weeks, then progress might be made in strengthening, potentially reversing the process that caused the initial muscle injury, and providing necessary positive feedback for an individual to increase overall activity and reduce kinesophobia. Unfortunately, the current state of the literature is such that high-quality studies that compare needling to placebo have not been performed, and the benefit of concurrent exercise along with any needling therapy has yet to be empirically evaluated (32).

A very similar argument may be made for injections of cervical and lumbar nerve roots, zygapophysial joints, and epidural steroid administration. Individuals who have suffered back or neck injuries may have dysfunction and/or irritation of nerve roots or specific joints of the cervical and lumbar spine. These disorders may be central to an injury or may be secondary to disordered movement. A plethora of evidence suggests that these procedures have short-term efficacy (33–38). However, if such an injection reduces pain temporarily without reversing spinal motion dysfunction or having an impact upon underlying weakness, these interventions may be short-lived. If, however, these procedures are used in the context of reparative treatment such as graded, isometric exercise, spinal manipulation, and/or proprioceptive retraining, long-lasting effects may be forthcoming. For example, the zygapophysial joints (L-z joints) in the lumbar spine assist in weight bearing of the trunk. Often, if there is excessive hyperextension force on the low back resulting from tightness in the hip flexors, these joints may become overstressed and highly painful (39). Injections of the L-z joints may reduce pain from hyperextension of the lumbosacral spine, but if the underlying mechanism of continued stress on the back is not relieved, the duration of action of an L-z joint injection will be short-lived. Approaches to rehabilitation of the lumbosacral spine that include adequate flexibility of the hips as one definitive treatment for disorders of and pain emanating from the L-z joints have been empirically supported (40). It would then stand to reason that any therapeutic maneuver that was to attempt to increase the flexibility of the hips and thighs to reduce stress on the z joints would likely be hampered by L-z-joint pain. Injections of the L-z joints would be an ideal adjunct to rehabilitation of hips and thighs as a combination approach. Dreyer and Dreyfus (39), in fact, comment that "the analgesic effects of L-z-joint injections serve as a 'window of opportunity' for the patient to progress through a previously intolerable active conservative treatment." The literature, however, is surprisingly replete in research that assesses the effectiveness of L-z joint interventions used as an adjunct to reparative therapies. This is a common theme in the overall study of interventions used in the context of the associated definitive rehabilitation therapies.

The empirical support for functional restoration through therapeutic exercise as an effective treatment for chronic pain is strong (41–56), with outcomes measured using a variety of dependent variables. Since therapeutic exercise programs have strong support for long-term success in the treatment of chronic pain, it follows that interventions that can increase patient enrollment and help maintain participation in these programs will produce the highest yield outcome. In many cases, the barrier for the individual with chronic pain to remain engaged in a multidisciplinary rehabilitation program is the pain and discomfort experienced when performing the necessary reconditioning exercises. This, coupled with an uncertain association between the exercise and a positive therapeutic outcome in the patient's mind, makes the development of adherence a challenging task. Pfingsten and colleagues (57) determined that pain anticipation and fear–avoidance beliefs significantly influence the behavior of patients with low back pain in that they motivate avoidance behavior. Given the impact of fear–avoidance beliefs on pain-related disability among chronic pain patients (58–70) as well as patient self-report of pain (59,71), the importance of altering these beliefs in a multidisciplinary treatment program is obvious. Traditionally, cognitive-behavioral therapy has been used in MPRCs to address fear–avoidance beliefs (72,73). However, if a trigger-point injection or a spinal injection procedure, for example, reduce discomfort and fear temporarily, to the extent that an individual can make therapeutic gains while simultaneously providing a sense that his or her pain is treatable, the treatment team has successfully leveraged a short-lived procedure to accomplish long-term goals. This technique is employed by many practitioners to engage individuals who may have a sense that there may be little they can do to tackle a difficult and chronically painful condition. Clearly, this approach is applicable to multidisciplinary chronic pain management programs that are heavily exercise-based.

NONSPECIFIC EFFECTS

Much of the overall benefit associated with using interventional measures within the context of a comprehensive multidisciplinary chronic pain management program is likely at least partially due to a placebo effect. By definition, a placebo is "an inert substance given as a medicine for its suggestive effect" (74). However, in addition to providing the positive short-term benefit of pain relief, limited interventional approaches in MPRCs can also have a profound impact on the physician–patient relationship. The interaction between a patient and a provider is far from "inert," and research support for the positive suggestive impact of procedures or the suggestive effect of an empathetic physician in decreasing pain is strong (75–80) and may offer some insight as to why individuals may feel more psychologically engaged when interventions are used successfully in the context of a multidisciplinary chronic pain management program. Some go as far as to regard this prescription of placebo as an important and exploitable phenomenon that should be used to assist a practitioner in achieving important end points, and some actually consider it an ethical imperative (81–83). Additionally, Seeley (84) has noted that among chronic pain patients, placebos can therapeutically empower patients to stimulate their psychophysiologic self-regulation abilities. Helping patients with chronic pain to enhance their psychophysiologic self-regulation skills has been determined to be an important aspect of the comprehensive treatment of this group of patients (85–92).

The extent to which the therapeutic effect of interventional techniques in the treatment of chronic pain is due to placebo has not been adequately addressed. Regardless, a well-timed pain-reducing injection can potentially increase a chronic pain patient's motivation. If any field of medicine exists in which the effect of motivation is critical, it is in dealing with chronic pain. For example, Friedrich and colleagues (93) determined that the long-term positive effect of a motivational program used in conjunction with a therapeutic exercise program for decreasing disability was more than twice that of the standard exercise program alone. Numerous other investigators (94–99) have also found empirical support for the crucial role of motivation in the management of chronic pain. Despite the fact that multidisciplinary chronic pain programs have a reputation for attributing patients' physical symptoms primarily to psychological causes and teaching patients not to dwell on their pain, the astute clinician recognizes the potential motivational impact of providing the suffering individual with a "holiday" from his or her discomfort.

Trust in health-care providers has been found to be positively related to health-care adherence and beneficial outcomes (100–105), and while not specifically studied, there is no reason to believe that these findings do not apply to multidisciplinary pain management. As the provision of pain relief is likely to be enhanced by patient trust, it follows that the short-term relief obtained through an interventional technique will potentially increase patient adherence to what is often considered a physically and emotionally demanding multidisciplinary chronic pain management program. Over the past several decades, studies regarding patient adherence have begun appearing in the literature, as empirically supported treatments for chronic conditions are only effective to the degree that patients follow the advice of health-care providers. Issues of adherence have been studied in regard to hyperlipidemia (106), antiretroviral therapy (107,108), diabetes (109), multiple sclerosis (110), upper extremity impairments (111), drug rehabilitation (112), and depression (113), among a host of other treatments and disease states. Estimates of the degree of adherence to long-term medical regimens have been estimated to be, on average, between 50% and 65% (114). Given the commonalities of chronic disease states, there is reason to consider that this paradigm may also be used to influence treatment adherence in patients with chronic pain who are treated through multidisciplinary programs. When the pain practitioner applies interventions aimed at optimizing characteristics of the patient, the environment of care and characteristics of the specific treatment modality appear to have a positive impact on treatment adherence.

Patient expectations regarding the efficacy of a multidisciplinary chronic pain management program are also thought to be related to outcomes, and these can be positively affected through the use of interventional techniques. In fact, results of a study by Kalauokalani and colleagues (115) suggested that patient expectations may influence the outcome of treatment for chronic pain independently of the treatment itself. Other investigators (116,117) have also found that patient expectations play a crucial role in outcome determination. Typically, by the time a patient enters a multidisciplinary program for chronic pain management, he or she has been symptomatic for an average of 7 years (5). Hopelessness is commonly evidenced among chronic pain patients (118–123), as they perceive the medical system as having failed them, and/or they see *themselves* as the locus of their failure to achieve relief. Additionally, repeated perceived failures can result in catastrophization, which has also been empirically linked to reports of higher pain levels (116,117,124–130), depression (126,131–137), risk of suicidality (138), activity interference (117,130–139), and a perceived lack of spousal/partner support (140–142). Reductions in catastrophization are associated with positive multidisciplinary chronic pain treatment outcomes (143–146). Through a pain-reducing injection early in a chronic pain management program, the physician has the opportunity of providing the patient with a "taste of success," albeit a likely temporary one. Despite its probable short-lived efficacy, a therapeutic injection has the potential to alter a patient's expectations, which, in turn, can have a positive influence on his or her emotional, as well as physical, outcomes.

Practitioners involved in the multidisciplinary treatment of individuals with chronic pain face significant challenges in causing their patients to adopt life-changing habits in order to assist them in reducing the disabling impact of symptoms. These include, but are not limited to, exercise, smoking cessation, dietary changes, and sometimes change of vocation. Similar issues are faced by the practitioner treating other chronic disease states such as obesity, diabetes, mental illness, and heart disease. If it is true that subtle characteristics of the physician–patient interaction will optimize the level of engagement and the degree of adherence to pain-altering treatments, then there is an obligation on the part of pain practitioners to understand and utilize them whenever possible. Meichenbaum and Turk define adherence as "the extent to which a person's behavior (in terms of taking medication, following diets, or executing lifestyle change) coincides with medical or health advice" (147). Because management of many chronic illnesses such as diabetes and hypertension commonly involves lifestyle changes, the literature on medication adherence may be applicable to the treatment of chronic pain conditions such as fibromyalgia and low back pain, which also involves adhering to programs including routine exercise and weight loss. The literature on adherence to treatment of other chronic diseases is replete with lessons that may help guide the practitioner treating chronic pain to maximize his or her effectiveness in treating the patient. Given that the primary interest of chronic pain sufferers is generally pain relief (148–150), the use of interventional techniques as a *means* of enhancing adherence to other aspects of the treatment program is certainly supported.

The importance of enhancing the self-efficacy of chronic pain patients is a common theme in the literature (130,151–170). To improve the individual's sense of self-efficacy, positive outcomes from injections such as incremental improvements in strength or range of motion through exercise should be clearly identified for a patient in a treatment program in order to capitalize on these gains; doing so serves to maximize self-efficacy and the expectation that treatments will be effective and reduced pain and increased function are possible. Restoration of one's sense of self-efficacy is thought to be a key contributor to the reduction of depression that is generally evidenced through involvement in a multidisciplinary chronic pain management program (171,172).

PRECAUTIONS IN USING INTERVENTIONAL TECHNIQUES WITHIN THE CONTEXT OF MPRCs

Caution should be taken to educate the patient that an isolated intervention is not a panacea. Because many chronic pain sufferers perpetuate their symptoms through behavioral overpacing (130,171,173–176), it is important to distinguish between "relief" and "repair." While patients in multidisciplinary treatment programs are likely to be appreciative of the short-term relief that they achieve through an injection, they should be educated regarding the likely temporary nature of the relief and the notion that therapeutic exercise is the key to recovery. Because of the risk of analgesia-induced overpacing, treatment team members should be warned to be vigilant following the provision of an interventional injection to a MPRC patient. If the treatment team *and* the patient are not fully aware of the significance and the limitations of an injection provided within the context of a multidisciplinary chronic pain management program, then all involved run the same risks associated with providing invasive interventions in isolation; the treatment team may potentially lose sight of the "big picture" of functional restoration, and the patient may erroneously consider himself or herself "fixed," potentially resulting in self-destructive behavioral overpacing or other forms of reduced adherence to other components of the prescribed treatment regimen. One effective way of educating patients regarding the limitations of a pain-reducing injection is to present it as representing only one "piece of the puzzle," suggesting that even the most telling puzzle piece in a collection does not provide one with a coherent vision of the whole picture.

However, if a patient is reluctant to undergo an intervention that the physician believes will facilitate his or her overall rehabilitative efforts, the physician can remind the patient that the puzzle will never be "whole" without the inclusion of all of the pieces.

While Drs. Kulich and Adolph have covered financial issues associated with multidisciplinary chronic pain management in chapter 15 in this volume, one cautionary note regarding the practice of providing therapeutic injections within the context of a MPRC should be provided. As numerous authors in this book discuss, the health-insurance industry, as a whole, is more concerned with cost containment and profitability than with the well-being of patients with chronic pain [see (20,21) for in-depth analyses of this ethical conflict]. Decision makers at health-insurance companies typically lack the training and sophistication to appreciate the complexity of effective chronic pain management, and therefore billing simultaneously for interventional techniques and multidisciplinary treatment will potentially result in only the *smaller* of the two charges being paid. Accordingly, it will behoove the practitioner (and, ultimately, the patient) to take measures to gain preapproval for any therapeutic injections that may be provided within the context of a MPRC.

CONCLUSIONS

Chapters in this book provide strong support for the efficacy and cost-efficiency of multidisciplinary chronic pain management. As mentioned earlier in this chapter, MPRCs unfairly gained the reputation of ignoring pathophysiology, and for only focusing on the psychological "causes" of chronic pain and related dysfunction. Arguments have been made (177–181) that the mind–body dualism historically associated with traditional medicine does not result in the effective treatment of chronic pain, given that pain affects every aspect of the patient's existence. Without a doubt, the Cartesian model is too restrictive to capture the essence of the chronic pain patient's dilemma. Reliance upon interventional techniques *in isolation* for the treatment of chronic pain is certainly not supported empirically in terms of clinical efficacy or cost-efficiency and is ethically questionable (19). However, within the context of a multidisciplinary chronic pain management program, therapeutic injections can be "therapeutic," although not necessarily curative. Whether the beneficial effects of interventional techniques in this context are direct or indirect, the complexity of chronic pain conditions and their profound effects on people who suffer from them necessitate approaches that may have once been considered "outside the box." As holistic as multidisciplinary chronic pain management is considered to be, the coordinated inclusion of interventional techniques, in certain cases, serves to further broaden the scope of the approach. Clearly, in the context of multidisciplinary chronic pain rehabilitation, the whole is far greater than the sum of the individual parts.

REFERENCES

1. Ridley MG, Kingsley GH, Gibson T, et al. Outpatient lumbar epidural corticosteroid injection in the management of sciatica. Br J Rheumatol 1988; 27(4):259–295.

2. Maniadakis N, Gray A. The economic burden of back pain in the UK. Pain 2000; 84:95–103.
3. National Academies of Sciences and Institute of Medicine. Musculoskeletal Disorders and the Workplace: Low Back Pain and Upper Extremities. Washington, DC: National Academies Press; 2001.
4. Luo X, Pietrobon R, Sun SX, et al. Estimates and patterns of direct health care expenditures among individual with back pain in the United States. Spine 2003; 29:79–86.
5. Flor H, Fydrich T, Turk DC. Efficacy of multidisciplinary pain treatment centers: a meta-analytic review. Pain 1992; 49:221–230.
6. Hoffman BM, Papas RK, Chatkoff KD, et al. Meta-analysis of psychological interventions for chronic low back pain. Health Psychol 2007; 26:1–9.
7. Jensen MK, Thomsen AB, Hojsted J. 10-year follow-up of chronic non-malignant pain patients: opioid use, health related quality of life and health care utilization. Eur J Pain 2006; 10:423–433.
8. Okifuji A, Turk DC, Kalauoklani D. Clinical outcome and economic evaluation of multidisciplinary pain centers. In: Block AR, Kramer EF, Fernandez E, eds. Handbook of Pain Syndromes: Biopsychosocial Perspectives. Mahwah, NJ: Lawrence Erlbaum Associates; 1999:77–97.
9. Schonstein E, Kenny DT, Keating J, et al. Work conditioning, work hardening and functional restoration for workers with back and neck pain. Cochrane Database Syst Rev 2003; 1:CD001822.
10. Turk DC. Transition from acute to chronic pain: role of demographic and psychosocial factors. In: Jensen TS, Turner JA, Wiesenfeld-Hallin Z, eds. Proceedings of the 8th World Congress on Pain, Progress in Pain Research and Management. Seattle, WA: IASP Press; 1997:185–213.
11. Marketdata Enterprises. Chronic Pain Management Programs: A Market Analysis. Marketdata Enterprises, Valley Stream, New York; 1995.
12. Rozenberg S, Dubourg G, Khalifa P, et al. Efficacy of epidural steroids in low back pain and sciatica. A critical appraisal by a French Task Force of randomized trials. Critical Analysis Group of the French Society for Rheumatology. Rev Rhum Engl Ed 1999; 66:79–85.
13. Nelemans P, Bie RA de, Vet HCW de, et al. Injection therapy for subacute and chronic benign low back pain. Cochrane Database Syst Rev 2000; 2:CD001824.
14. Niemisto L, Kalso E, Malmivaara A, et al. Radiofrequency denervation for neck and back pain. A systematic review of randomized controlled trials. Cochrane Database Syst Rev 2003; 1:CD004058.
15. McLain RF, Kapural L, Mekhail NA. Epidural steroid therapy for back and leg pain: mechanisms of action and efficacy. Spine J 2005; 5:191–201.
16. Freeman BJ. IDET: a critical appraisal of the evidence. Eur Spine J 2006; 15(Suppl 15):448–457.
17. Leonardi M, Pfirrmann CW, Boos N. Injection studies in spinal disorders. Clin Orthop Relat Res 2006; 443:168–182.
18. Lebovitz A. Ethics and pain: why and for whom? Pain Med 2001; 2:92–96.
19. Schatman ME, Giordano J. The ethical obligation of the physiatrist to treat chronic pain and suffering: the primacy of the person. Manuscript submitted for review.
20. Schatman ME. The demise of multidisciplinary pain management clinics? Practical Pain Manage 2006; 6:30–41.
21. Schatman ME. The demise of the multidisciplinary chronic pain management clinic: bioethical perspectives on providing optimal treatment when ethical principles collide. In: Schatman ME, ed. Ethical Issues in Chronic Pain Management. New York: Informa Healthcare; 2007:43–62.
22. Eccleston C. Chronic pain and attention: a cognitive approach. Br J Clin Psychol 1994; 33:535–547.
23. Snider BS, Asmundson GJ, Wiese KC. Automatic and strategic processing of threat cues in patients with chronic pain: a modified stroop evaluation. Clin J Pain 2000; 16:144–154.

24. Asmundson GJ, Wright KD, Hadjistavropoulos HD. Hypervigilance and attentional fixedness in chronic musculoskeletal pain: consistency of findings across modified stroop and dot-probe tasks. J Pain 2005; 6:497–506.
25. Harman K, Ruyak P. Working through the pain: a controlled study of the impact of persistent pain on performing a computer task. Clin J Pain 2005; 21:216–222.
26. Vangronsveld K, Van Damme S, Peters M, et al. An experimental investigation on attentional interference by threatening fixations of the neck in patients with chronic whiplash syndrome. Pain 2007; 127:121–128.
27. Simons DG, Travell JG. Myofascial origins of low back pain. 1. Principles of diagnosis and treatment. Postgrad Med 1983; 73:66, 68–70, 73.
28. Simons DG, Travell JG. Myofascial origins of low back pain. 2. Torso muscles. Postgrad Med 1983; 73:81–92.
29. Simons DG, Travell JG. Myofascial origins of low back pain. 3. Pelvic and lower extremity muscles. Postgrad Med 1983; 73:99–105, 108.
30. Simons DG. Myofascial pain syndrome due to trigger points. In: Goodgold J, ed. Rehabilitation Medicine. St. Louis, MO: C.V. Mosby Co.; 1988:686–723.
31. Hagberg M, Kvarnstrom S. Muscular endurance and electromyographic fatigue in myofascial shoulder pain. Arch Phys Med Rehab 1984; 65:522–525.
32. Cummings MT, White AR. Needling therapies in the management of myofascial trigger point pain: a systematic review. Arch Phys Med Rehab 1996; 82: 986–992.
33. Watts RW, Silagy CA. A meta-analysis on the efficacy of epidural corticosteroids in the treatment of sciatica. Anaesth Intensive Care 1995; 23:564–569.
34. Blair B, Rokito AS, Cuomo F, et al. Efficacy of injections of corticosteroids for subacromial impingement syndrome. J Bone Joint Surg Am 1996; 78:1685–1689.
35. McColl GJ, Dolezal H, Eizenberg N. Common corticosteroid injections. An anatomical and evidence based review. Aust Fam Physician 2000; 29:922–926.
36. Karppinen J, Ohinmaa A, Malmivaara A, et al. Cost effectiveness of periradicular infiltration for sciatica: subgroup analysis of a randomized controlled trial. Spine 2001; 26:2587–2595.
37. Karabacakoglu A, Karakose S, Ozerbil OM, et al. Fluoroscopy-guided intraarticular corticosteroid injection into the sacroiliac joints in patients with ankylosing spondylitis. Acta Radiol 2002; 43:425–427.
38. Pneumaticos SG, Chatzioannou SN, Hipp JA, et al. Low back pain: prediction of short-term outcome of facet joint injection with bone scintigraphy. Radiology 2006; 238:693–698.
39. Dreyer SJ, Dreyfus PH. Low back pain and the zygapophysial (facet) joints. Arch Phys Med Rehab 1996; 77:290–300.
40. Geraci M. Rehabilitation of pelvis, hip and thigh injuries in sports. Phys Med Rehabil Clin North Am 1994; 5:157–173.
41. Timm KE. A randomized-control study of active and passive treatments for chronic low back pain following L5 laminectomy. J Orthop Sports Phys Ther 1994; 20:276–286.
42. Faas A. Exercises: which ones are worth trying, for which patients, and when? Spine 1996; 21(15):2874–2878.
43. O'Sullivan PB, Phyty GD, Twomey LT, et al. Evaluation of specific stabilizing exercise in the treatment of chronic low back pain with radiologic diagnosis of spondylolysis or spondylolisthesis. Spine 1997; 22(15):2959–2967.
44. Carpenter DM, Nelson BW. Low back strengthening for the prevention and treatment of low back pain. Med Sci Sports Exerc 1999; 31:18–24.
45. Kankaanpaa M, Taimela S, Airaksinen O, et al. The efficacy of active rehabilitation in chronic low back pain. Effect on pain intensity, self-experienced disability, and lumbar fatigability. Spine 1999; 24(15):1034–1042.
46. Bronfort G, Assendelft WJ, Evans R, et al. Efficacy of spinal manipulation for chronic headache: a systematic review. J Manipulative Physiol Ther 2001; 24:457–466.
47. Philadelphia Panel. Philadelphia Panel evidence-based clinical practice guidelines on selected rehabilitation interventions for neck pain. Phys Ther 2001; 81:1701–1717.

48. Jentoft ES, Kvalvik AG, Mengshoel AM. Effects of pool-based and land-based aerobic exercise on women with fibromyalgia/chronic widespread muscle pain. Arthritis Rheum 2001; 45:42–47.
49. Ylinen J. Analysis of strength measures of different sexes. Clin Rehabil 2003; 17:691.
50. Maher CG, Sherrington C, Elkins M, et al. Challenges for evidence-based physical therapy: accessing and interpreting high-quality evidence on therapy. Phys Ther 2004; 84:644–654.
51. Rainville J, Hartigan C, Jouve C, et al. The influence of intense exercise-based physical therapy program on back pain anticipated before and induced by physical activities. Spine J 2004; 4:176–183.
52. Shirado O, Ito T, Kikumoto T, et al. A novel back school using a multidisciplinary team approach featuring quantitative functional evaluation and therapeutic exercises for patients with chronic low back pain: the Japanese experience in the general setting. Spine 2005; 30:1219–1225.
53. Koumantakis GA, Watson PJ, Oldham JA. Supplementation of general endurance exercise with stabilisation training versus general exercise only: physiological and functional outcomes of a randomised controlled trial of patients with recurrent low back pain. Clin Biomech 2005; 20:474–482.
54. Hayden JA, van Tulder MW, Malmivaara A, et al. Exercise therapy for treatment of non-specific low back pain. Cochrane Database Syst Rev 2005; 3:CD000335.
55. Rydeard R, Leger A, Smith D. Pilates-based therapeutic exercise: effect on subjects with nonspecific chronic low back pain and functional disability: a randomized controlled trial. J Orthop Sports Phys Ther 2006; 36:472–484.
56. Falla D, Farina D. Neuromuscular adaptation in experimental and clinical neck pain. J Electromyogr Kinesiol 2006 Dec 28; epub ahead of print.
57. Pfingsten M, Leibing E, Harter W, et al. Fear-avoidance behavior and anticipation of pain in patients with chronic low back pain: a randomized controlled study. Pain Med 2001; 2:259–266.
58. Waddell G, Newton M, Henderson I, et al. A Fear-Avoidance Beliefs Questionnaire (FABQ) and the role of fear-avoidance beliefs in chronic low back pain and disability. Pain 1993; 52:157–168.
59. McCracken LM, Gross RT, Aikens J, et al. The assessment of anxiety and fear in persons with chronic pain: a comparison of instruments. Behav Res Ther 1996; 34:927–933.
60. Crombez G, Vlaeyen JW, Heuts PH, et al. Pain-related fear is more disabling than pain itself: evidence on the role of pain-related fear in chronic back pain disability. Pain 1999; 80:329–339.
61. Mannion AF, Junge A, Taimela S, et al. Active therapy for chronic low back pain: part 3. Factors influencing self-rated disability and its change following therapy. Spine 2001; 26:920–929.
62. Al-Obaidi SM, Al-Zoabi B, Al-Shuwaie N, et al. The influence of pain and pain-related fear and disability beliefs on walking velocity in chronic low back pain. Int J Rehabil Res 2003; 26:101–108.
63. Vowles KE, Gross RT. Work-related beliefs about injury and physical capability for work in individuals with chronic pain. Pain 2003; 101:291–298.
64. Denison E, Åsenlöf P, Lindberg P. Self-efficacy, fear avoidance, and pain intensity as predictors of disability in subacute and chronic musculoskeletal pain patients in primary health care. Pain 2004; 111:245–252.
65. Grotle M, Vollestad NK, Veierod MB, et al. Fear-avoidance beliefs and distress in relation to disability in acute and chronic low back pain. Pain 2004; 112:343–352.
66. Woby SR, Watson PJ, Roach NK, et al. Are changes in fear-avoidance beliefs, catastrophizing, and appraisals of control, predictive of changes in chronic low back pain and disability? Eur J Pain 2004; 8:201–210.
67. Woby SR, Watson PJ, Roach NK, et al. Adjustment to chronic low back pain–the relative influence of fear-avoidance beliefs, catastrophizing, and appraisals of control. Behav Res Ther 2004; 42:761–774.

68. Al-Obaidi SM, Beattie P, Al-Zoabi B, et al. The relationship of anticipated pain and fear avoidance beliefs to outcome in patients with chronic low back pain who are not receiving workers' compensation. Spine 2005; 30:1051–1057.
69. George SZ, Fritz JM, McNeil DW. Fear-avoidance beliefs as measured by the fear-avoidance beliefs questionnaire: change in fear-avoidance beliefs questionnaire is predictive of change in self-report of disability and pain intensity for patients with acute low back pain. Clin J Pain 2006; 22:197–203.
70. Grotle M, Vollestad NK, Veierod MB Fear-avoidance beliefs and distress in relation to disability in acute and chronic low back pain. Pain 2004; 112:343–352.
71. George SZ, Fritz JM, McNeil DW. Fear-avoidance beliefs as measured by the Fear-Avoidance Beliefs Questionnaire: change in Fear-Avoidance Beliefs Questionnaire is predictive of change in self-report of disability and pain intensity for patients with acute low back pain. Clin J Pain 2006; 22:197–203.
72. Walsh DA, Radcliffe JC. Pain beliefs and perceived physical disability of patients with chronic low back pain. Pain 2002; 97(1–2):23–31.
73. Wittink HM, Rogers WH, Lipman AG, et al. Older and younger adults in pain management programs in the United States: differences and similarities. Pain Med 2006; 7:151–163.
74. Stedman TL. Stedmans Medical Dictionary, 25th edn. Baltimore, MD: Williams and Wilkins; 1990.
75. Nabeta T, Kawakita K. Relief of chronic neck and shoulder pain by manual acupuncture to tender points—a sham-controlled randomized trial. Complement Ther Med 2002; 10:217–222.
76. Johansen I, Henriksen G, Demkjaer K, et al. Quality assurance and certification of health IT-systems communicating data in primary and secondary health sector. Stud Health Technol Inform 2003; 95:601–605.
77. Wager E. BMJ ethics committee. Experiences of the BMJ ethics committee. BMJ 2004; 329:510–512.
78. Kaptchuk TJ, Stason WB, Davis RB, et al. Sham device v inert pill: randomised controlled trial of two placebo treatments. BMJ 2006; 332:391–397.
79. Matre D, Casey KL, Knardahl S. Placebo-induced changes in spinal cord pain processing. J Neurosci 2006; 26:559–563.
80. Wager TD, Matre D, Casey KL. Placebo effects in laser-evoked pain potentials. Brain Behav Immun 2006; 20:219–230.
81. Cheyne C. Exploiting placebo effects for therapeutic benefit. Health Care Anal 2005; 13:177–188.
82. Szawarski Z. The concept of placebo. Sci Eng Ethics 2004; 10:57–64.
83. Biller-Andorno N. The use of placebo effect in clinical medicine—ethical blunder or ethical imperative? Sci Eng Ethics 2004; 10:43–50.
84. Seeley D. Selected nonpharmacological therapies for chronic pain: the therapeutic use of the placebo effect. J Am Acad Nurse Pract. 1990; 2:10–16.
85. Gottlieb H, Strite LC, Koller R, et al. Comprehensive rehabilitation of patients having chronic low back pain. Arch Phys Med Rehabil 1977; 58:101–108.
86. Aronoff GM. The use of non-narcotic drugs and other alternatives for analgesia as part of a comprehensive pain management program. J Med 1982; 13:191–202.
87. Gottlieb HJ, Koller R, Alperson BL. Low back pain comprehensive rehabilitation program: a follow-up study. Arch Phys Med Rehabil 1982; 63:458–461.
88. Ruoff GE, Beery GB. Chronic pain. Postgrad Med 1985; 78:91–97.
89. Stenger EM. Chronic back pain: view from a psychiatrist's office. Clin J Pain 1992; 8:242–246.
90. Harden RN, Cole PA. New developments in rehabilitation of neuropathic pain syndromes. Neurol Clin 1998; 16:937–950.
91. Bruehl S, Chung OY. Psychological and behavioral aspects of complex regional pain syndrome management. Clin J Pain 2006; 22:430–437.
92. Stanos S, Houle TT. Multidisciplinary and interdisciplinary management of chronic pain. Phys Med Rehabil Clin N Am 2006; 17:435–50, vii.

93. Friedrich M, Gittler G, Arendasy M, et al. Long-term effect of a combined exercise and motivational program on the level of disability of patients with chronic low back pain. Spine 2005; 30:995–1000.
94. Elkayam O, Ben Itzhak S, Avrahami E, et al. Multidisciplinary approach to chronic back pain: prognostic elements of the outcome. Clin Exp Rheumatol 1996; 14:281–288.
95. Tan V, Cheatle MD, Mackin S, et al. Goal setting as a predictor of return to work in a population of chronic musculoskeletal pain patients. Int J Neurosci. 1997; 92:161–170.
96. Habib S, Morrissey S, Helmes E. Preparing for pain management: a pilot study to enhance engagement. J Pain 2005; 6:48–54.
97. Heapy A, Otis J, Marcus KS, et al. Intersession coping skill practice mediates the relationship between readiness for self-management treatment and goal accomplishment. Pain 2005; 118(5):360–368.
98. Sullivan MJ, Adams H, Rhodenizer T, et al. A psychosocial risk factor–targeted intervention for the prevention of chronic pain and disability following whiplash injury. Phys Ther 2006; 86:8–18.
99. Zenker S, Petraschka M, Schenk M, et al. Adjustment to chronic pain in back pain patients classified according to the motivational stages of chronic pain management. J Pain 2006; 7:417–427.
100. Mostashari F, Riley E, Selwyn PA, et al. Acceptance and adherence with antiretroviral therapy among HIV-infected women in a correctional facility. J Acquir Immune Defic Syndr Hum Retrovirol 1998; 18:341–348.
101. Safran DG, Kosinski M, Tarlov AR, et al. The Primary Care Assessment Survey: tests of data quality and measurement performance. Med Care 1998; 36:728–739.
102. Thom DH, Kravitz RL, Bell RA, et al. Patient trust in the physician: relationship to patient requests. Fam Pract 2002; 19:476–483.
103. Bonds DE, Camacho F, Bell RA, et al. The association of patient trust and self-care among patients with diabetes mellitus. BMC Fam Pract 2004; 5:26.
104. O'Malley AS, Sheppard VB, Schwartz M, et al. The role of trust in use of preventive services among low-income African-American women. Prev Med 2004; 38:777–785.
105. Franks P, Fiscella K, Shields CG, et al. Are patients' ratings of their physicians related to health outcomes? Ann Fam Med 2005; 3:229–234.
106. Kiortsis DN, Giral P, Bruckert E, et al. Factors associated with low compliance with lipid-lowering drugs in hyperlipidemic patients. J Clin Pharm Ther 2000; 25:445, 51.
107. Ammassari A, Trotta MP, Murri R, et al. Correlates and predictors of adherence to highly active antiretroviral therapy: overview of published literature. J Acquir Immune Defic Syndr 2002; 31(Suppl 3):S123–S127.
108. Goujard C, Bernard N, Sohier N, et al. Impact of a patient education program on adherence to HIV medication. J Acquir Immune Defic Syndr 2003; 34:191–194.
109. Lee WC, Balu S, Cobden D, et al. Medication adherence and the associated health-economic impact among patients with type 2 diabetes mellitus converting to insulin pen therapy: an analysis of third-party managed care claims data. Clin Ther 2006; 28:1712–1725.
110. Fraser C, Hadjimichael O, Vollmer T. Predictors of adherence to Copaxone therapy in individuals with relapsing remitting multiple sclerosis. J Neurosci Nurs 2001; 33:231–239.
111. Chen C, Neufeld PS, Skinner CS, et al. Factors Influencing compliance with home exercise programs among patients with upper extremity impairment. Am J Occup Ther 1999; 53:171–180.
112. Demas P, Schoenbaum EE, Hirky AE, et al. The relationship of HIV treatment acceptance and adherence to psychosocial factors among injecting drug users. AIDS Behav 1998; 2:283–292.
113. Masand PS. Tolerability and adherence issues in antidepressant therapy. Clin Ther 2003; 25:2289–2304.
114. Melnikow J, Kiefe C. Patient compliance and medical research: issues in methodology. J Gen Intern Med 1994; 9:96–105.

115. Kalauokalani D, Cherkin DC, Sherman KJ, et al. Lessons from a trial of acupuncture and massage for low back pain: patient expectations and treatment effects. Spine 2001; 26:1418–1424.
116. Tan V, Cheatle MD, Mackin S, et al. Goal setting as a predictor of return to work in a population of chronic musculoskeletal pain patients. Int J Neurosci 1997; 92:161–170.
117. Turner JA, Jensen MP, Warms CA, et al. Blinding effectiveness and association of pretreatment expectations with pain improvement in a double-blind randomized controlled trial. Pain 2002; 99:91–99.
118. Peek LA, Sawyer JP. Utilization of the Family Drawing Depression Scale with pain patients. Art Psychother 1988; 15:207–210.
119. Varma VK, Chaturvedi SK, Malhotra A, et al. Psychiatric symptoms in patients with non-organic chronic intractable pain. Indian J Med Res 1991; 94:60–63.
120. Hitchcock LS, Ferrell BR, McCaffery M. The experience of chronic nonmalignant pain. J Pain Symptom Manage 1994; 9:312–328.
121. Anderson KO, Dowds BN, Pelletz RE, et al. Development and initial validation of a scale to measure self-efficacy beliefs in patients with chronic pain. Pain 1995; 63:77–84.
122. Hallberg LR, Carlsson SG. Psychosocial vulnerability and maintaining forces related to fibromyalgia. Scand J Caring Sci 1998; 12:95–103.
123. Koleck M, Mazaux JM, Rascle N, et al. Psycho-social factors and coping strategies as predictors of chronic evolution and quality of life in patients with low back pain: a prospective study. Eur J Pain 2006; 10:1–11.
124. Turner JA, Clancy S. Strategies for coping with chronic low back pain: relationship to pain and disability. Pain 1986; 24:355–364.
125. Keefe FJ, Brown GK, Wallston KA, et al. Coping with rheumatoid arthritis pain: catastrophizing as a maladaptive strategy. Pain 1989; 37:51–56.
126. Severeijns R, Vlaeyen JW, van den Hout MA, et al. Pain catastrophizing predicts pain intensity, disability, and psychological distress independent of the level of physical impairment. Clin J Pain 2001; 17:1651–1672.
127. Picavet HS, Vlaeyen JW, Schouten JS. Pain catastrophizing and kinesiophobia: predictors of chronic low back pain. Am J Epidemiol 2002; 156(1):1028–1034.
128. Giardino ND, Jensen MP, Turner JA, et al. Social environment moderates the association between catastrophizing and pain among persons with a spinal cord injury. Pain 2003; 106:19–25.
129. Litt MD, Shafer D, Napolitano C. Momentary mood and coping processes in TMD pain. Health Psychol 2004; 23:354–362.
130. Turner JA, Brister H, Huggins K, et al. Catastrophizing is associated with clinical examination findings, activity interference, and health care use among patients with temporomandibular disorders. J Orofac Pain 2005; 19:291–300.
131. Sullivan MJ, D'Eon JL. Relation between catastrophizing and depression in chronic pain patients. J Abnorm Psychol 1990; 99:260–263.
132. Swimmer GI, Robinson ME, Geisser ME. Relationship of MMPI cluster type, pain coping strategy, and treatment outcome. Clin J Pain 1992; 8:131–137.
133. Geisser ME, Robinson ME, Keefe FJ, et al. Catastrophizing, depression and the sensory, affective and evaluative aspects of chronic pain. Pain 1994; 59:79–83.
134. Hassett AL, Cone JD, Patella SJ, et al. The role of catastrophizing in the pain and depression of women with fibromyalgia syndrome. Arthritis Rheum 2000; 43:2493–2500.
135. Turner JA, Jensen MP, Romano JM. Do beliefs, coping, and catastrophizing independently predict functioning in patients with chronic pain? Pain 2000; 85:115–125.
136. Turner JA, Dworkin SF, Mancl L, et al. The roles of beliefs, catastrophizing, and coping in the functioning of patients with temporomandibular disorders. Pain 2001; 92:41–51.
137. Hirsh AT, George SZ, Riley JL, III, et al. An evaluation of the measurement of pain catastrophizing by the coping strategies questionnaire. Eur J Pain 2007; 11:75–81.

138. Edwards RR, Smith MT, Kudel I, et al. Pain-related catastrophizing as a risk factor for suicidal ideation in chronic pain. Pain 2006; 126:272–279.
139. Turner JA, Cardenas DD, Warms CA, et al. Chronic pain associated with spinal cord injuries: a community survey. Arch Phys Med Rehabil 2001; 82:501–509.
140. Boothby JL, Thorn BE, Overduin LY, et al. Catastrophizing and perceived partner responses to pain. Pain 2004; 109:500–506.
141. Cano A. Pain catastrophizing and social support in married individuals with chronic pain: the moderating role of pain duration. Pain 2004; 110:656–664.
142. Buenaver LF, Edwards RR, Haythornthwaite JA. Pain-related catastrophizing and perceived social responses: inter-relationships in the context of chronic pain. Pain 2007; 127:234–242.
143. Jensen MP, Turner JA, Romano JM. Changes in beliefs, catastrophizing, and coping are associated with improvement in multidisciplinary pain treatment. J Consult Clin Psychol 2001; 69:655–662.
144. Burns JW, Kubilus A, Bruehl S, et al. Do changes in cognitive factors influence outcome following multidisciplinary treatment for chronic pain? A cross-lagged panel analysis. J Consult Clin Psychol 2003; 71:81–91.
145. Spinhoven P, Ter Kuile M, Kole-Snijders AM, et al. Catastrophizing and internal pain control as mediators of outcome in the multidisciplinary treatment of chronic low back pain. Eur J Pain 2004; 8:211–219.
146. Smeets RJ, Vlaeyen JW, Kester AD, et al. Reduction of pain catastrophizing mediates the outcome of both physical and cognitive-behavioral treatment in chronic low back pain. J Pain 2006; 7:261–271.
147. Meichenbaum D, Turk DC. Facilitating Treatment Adherence: A Practitioner's Guidebook. New York: Plenum; 1987.
148. Verbeek J, Sengers MJ, Riemens L, et al. Patient expectations of treatment for back pain: a systematic review of qualitative and quantitative studies. Spine 2004; 29:2309–2318.
149. Petrie KJ, Frampton T, Large RG, et al. What do patients expect from their first visit to a pain clinic? Clin J Pain 2005; 21:297–301.
150. Robinson ME, Brown JL, George SZ, et al. Multidimensional success criteria and expectations for treatment of chronic pain: the patient perspective. Pain Med 2005; 6:336–345.
151. Dolce JJ. Self-efficacy and disability beliefs in behavioral treatment of pain. Behav Res Ther 1987; 25:289–299.
152. Kores RC, Murphy WD, Rosenthal TL, et al. Predicting outcome of chronic pain treatment via a modified self-efficacy scale. Behav Res Ther 1990; 28:165–169.
153. Jensen MP, Turner JA, Romano JM. Self-efficacy and outcome expectancies: relationship to chronic pain coping strategies and adjustment. Pain 1991; 44:263–269.
154. Nicholas MK, Wilson PH, Goyen J. Comparison of cognitive-behavioral group treatment and an alternative non-psychological treatment for chronic low back pain. Pain 1992; 48:339–347.
155. Lacker JM, Carosella AM, Feuerstein M. Pain expectancies, pain, and functional self-efficacy expectancies as determinants of disability in patients with chronic low back disorders. J Consult Clin Psychol 1996; 64:212–220.
156. Lin CC, Ward SE. Perceived self-efficacy and outcome expectancies in coping with chronic low back pain. Res Nurs Health 1996; 19:299–310.
157. Robbins RA, Moody DS, Hahn MB, et al. Psychological testing variables as predictors of return to work by chronic pain patients. Percept Mot Skills 1996; 83:1317–1318.
158. Arnstein P, Caudill M, Mandle CL, et al. Self efficacy as a mediator of the relationship between pain intensity, disability and depression in chronic pain patients. Pain 1999; 80:483–491.
159. Arnstein P. The mediation of disability by self efficacy in different samples of chronic pain patients. Disabil Rehabil 2000; 22:794–801.

160. Coughlin AM, Badura AS, Fleischer TD, et al. Multidisciplinary treatment of chronic pain patients: its efficacy in changing patient locus of control. Arch Phys Med Rehabil 2000; 81:739–740.
161. Asghari A, Nicholas MK. Pain self-efficacy beliefs and pain behaviour. A prospective study. Pain 2001; 94:85–100.
162. Lumley MA, Smith JA, Longo DJ. The relationship of alexithymia to pain severity and impairment among patients with chronic myofascial pain: comparisons with self-efficacy, catastrophizing, and depression. J Psychosom Res 2002; 53:823–830.
163. Wells-Federman C, Arnstein P, Caudill M. Nurse-led pain management program: effect on self-efficacy, pain intensity, pain-related disability, and depressive symptoms in chronic pain patients. Pain Manag Nurs 2002; 3:131–140.
164. Barry LC, Guo Z, Kerns RD, et al. Functional self-efficacy and pain-related disability among older veterans with chronic pain in a primary care setting. Pain 2003; 104:131–137.
165. Rahman A, Ambler G, Underwood MR, et al. Important determinants of self-efficacy in patients with chronic musculoskeletal pain. J Rheumatol 2004; 31:1187–1192.
166. Oliver K, Cronan TA. Correlates of physical activity among women with fibromyalgia syndrome. Ann Behav Med 2005; 29:44–53.
167. Marks R, Allegrante JP, Lorig K. A review and synthesis of research evidence for self-efficacy-enhancing interventions for reducing chronic disability: implications for health education practice (part II). Health Promot Pract 2005; 6:148–156.
168. Brister H, Turner JA, Aaron LA, et al. Self-efficacy is associated with pain, functioning, and coping in patients with chronic temporomandibular disorder pain. J Orofac Pain 2006; 20:115–124.
169. Nicholas MK. The pain self-efficacy questionnaire: Taking pain into account. Eur J Pain 2007; 11:153–163.
170. Turner JA, Holtzman S, Mancl L. Mediators, moderators, and predictors of therapeutic change in cognitive-behavioral therapy for chronic pain. Pain 2007; 127:276–286.
171. Williams AC, Nicholas MK, Richardson PH, et al. Evaluation of a cognitive behavioural programme for rehabilitating patients with chronic pain. Br J Gen Pract 1993; 43:513–518.
172. Keller S, Ehrhardt-Schmelzer S, Herda C, et al. Multidisciplinary rehabilitation for chronic back pain in an outpatient setting: a controlled randomized trial. Eur J Pain 1997; 1:279–292.
173. Sternbach RA. Treatment of the chronic pain patient. J Human Stress 1978; 4:11–15.
174. Nielson WR, Jensen MP, Hill ML. An activity pacing scale for the chronic pain coping inventory: development in a sample of patients with fibromyalgia syndrome. Pain 2001; 89:111–115.
175. Turner-Stokes L, Erkeller-Yuksel F, Miles A, et al. Outpatient cognitive behavioral pain management programs: a randomized comparison of a group-based multidisciplinary versus an individual therapy model. Arch Phys Med Rehabil 2003; 84:781–788.
176. Dudgeon BJ, Tyler EJ, Rhodes LA, et al. Managing usual and unexpected pain with physical disability: a qualitative analysis. Am J Occup Ther 2006; 60:92–103.
177. Novy DM, Nelson DV, Francis DJ, et al. Perspectives of chronic pain: an evaluative comparison of restrictive and comprehensive models. Psychol Bull 1995; 118:238–247.
178. Bates MS, Rankin-Hill L, Sanchez-Ayendez M. The effects of the cultural context of health care on treatment of and response to chronic pain and illness. Soc Sci Med 1997; 45:1433–1447.
179. Grace VM. Mind/body dualism in medicine: the case of chronic pelvic pain without organic pathology: a critical review of the literature. Int J Health Serv 1998; 28:127–151.
180. Nicholson K, Martelli MF. The problem of pain. J Head Trauma Rehabil 2004; 19:2–9.
181. Martelli MF, Zasler ND, Bender MC, et al. Psychological, neuropsychological, and medical considerations in assessment and management of pain. J Head Trauma Rehabil 2004; 19:10–28.

8 Who Can Help Me? A Chronic Pain Patient's View of Multidisciplinary Treatment

Debra E. Benner
Hershey Medical Center, Hershey, Pennsylvania, U.S.A.

> The desert experience of pain is an enforced sojourn away from the familiar landscape of life-as-usual. It narrows the field of vision while it sharpens what remains in the sights. Gone are the things you thought you needed. You are thrust into an environment that has ruthlessly pared them away. There are only a few things necessary: enough relief from the pain so that you can develop the ability to cope with it; help from those who know how to guide you toward healing; and sufficient personal support to keep you traversing this alien landscape instead of dropping in your tracks from exhaustion and discouragement.
>
> - Erv Hinds, MD, in *A Life Larger Than Pain*

INTRODUCTION

I vividly remember the day my surgeon told me that he could do nothing more to ease my pain. I had experienced year after year of scheduling preoperative appointments, spinal surgery dates, and a myriad of postoperative follow-up appointments and radiographs, but this day I left without any further appointments to schedule. I was discarded by the traditional medical system. Instead of another interventional procedure, my surgeon told me to contact a pain management clinic to learn to handle the pain that his medical science could not heal. As he wrote the recommendation for a pain management consultation on the fee sheet, I could feel a sense of defeat permeate the room. He was a good man, and I believe he was truly sorry that my case had come to this. As I presented my sheet to his front office staff, there was none of the usual friendly banter between myself and the staff. All was quiet. Eyes that were normally warm and friendly looked away as I presented my fee sheet which held that equivalent of a failing grade. I felt defeated and they felt defeated too. I was being sent to the land of the broken—the place where patients go when pain has become a permanent reality of life.

I was skeptical regarding this referral to a physician who specialized in pain management. But, by this time, my former life was in total disarray, and I really had no other option than to test the waters of this new experience. I called and set up the appointment. My records were to be transferred from my surgeon's office. As I signed in upon my arrival, the receptionist told me they had indeed received all of my information. I guess it was particularly memorable to her as she told me that the fax machine had taken two full hours to accomplish the task. As I took a seat to await that first appointment, I surveyed my surroundings. What was I doing here in the middle of the afternoon with all of these broken people? Up to the time of the automobile accident, which marked the beginning of my medical journey, I had always had control over my life. I already had one doctoral degree in veterinary medicine and was working on another doctoral degree in theology. I had had a successful veterinary career before deciding to explore options in the ministerial field. I had taught physiology and pathophysiology for several years at a local university as I transitioned into full-time ministry. Immediately prior to the accident that brought me to this waiting room, I had been the executive director of a 2000-member nonprofit ministry organization. Again I asked myself, what was *I* doing *here* in the middle of a workday with people in wheelchairs and others who grimaced every time they adjusted their bodies into a more comfortable position?

MY LIFE WITH CHRONIC PAIN

I had compassion for the others who were waiting, but I did not want to find commonality with them beyond the universal suffering we all experience at times as limited human beings. I did not want to accept that my life would now revolve around my pain. But, then I began to think about all of the changes that had been thrust upon me over the past 3–4 years of coping with chronic pain. I knew I had been dealing with declining functioning for several years at this point, but there was still a large part of myself that remained unable to grasp the reality of its permanence. I did not want to be here. I wanted to be working and productive. There was a surreal feeling about where I found myself. I considered myself to be a strongly spiritual person, and felt I had worked through the "why me?" question, but now the question returned as I awaited this first appointment. I did not know what to expect. I had long ago decided to stop talking about my pain with my friends or family. This was not out of a sense of stoicism as much as self-protection. Unless someone has experienced a chronic pain or chronic illness problem that has totally disrupted one's life, it is pointless to expect any degree of true understanding from even those who are closest to you. All one will hear is platitudes as they struggle with how to be a supportive influence. What too often goes unrealized is how deeply these platitudes can injure the patient who so desperately desires understanding from another human being. What is a sincere effort by others to be supportive often strikes the chronic pain sufferer as dismissive or minimizing of the experience and its multitude of subsequent losses.

What were these losses for me? My life had changed dramatically, and I was having a lot of difficulty making healthy adjustments to my new situation. Pain had become a permanent and unwelcome companion. It was with me every second of every day. I had always been a high-energy person, but now coping with the constant pain was draining both my motivation and hopes for the future. On "good pain" days, my ability to enjoy many parts of my former life was lacking; on "bad pain" days, even my ability to concentrate enough to read or watch a movie had been taken away. The routine physical actions I had always taken for granted were now difficult. Whether it was getting dressed, driving a car, doing small chores around the house, or any of the hundreds of things we do in an average day, every activity now had a price. It was as if I had been given a small budget of energy to spend at the beginning of each day and it was up to me to determine how I wanted to spend it. There were no reserves. If I wanted to do something later in the day, I had to learn to expend a minimum of energy earlier in the day. As one who always had an overabundance of energy, I was not adjusting well to this new lifestyle. In fact, I absolutely detested it. I had been started on an opioid pain reliever which, like many pain patients, I had initially hoped would remove the pain. It was not long before I realized that the best this medication could do was to dial down the pain enough to function in some limited way. As I would somewhat naively ask my surgeon when my situation might improve, he would change the topic. It seems that the traditional medical community is fairly uninformed regarding dealing with people in chronic pain. As I eventually progressed through a more multidisciplinary approach, I came to see that this initial assessment was correct.

Both the pain and multiple cervical and thoracic vertebral surgeries had prevented my return to work. I had no disability insurance through the ministry; therefore, I was forced to apply for Social Security Disability. After a 5-month waiting period, I received my first payment. That was a very sad day for me. I felt shame, even though I knew I was fully eligible to join the ranks of the unemployed for very legitimate reasons. The acceptance of assistance from the Social Security system meant I had officially joined the ranks of the poor in this country. I dealt with this by assuring myself that I would figure out some way to financially support myself in the future. I realized I was more fortunate than many because I had only myself to support and my needs (other than medical) were relatively simple. However, that also meant I had no one else to assist me—either now or in the future. My savings had already been consumed by the cost of prescription medications and the household living expenses of a more than 3-year period of multiple surgical interventions which precluded employment. I could not imagine the strain and desperation that unemployment places on those chronic pain patients who have families to support. I was also fortunate in having a varied educational background. I could no longer physically return to the practice of veterinary medicine, but I could continue to work on my theology degree in preparation for a more sedentary career. I drew solace from my hopes for a future in some form of ministry. However, doubt of returning to gainful employment did remain in the back of my mind as I knew that each day had become a physical ordeal.

Becoming unemployed took so much more than just a financial toll on my life. I had been working since the age of 14. I derived fulfillment and self-esteem from my work—whether it was as an owner/veterinarian, college professor, or as a minister. I had never been granted the privilege of parenthood, and therefore my time, energy, and commitment had gone fully into my work. Even though my spiritual life told me that my identity was much more than what I accomplished each day, I could not transfer that knowledge to my emotional well-being. When my work was fully gone, I realized exactly how much of my identity was tied to my career roles. Now how was I to define myself? I had thought my best career years were ahead of me, but now there was the possibility that I may never be able to work again. My self-confidence and self-esteem plummeted. I felt useless and hopeless about prospects for my future. This sense of hopelessness began to erode my emotional well-being.

Another major loss that accompanied unemployment for me was my social life. I am an admitted workaholic. My social companions for the most part were my work companions. Even the best group of people will move on with their lives when a coworker/friend disappears from the scene for too long. People generally know how to respond to an acute crisis. They accept and respond to an acute injury or illness with love and care. This response carries with it the expectation that the person will get well and be able to return to normal activity. With my first two surgeries, I had much more assistance than I needed. My friends invaded my hospital room at all hours, until I could not even keep track of how many visitors I had had that day. When I was recuperating at home, my refrigerator was loaded with prepared meals and snacks. There was a steady stream of well-wishers who would help me pass the time and assist me with chores around the house and other assorted errands. Since I lived alone at the time, various friends offered to stay round-the-clock with me, as that was a medical necessity in the first few weeks following surgery.

As weeks turned into months and the only progress was toward the next surgery date, the response of friends and coworkers became very different. With each further surgery and recovery, there were fewer and fewer visitors. My world became very small. I will always be grateful for the one or two friends who remained by my side through these times, but I was embittered for quite a while by the response of the majority. I had fallen off of their radar screen. The visits and telephone calls stopped. I would receive the occasional card telling me that they were thinking of me or some other nonsense that I no longer felt was true. Therefore, as with many chronic pain patients, as my physical and emotional needs grew larger, my social support network grew smaller. Even after I had passed through the acute recovery phases from each surgery and was again able to drive and enjoy outings, I noticed that something had changed in my relationship with my friends. When one is viewed as a chronic patient by others, the assumptions attached to that role are very difficult to overcome. It is a battle to establish oneself as the responsible and equal adult one was before the ordeal began. People's minds become fixated on uninformed stereotypes of what they conceive a permanent patient's role in life to be. This is expressed to the chronic pain sufferer as a lack of respect or regard in making social decisions. The end result is a form of social ostracism, even if the activity or outing would be well within the person's physical tolerance. I began to feel very alone and isolated, which added greatly to my suffering.

To summarize my situation in life the day I walked into the pain management physician's waiting room: I was in a lot of pain, unemployed, discouraged, isolated, hopeless, tense, and spiritually dry. I thought that this appointment was my last resort for regaining any semblance of normalcy in my life. My expectations were low, but I had nowhere else to go. I had been through surgeries, epidural injections, rhizotomies, and endless rounds of physical therapies of various types. I did not know what else could possibly be done to help me, but I had nothing at all to lose in following my surgeon's recommendation. Therefore, here I was in the middle of a "normal" workday in a waiting room full of physically broken people. I was sure that each of them had a story to tell. Some of the stories would be far more grim than my own story, and some would be better. That did not matter. We were all traveling with that same unwelcome and uninvited companion—chronic pain.

PAIN MANAGEMENT AT LAST

All of these thoughts were swirling through my mind as I entered the consulting room of the physician. As we spoke and the doctor actually *listened* intently to my journey through the past few years, I could feel a small hope beginning to return. Having a health-care professional spend the time to listen fully to a patient's concerns had been a rarity for me up to this time. I had always felt rushed as I knew they were busy, and as they very quickly focused in on their subspecialty.

I remembered reading that the average time a patient speaks to a doctor before the doctor begins to offer his or her opinion is 18 seconds. It had always seemed that I, as a person, was just along as transportation for whatever body part was the focus of the appointment that day. This appointment was going differently. The physician was asking about my coping strategies and how my life had changed. Only after this extended discussion did the physical examination begin. After the completion of this examination, I was asked to get dressed and wait in the physician's office. A series of recommendations were offered to me. First, she explained that it would be necessary to increase the opioid dosage so that I could function at a lower level of pain. Although I was reluctant, I knew that changes had to be made if I were ever to leave my living room. Second, she promised to work with me to find medical approaches that could be helpful in my situation. She told me *we* would work together to return some quality of life to me. There was great power in her use of the word "we." I wondered if the physician fully realized what this statement meant to me at that time. It felt like I had been abandoned by the surgeon on whom I had grown to rely and trust. Now I was being told that this doctor would actually stay with me and work with me. I could feel tears well up in my eyes at this simple statement and the sentiment it represented. Third, she recommended that I contact the chronic pain management clinic to whom she made regular referrals. I did not know much about this type of program; therefore she explained that it was a multidisciplinary approach to pain control techniques. She told me that she would continue to handle the medical aspects of my case but felt that I would also benefit at this point from learning other pain control techniques. I readily agreed to try this approach and the office staff assisted me in setting up my first consultation with the head of the program.

MY EXPERIENCE WITH A MULTIDISCIPLINARY CHRONIC PAIN MANAGEMENT PROGRAM

The pain management clinic to which I was referred was led by a licensed psychologist who had a long clinical history of working with chronic pain patients. He introduced me to the mission of the program, which was to assist people suffering from chronic pain to regain a better quality of life by learning various techniques to restore the body and mind. He explained that the first step was to complete a battery of tests to uncover any signs of hidden depression or anxiety and to begin to understand how my personality might both assist and hinder my recovery. The staff I would be working with included the psychologist, a vocational counselor, a registered nurse, a biofeedback therapist, and a variety of specialized physical therapists. There would be time for relaxation and meditation techniques, stretching exercises, aerobic conditioning, deep heat massage, aquatic exercises, individual physical therapy, group educational programs, individual cognitive therapy, biofeedback training, and vocational counseling. The program required much commitment on my part, as it began at eight o'clock in the morning and ended at four o'clock in the evening each day. I was expected to be in attendance every weekday regardless of what my pain level was in the morning. The psychologist reminded me that the treatment team could do more to help me with my pain at the clinic than I could do for myself at home at that point. The program varied in length depending on progress and need, but I could expect to be there for approximately 6 weeks.

I appreciated this approach, as I finally felt understood. I had long ago realized that my pain had affected every aspect of my life. I knew that I had found a pain management physician to help me with the medical aspects of chronic pain, but I also knew that would not be enough. I was depleted physically, emotionally, and spiritually from my battles with pain. I knew nothing about pain management clinics prior to that day; therefore my initial impression was that a program such as this one really focused on a multidisciplinary approach to restoring wholeness. I knew it would take such a holistic view to bring any healing into my life, since I was beginning to accept that pain would remain a lifelong companion. I was not expecting my pain to miraculously disappear; therefore, I knew I had to somehow and in some way "make friends" with it. I wanted to control the pain. I did not want to continue to let the pain control me. It seemed to me that this was the difference between pain and suffering. I may have needed to accept the first, but I did not need to live the remainder of my life with the second. I remember expressing these issues to the program's director during our first meeting. I also told him that I was strongly motivated to return to work in some useful capacity, but that I was so depleted that I would need assistance to sort out reasonable options. I needed restoration of my self-confidence and self-esteem. I was in my mid-forties and was tired of feeling like my life was essentially over as far as being able to contribute to society in any significant way.

The director scheduled me to begin the following week. There were eight other people who were currently enrolled in the same program. We came from a very wide range of backgrounds and vocational fields. We also varied greatly in the nature and duration of our chronic pain conditions. There were individuals present who had been assigned to the program by their employers, others who were recommended by their physicians, and others, like myself, who had tried all of the traditional medical approaches and who were now ready to determine whether a more varied approach would help. After spending several years in the very isolated environment of my living room, it felt very good to be around people again. It also felt very good to have some kind of a schedule again. Although I am an introvert who is not particularly fond of tight schedules, I discovered that one can definitely have way too much of a good thing. I had become accustomed to people telling me how much they envied the time I now had to read and do what I wanted. I challenge anyone who says such a thing to a chronic pain patient to spend a year or more in that pattern of living. I believe that they would no longer see it as enviable freedom, but rather as the kind of purgatory it really is.

Before the various physical therapy protocols were instituted, biometric measurements were taken and recorded. The primary goal was to strengthen the unaffected areas of the body so that the injured areas would not be taking as much of the strain. I was taught the difference between hurt and harm. For the chronic pain patient, many activities and motions will increase the pain that is experienced; however, these same activities and motions will not necessarily bring harm in the form of increased damage to the joints, muscles, or tissues. It is critical to develop an understanding of the difference. Not only will knowing the difference protect against further injury, but this kind of knowledge will also remove much of the fear that restricts maximizing motion. With reduced fear comes more and more tolerance of the motion, thus increasing strength and mobility, which serves to reduce the amount of pain that is experienced. It was amazing to me to see how simple things like proper breathing and proper posture could decrease my pain levels. As I worked throughout the day, the staff would provide constant reminders regarding breathing and posture in an effort to make them habitual behaviors.

The staff would also provide constant reminders regarding exhibited pain behaviors. "Pain behaviors" are those facial expressions or body motions that let the world know that you are hurting. They may be grimaces or groans upon arising from a chair or a few limping steps while leaving a room. These types of body cues serve no useful function. They *seem* natural, but they are also unproductive. Many chronic pain patients turn early pain behaviors into habits. Perhaps they began as attempts to receive secondary gains like sympathy from family and friends, or perhaps they are familial patterns of handling pain. Regardless, they will eventually become irritating and frustrating to other people who are around the chronic pain sufferer and will serve to perpetuate a permanent state of "patienthood." It was very interesting to notice the variation in pain behaviors exhibited by different members of the group. There were times that the reminders would be almost comical, as group members became aware of the absurdity of exhibiting pain behaviors in front of others with chronic pain.

The most difficult aspect of the physical portion of the pain management program for a high-energy workaholic person like me was the constant reminder about pacing. The exercise program was designed to be interspersed with periods of stretching and rest. This seemingly simple concept was not readily translatable to my work style. Yet, it was a critical element for me to learn, as it would be a necessary component of performing tasks for the remainder of my life. My tendency had been to push myself for as long and hard as I could while trying to override any pain that I experienced until it was too late and I could no longer regain control over the pain. I knew I was going to have trouble with pacing when I finished the aerobic and strengthening exercises in 30 minutes rather than the designated 3 hours. It took me weeks to really see any improvement in this area, and it remained a significant source of frustration for me (and the staff).

Relaxation and meditation techniques were taught every morning and practiced throughout the day. Positive imagery training and progressive relaxation created greater awareness of my physical self. Prior to this pain management program, my main pain control technique was distraction. I would try to keep my mind intellectually engaged to override the pain signals. This would work for a while, but it was not a technique I could access when I was fatigued. In our Western medical system, there is such an intense Cartesian mind–body dualism. I would often picture riding my body as if I were riding a horse. It was as if my mind and body were only remotely connected as I practiced a kind of mind-over-matter style of coping with pain. This kind of extreme disconnect of mind from body would only lead to extreme bouts of pain when fatigue set in. This would often happen as I began to relax in the first stages of sleep. My sleep pattern was then disrupted to the point that I could neither fall asleep nor stay asleep. The relaxation, meditation, and biofeedback training gave me back the awareness that I was lacking. Instead of overriding pain signals, I learned to interpret them. I began to feel the tension I held in my shoulders, neck, and upper back. Initially, this was not a pleasant experience. I became even more aware of the constant muscle spasms that resulted from damage to spinal nerve roots. The biofeedback training helped me learn to begin to relax the muscles and break the repetitive loop of tension to spasm to resultant pain.

A major aspect of this pain management program was the individual cognitive therapy offered by the director of the program. Our therapeutic alliance developed quickly and we worked well together. I came into the program struggling with a moderate situational depression. I was particularly dispirited by my loss of employment and all of the areas of my life attached to that loss. It was going to take much reversal of negative thinking if I was going to be able to regain my former levels of self-confidence and self-esteem. Although not an expert by any means, I was not unaware of cognitive techniques due to my vocational and educational background as a pastoral counselor. I was concerned that my knowledge of the techniques would impede my progress. The skill of the psychologist quickly dispelled this concern. I met with him two or three times each week during the program. It was so therapeutic to be able to express all that I had held within myself for the past 3–4 years. I could speak about my disappointment, anger, and frustration with what I felt was my ruined life. I could also analyze the successes I was having in the program and how they were rebuilding the foundation of my future. I began to realize how much chronic pain and its many consequences had affected my outlook on everything in my life. I did not want to give in to the pain or allow it to have that kind of control over me. My former modes of coping were no longer working for me. We spent much time talking about new ways of coping and reframing the power that pain had in my life. These techniques helped me gain a sense of control over my life again. I no longer felt like an empty boat being tossed about by the waves. I was acquiring tools to help steer the boat through what I knew would remain turbulent waters.

Much of our time together was also spent discussing my concerns about vocational possibilities. The physical therapists could measure my progress with strength and conditioning, but the structural and mechanical problems of extensive spinal fusions limited my abilities to perform any tasks that involved lifting or stretching with my upper body. I had permanent sensory nerve damage in my hands that would worsen as the day progressed. Even though I had made the choice to leave veterinary medicine and enter into ministry as a career, I always knew that I could return to my first career if necessary, or use it to supplement a possibly less-than-lucrative ministerial position. I did not want to accept that this path was closed to me. The ability to speak about these concerns with someone who was experienced and skilled in dealing with people who struggle with chronic pain was life transforming. I do not believe that any psychologist without the expertise required in effectively counseling chronic pain or chronic illness patients should engage in this type of therapy. I fear the harm that could come from uninformed or underinformed training and experience. By the time a chronic pain patient has accepted the fact that his or her life has changed to the point of requiring the specialized assistance offered by a multidisciplinary pain management program, he or she has already battled with the traditional health-care system. Many physicians who may not understand or appreciate chronic pain and its ramifications have probably already seen the patient. It is common that a referral is made to see a mental-health therapist. The patient is sent to someone in his or her geographic vicinity who probably has little or no expertise in dealing with chronic pain. Instead of effective therapy, patients are at risk of receiving more platitudes that are merely couched in sophisticated psychological terminology. Or, even worse, there are intimations of malingering or somatic exaggeration. The effect on the patient may be the antithesis of what the professional (and the patient) desires. The patient may grow more despondent and discouraged. He or she may even begin to sense that no one believes them. The pain experience is an admittedly subjective experience. Only the patient really knows what is being experienced, but any chronic pain condition is negatively compounded by attitudes of doubt or disbelief. It takes a trained professional to make any kind of accurate diagnostic assessment. Without this, a cycle of treatment for depression begins without sorting out the underlying causes that are brought about by dealing ineffectively with chronic pain. It takes a professional who recognizes and understands the underlying causes to stop this cycle. Unfortunately, I have had the experience of meeting and speaking with too many chronic pain patients who were caught up in the traditional mental-health system rather than being referred to a multidisciplinary pain management program.

When I reached the point in the pain management program at which I was more able to consider possible vocational options, I began meeting with the treatment team's vocational counselor. As a certified rehabilitation counselor, this therapist could answer many of my questions regarding employment. I was assessed for a return to work on a limited part-time basis. I was quite anxious about this plan, as I knew I would require a position that included health benefits. After spending some time discussing this with the vocational counselor, I hit an emotional low point in my journey through the program. I felt defeated by the Social Security and American health care systems. Even with my varied professional and educational background, it seemed that my options were actually quite limited. There is a very low ceiling for earned income while remaining eligible for health-care benefits from the Social Security Administration. Accordingly, it seemed that in order to afford individual health care insurance, I would need to ignore medical clearance for limited part-time work. The vocational counselor assisted me in attempting to find a part-time position that offered group health insurance, but without much success. My only option for part-time employment that would produce sufficient income to purchase individual health care was a return to veterinary practice. Because of my medical limitations, no one was in agreement with this option, including me. I decided to keep working with the vocational counselor through the end of the program to see if other possibilities would arise, but I spent quite a few nights sleepless with anxiety regarding financial and health-care security for my future.

It was amazing how quickly this increased emotional stress impacted my pain levels. With stress and fatigue, muscles tighten and spasms become more widespread and more intense. I no longer needed convincing about the mind–body connection, but I experienced this added reinforcement. There is also an increased energy drain when functioning with stress and fatigue. Since chronic pain creates its own energy expenditures, I became tired more easily. I continued to force myself through the reconditioning aspect of the program, but it was not long until I also suffered a physical setback. I had strained some tight muscles while performing mild stretching in the therapeutic pool. This added pain took several weeks to overcome. I worked more diligently with relaxation and biofeedback to control my body's reaction to the emotional stress and added pain. I learned a difficult but valuable lesson for the future about allowing emotional stressors to dominate my thinking.

As multidimensional as this pain management program was, I believe that there was one vital aspect of self that was overlooked and should be an essential part of every pain management program. As opposed to traditional Western medicine, this program succeeded in removing the false dichotomy between the body and the mind. However, as a spiritual person, I believe that there is also a strong soul component to wholeness and health. Carl Jung believed that every question that is asked over the age of 40 is really a spiritual question. I would like to add to that and say that every question asked by someone struggling with chronic pain is really a spiritual question. Chronic pain attacks the core of what it means to be human. It is no respecter of education, social standing, or religious affiliation. Whether phrased in this particular way or not, every chronic pain patient will eventually be required to deal with his or her own existential abyss. Those who do not will never be able to reach the same level of healing as those who do. Pain is too strong of a reminder of our human frailty and mortality to be overlooked. It returns us to the primitive state of daily survival. It is not coincidental that suicidal ideation is high in the chronic pain population. What drives this ideation? I am sure it varies for each person. But, if one is forced to deal on a daily basis with his or her own built-in reminder of the suffering this life can bring, then he or she must develop a reason for choosing to remain in this life. This reason comes from neither the body nor the mind, but from the soul. It does not matter if someone has never stepped one foot into a church, cathedral, synagogue, or mosque. Every human being is endowed with some understanding of permanence or impermanence. Therefore, every human being must develop his or her own sense of spiritual reality. Even a denial of the spiritual realm is a belief system devised by that individual. Those professionals who have dedicated their lives to working with people who have chronic pain do not want to see their work fail because the patient chooses not to live. I believe that an essential team member to add to any interdisciplinary pain management program is a professional chaplain who, by training, has dealt with the kinds of existential questions about life's meaning and purpose that go along with the realization of our own limited humanity.

CONCLUSIONS

It has been almost 3 years since I began the multidisciplinary chronic pain management program. At this point, my experiences there occurred at about the halfway point on my journey with chronic pain. My life continues to change and evolve, but now my chronic pain is along for the ride and no longer doing the driving. I have reclaimed that right. That is not to say that I have been physically healed. In fact, due to ongoing spinal deterioration, I probably deal with more intense pain now than I did while in the program. But I came out of the pain management program with tools to cope with chronic pain that I never had before. The tools that I acquired and the resources that were made available to me have proven to be the foundations on which I have begun to rebuild my life in a positive way. I have expanded what it means to pace each day into what it means to pace my life. When I choose to expend energy on something, it is an item of priority. There is so much of what we do each day that is an unnecessary waste of energy. I continue to try to uncover those aspects of my life in an attempt to minimize or discard them so that I can focus on the path which I have chosen.

As my life has gotten busier, I must sometimes stop and remind myself about such basics as good breathing and good posture. I have tried to incorporate these techniques into my subconscious so that they are habitual, but I am not always successful. Under times of stress, I must focus on many of the meditative, biofeedback, and relaxation techniques that I began to learn during the program and to which I have added other techniques that I have learned along the way. My personality and familial influences are two of my biggest obstacles to proper self-care. I am much too goal and task driven. I often know what it is I should do to care for myself, but I still have the tendency to push myself first and relax later. When this begins to become a pattern, I pay a heavy price. I am still hopeful that I will someday have the wisdom to do those things I know to be correct.

Looking back, I realize that there was much that I learned during that period of time that was not necessarily an intentional aspect of learning about chronic pain management. For example, that 6-week period of time taught me how to be in relationships again. I still shudder when I remember how isolated I had become prior to that program. As the program required the necessary commitment of time and energy, I was forced to break out of the rut of staying at home and becoming more despondent about what my life had become. In doing so, I found some of the energy that I had lost during my surgical recoveries. I also discovered the self-confidence that I needed to take the next steps in my life so that I could once again contribute to helping others, which has always been so very important to me. With this change, my internal focus on my health became less important as my outward focus on others expanded. For me, this was a large component of becoming more whole again. I do admit that I choose my friends more carefully now than I did before I dealt with chronic pain. That is a matter of necessity, as I no longer have the energy level to foster a multitude of new relationships. Instead, I focus on those people and relationships that are most vital to me in a positive way. I am in a career in which I am around many people for many hours each day. The time I spend alone when my workweek is finished is chosen solitude, not forced loneliness.

Since my spiritual beliefs deny mere luck, I remain forever grateful for the opportunity that opened up to me when I was presented with the option of being a patient in that particular chronic pain management program at that particular time. I came into contact with several individuals who drastically altered, and possibly saved, my life. I hold the utmost respect, love, and admiration for these individuals including my pain management physician and the person who was the director of the pain management program during my time there as a patient. These two dedicated and loving people instilled the sense of hope, human caring, and courage that I so badly needed at that critical juncture in my journey.

How does a person who deals with daily chronic pain know when healing has begun? I can answer this question only for myself. It goes back to the difference between pain and suffering. These two terms, which are too often used synonymously, will, if properly defined, stand as markers to healing. If definitions are confined only to physical pain and suffering, pain is the physical reaction to an insult in the body that triggers the pain pathway in the nervous system, while suffering is an emotional reaction to how that pain is perceived. Therefore, one can have physical pain without suffering from that pain. This kind of healing will happen if some of the negative connotations are removed from the pain experience. This happens when one learns to have chronic pain without anticipation. In order for this to happen, a chronic pain sufferer must find a place between hope and fear—hope that the pain will disappear and fear that one will not have the strength to endure it. It is paradoxical that as long as a person with chronic pain holds on to hoping that his or her life becomes pain free, he or she will never be free. Freedom comes only from the inner peace that knows whatever comes next will be tolerated. Chronic pain does not need to be seen as a series of closed doors. Healing begins when it is seen as an entryway into a deeper and more meaningful way of living.

9 Multidisciplinary Treatment of Chronic Pain in Vulnerable Populations

Raymond C. Tait and Laura Miller
Saint Louis University School of Medicine, St. Louis, Missouri, U.S.A.

INTRODUCTION

This chapter focuses on the multidisciplinary treatment of chronic pain in vulnerable patient populations. Some might argue that a focus on vulnerable patient populations is redundant, as the *general* population of patients with chronic pain is vulnerable to inadequate treatment. Indeed, there is no doubt that chronic pain patients present with a complex array of medical and psychosocial problems that render them vulnerable as a class (1). Further, there is evidence of prejudicial attitudes held by health-care providers toward patients with persistent pain (2), attitudes that render this entire patient group vulnerable to symptom discounting and undertreatment, both of which are common among patients with chronic pain (3–6).

While all of the above is true, selected groups are even more vulnerable than the general population of patients in pain to undertreatment and to poor treatment outcomes. In fact, the literature clearly shows that racial/ethnic minorities constitute such a group: treatment disparities have been found for Hispanics (7), Blacks (8–10), and other minorities (11). Similarly, treatment disparities have been demonstrated for patients at both ends of the age continuum, children (12–14) and older adults (15,16). Within the latter group, minorities (8), those with neurocognitive deficits (17), and those approaching the end of life (8) have been shown to be particularly vulnerable to unsatisfactory treatment. Other patient groups also have been identified by federal regulations as vulnerable, including patients with psychiatric disorders and those who reside within prisons (18). Finally, although more debatable, persons who sustain occupational injuries leading to persistent pain constitute another vulnerable group, secondary to prejudicial attitudes often held about them (19). Thus, even though the general class of patients in pain faces the risk of undertreatment, the patient groups described above deserve special attention as a distinctly vulnerable class.

Although these groups are disparate in regard to the factors that render them vulnerable, they generally present with more complex medical and psychosocial problems than those typical of patients in pain. Because multidisciplinary pain programs were developed to treat the complexities that attend persistent pain (20), they would appear ideally suited to these vulnerable populations. Nonetheless, there is scant literature specific to the incremental benefits of multidisciplinary versus single-discipline approaches to treatment of vulnerable populations with chronic pain. While empirical comparisons may be lacking, there is a reasonable body of literature that provides a rationale for multidisciplinary treatment of vulnerable groups. This chapter will focus primarily on the rationales for such treatment. When possible, we will provide data that speak to the incremental value of multidisciplinary care. Before moving to these topics, however, we briefly consider a term that is central to the discussion, vulnerability.

Vulnerability

Dictionary definitions are of little value when considering the concept of "vulnerability" as it is used in this chapter. Those definitions (21) are derived from the Latin word for wound (vulnus): "being susceptible to physical or emotional injury." This definition applies poorly for several reasons: (1) the precept to "do no harm" is well-accepted and widely practiced among health-care providers; (2) the threat of litigation for malpractice serves as a general deterrent to practices that might occasion injury; and (3) at the federal and local levels, there is a push to reduce medical errors that might eventuate in injury (22).

Rather than focus on injury, this chapter uses the term "vulnerability" to refer more broadly to risks shared by a group of patients. Relative to other groups of patients with comparable health conditions, a vulnerable group is at a greater risk for experiencing poor treatment and/or poor outcomes from treatment. From an ethical perspective, vulnerability represents a violation of the principle of justice; inadequate care is rendered disproportionately to members of a vulnerable group.

Although vulnerability is a social construct that refers to patient groups that share a common feature, it would be simplistic to assume that the group is vulnerable simply because of that feature. Instead, a group's risk of poor treatment and/or outcomes is multidetermined, a function of a set of factors that, together, militate against the provision of adequate treatment and/or against a good response to treatment. Conceptually, these multiple determinants constitute the strongest argument for approaching vulnerable populations in a multidisciplinary manner.

A stress–diathesis model (19,23) offers a useful framework within which to view the various determinants of vulnerability. According to this model, adjustment to chronic pain is a function of two sets of forces. One set of forces reflects the stressor, an event (e.g., illness, injury, degenerative changes, etc.) that causes pain and challenges an individual's customary adaptation. The other set of forces reflects the resources that an individual can muster in coping with the stressor or, alternatively, a predisposition toward a poor adaptation. According to this formulation, adaptation to pain is related not only to the magnitude of the stressor (e.g., pain severity, pain extent) but also to the strengths and weaknesses of the individual confronting the stressor. Thus, a less-resilient person is more likely to experience major life disruptions in response to persistent pain than a more resilient person.

The stress–diathesis model has been applied to the risk of disability following occupational injury (19). As Figure 1 indicates, the latter risk depends on several sources of vulnerability. Many are associated with features of the person who is injured, including his or her level of education, beliefs/expectancies, premorbid emotional status, race, etc. Others, however, involve situational factors surrounding the injury, including job flexibility, financial hardship, and presence of litigation.

Of course, some of the factors that constitute vulnerability reflect a complex interplay of forces. For example, race is listed as a vulnerability in Figure 1 because of the literature that has described disparities in treatment. It is unclear whether the disparities are a function of characteristics of the person (e.g., distrust of the health-care system), the provider (e.g., inadequate treatment secondary to negative racial stereotypes), the situation (e.g., less access to care secondary to place of residence

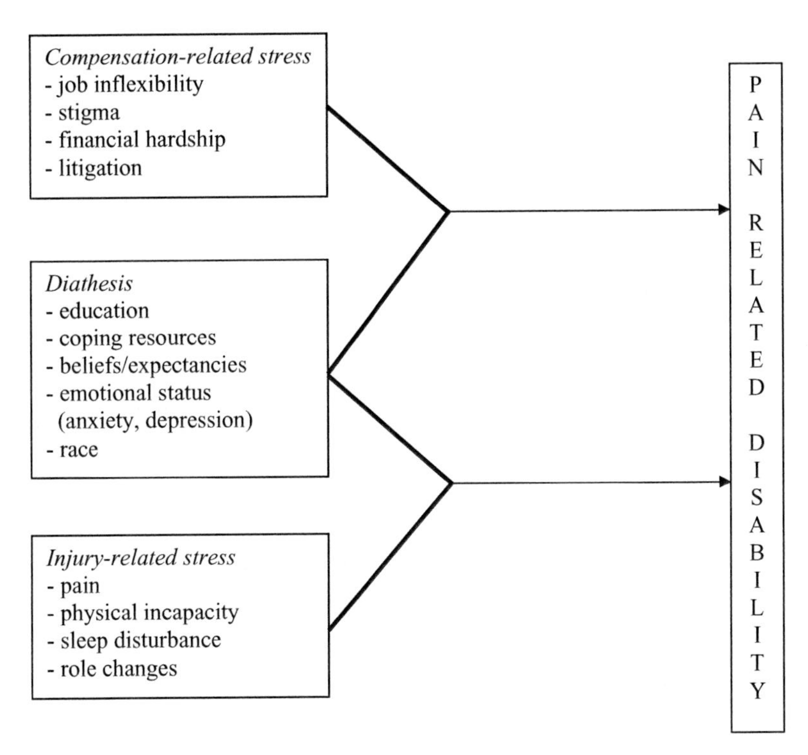

FIGURE 1 A stress-diathesis model for pain-related disability with compensable injury. (Reprinted with permission from Dworkin RH, Breitbart WS, eds. Psychosocial Aspects of Pain: A Handbook for Health Care Providers. Seattle, WA: IASP Press, 2004: 561.)

or insurance status), or a combination of all the above. Similarly, age (old or young) may represent a further set of vulnerabilities, as may psychiatric status or another comorbid health condition. In short, each of these vulnerabilities may represent an obstacle to successful adaptation to pain. Ideally, multidisciplinary treatment would address every obstacle in order to minimize roadblocks to successful outcomes.

RACIAL / ETHNIC MINORITIES

Sources of Vulnerability

As noted earlier, there is abundant evidence that racial/ethnic minorities are undertreated relative to nonminority patients (11). The evidence is particularly convincing for Blacks (9), although undertreatment has also been documented for Hispanics (7) and other minority groups (11). Similarly, there is evidence that minority patients may experience more pain-related disability than nonminorities (24–26). There is very little information on disparities in treatment outcomes, however, that is not confounded by such factors as differences in the level of treatment provided (24). In a study in which treatment was consistent across racial/ethnic groups, Gatchel and colleagues found that minority patients treated for pain following occupational injury were less successful in returning to the workforce than nonminority patients (27). The results, however, may have been confounded by other factors, such as differences in socioeconomic status (SES) and job opportunities that also differentiated the groups.

While the data presented above suggest possible differences in response to treatment associated with minority status, the research clearly does not justify such conclusions with any degree of confidence. Nonetheless, there are vulnerabilities linked with minority status that, if not addressed in treatment, may compromise adjustment to pain. For example, psychophysiologic research suggests that there may be differences in pain perception associated with minority status. Relative to Whites, Blacks appear to report more negative affective responses to pain when exposed to standard levels of noxious stimulation in laboratory studies (28). Similar patterns also have been described for patients seen in clinic settings for treatment of chronic pain. While the clinical and experimental differences between racial/ethnic groups have been small and the experimental evidence somewhat mixed (e.g., they appear to be affected by the nature of the experimental stimulus and, perhaps, by the race and gender of the experimenter), they certainly raise the possibility that Blacks react to pain somewhat differently than Whites.

Aside from differences in perception, Blacks may cope with pain differently than Whites. For example, prayer is a more common coping response to pain among Blacks (and Hispanics) than it is among Whites (29). Further, Blacks may favor passive (rather than active) coping strategies, a maladaptive approach to pain of a chronic nature (30). Similarly, Blacks appear to have lower expectations of treatment effectiveness, making them less likely to opt for surgical intervention (e.g., knee replacement), even when the data supporting the effectiveness of that treatment are sound (31).

Of course, some of the above results may be mediated by factors that operate at the patient–provider interface. Surveys indicate that both Blacks and Hispanics distrust the medical system more than Whites (32). They also may participate less actively in clinical decision-making than Whites (33). Clearly, each of these elements can militate against effective treatment of clinical conditions such as chronic pain, in which crucial aspects are largely subjective and require interactive communication for effective problem-solving (34).

Treatment Considerations

Of the above features that call for a multidisciplinary approach to treatment, probably the most important one involves the need to build trust and establish lines of communication between patients and providers. While crucial to successful treatment, establishing trust and communication are both time-consuming and costly, especially when they consume physician time. In multidisciplinary settings, others on the treatment team (at lower cost) can devote the time that is needed to build clear communication and to shape appropriate expectations for treatment (35). Multidisciplinary approaches to treatment have been shown to be particularly effective in shaping two important expectations (36): the expectation that patients must assume an active role in their care and the expectation that success in treatment will be measured not by pain cessation but by effective management and an increase in function. While all members of the treatment team must share the latter expectations, primary responsibility for cultivating these expectations commonly resides with nonphysician members of the team, including nurses, social workers, and psychologists (37).

Education is another time-consuming responsibility that often is borne by nonphysician members of a treatment team. The importance of education cannot be minimized, as it is often surprising to see how little patients know about a chronic condition such as pain. Indeed, patient education is one of the great casualties of the current health-care system's emphasis on productivity. Because Black patients often come from lower SES environments (38), they are particularly susceptible to knowledge deficits and/or dysfunctional beliefs regarding pain. Yet, the patient who understands mechanisms that underlie pain (and pain exacerbations) is often the most effective collaborator in treatment. Contrariwise, patients for whom pain is a mystery are more susceptible to a range of maladaptive responses that can undermine treatment effectiveness (39).

As noted above, Blacks may use more passive strategies to cope with pain than Whites. Because the evidence supports the adaptive value of more active coping responses to pain over the long term, there is reason to instruct minorities (indeed, all patients) in a range of more active techniques. Some techniques are psychological (e.g., self-hypnosis, problem-solving), and others are physical (e.g., stretching, conditioning). Psychologists and physical therapists often are best suited to provide such training. By the same token, patients who primarily rely on medication to cope with pain also can benefit from training; a recent study showed that, among patients in treatment for cancer pain, minorities demonstrated the greatest benefit (in terms of postintervention pain reduction relative to baseline) from tailored education and communication skills training (40). In the latter study, the training was provided by volunteers, rather than health-care professionals, suggesting the possible value of lay volunteers in multidisciplinary teams.

As noted earlier, Blacks and other minorities use prayer more often than Whites in their efforts to cope with pain. While many consider prayer to be a form of passive coping, that interpretation has been challenged by others who argue that prayer can be used to reinforce a host of approaches to coping with pain. Patients who rely strongly on prayer, therefore, may benefit from interactions that reinforce such coping; chaplains and other religious personnel may be another resource of potential benefit to teams that treat such patients. Such personnel may be of particular benefit for centers that treat patients approaching the end of life (41).

Of course, the vulnerabilities associated with race/ethnicity are not restricted to patient factors. A host of environmental factors are also likely to influence the success of pain management. For example, there may be inadequate access to pharmacies that stock opioid analgesics (42). Similarly, patients who face financial struggles may be unable to afford analgesic treatments necessary for them to maintain quality of life. For patients who face such problems in living, consultation with social services can be instrumental in acquiring access to needed services.

Finally, at the societal level, there is reason to believe that the stresses endemic to prejudice and racism exact a psychological toll on minorities that further complicates their efforts to cope with pain (38,43). When combined with the multiple stresses related to pain chronicity, the former stresses can undermine efforts at adaptive coping. Clearly, stresses related to racism call for intervention at the societal rather than provider level. Nonetheless, providers must be sensitive to the potential impact of racism on patient care. This sensitivity is likely to be enhanced when a treatment team is involved, some of whom are likely to be more sensitive than others to the poisonous effects of racism.

OLDER ADULTS

Sources of Vulnerability

Pain is widespread among older adults, both those who reside in the community and those who reside in assisted living facilities (44). Despite its prevalence, older adults are seldom referred to specialty pain clinics, even though a reasonable literature attests to the benefits that older adults can derive from multidisciplinary pain treatment (45). Not only is pain likely to be undertreated in the general population of older adults (46), but those with communication deficits (47) and those approaching the end of life (48) are especially vulnerable to undertreatment.

Ageism is possibly the single biggest obstacle to adequate pain care for the older adult in pain: "... a deep and profound prejudice against the elderly which ... allows the younger generations to see older people as different from themselves" (49). This attitude fosters beliefs that militate against effective pain control, including the belief that symptoms such as pain are to be tolerated when they occur among older adults, largely because such symptoms are seen as a natural consequence of aging. While there is considerable evidence to the contrary (50), such beliefs remain widespread. Not only are these beliefs widespread among younger adults, but they are often shared by older adults, including those who experience symptoms of pain. Older adults who entertain these beliefs may underreport symptoms, rather than seeking treatment, greatly complicating the provision of satisfactory care (51).

An interaction with an older adult candidate for a research study exemplifies the latter issue. To identify potentially appropriate study participants, we reviewed the medical records of recent admissions to a subacute care facility for injuries likely to cause pain and then interviewed patients to determine whether they reported pain (one of the inclusion criteria for study participation). A 90-year-old patient with widespread arthritis had suffered contusions but no fractures in a recent fall. The fall, however, had sufficiently compromised her ability to function independently that she was admitted to the subacute care facility. When questioned about the presence of pain, she denied any, rating it as a 0 on a 0–100 Likert-type scale, although she freely acknowledged "stiffness," rating it as "100" on a 0–100 scale. In light of the latter rating, she was asked to reconsider her rating of pain, but she adamantly refused to do so. While her refusal to acknowledge pain excluded her from the study, fortunately it did not preclude the administration of analgesics to facilitate her recovery of function.

Aside from ageism and underreporting, there are other elements that put older adults at risk for inadequate treatment, several of which reflect medical complications that can attend aging. For example, older adults are more likely than younger adults to experience a range of comorbid health conditions. In combination with chronic pain, the presence of multiple health problems greatly increases the risk of pain-related disability, potentially compromising the mobility required for independent living.

Of course, older adults are also likely to require multiple medications. The use of multiple medications increases the likelihood of drug–drug interactions. While this is less problematic for opioid medications (that have relatively few interactions), it is more so for the adjunctive medications often required for the treatment of intractable pain conditions. For example, neuropathic pain is common in older adults (52). While this can be effectively managed with a range of anticonvulsants and/or antidepressants, frequent side effects and/or drug–drug interactions include drowsiness and ataxia, secondary to their pharmacokinetics among older adults (53). Such complications can hinder effective treatment in this patient population, especially among providers without special expertise in the management of such complications.

As noted earlier, among older adults in pain, several subgroups are at particular risk for inadequate treatment. One such group involves those with cognitive deficits, often associated with dementing conditions or cardiovascular accidents. While not so problematic for older adults with mild-to-moderate deficits [who have been shown to have the capacity for accurate self-report (54)], those with more profound cognitive deficits lose the capacity for meaningful self-report, the primary channel for assessing pain intensity. Without meaningful assessment of pain intensity, it is difficult to initiate treatment and, subsequently, to evaluate the effectiveness of treatment. While a variety of observational strategies have been proposed to evaluate pain sequelae (e.g., agitation, passivity), their implementation is challenging, even for a multidisciplinary team (55).

The other group of older adults at great risk for inadequate treatment involves those near the end of life. The Study to Understand Prognoses and Preferences of Outcomes and Risks of Treatment (SUPPORT) clearly identified unsatisfactory levels of pain control for these patients, and it also demonstrated that education of health-care providers was not sufficient to significantly improve the quality of care (4). In the face of this and other evidence that raised concerns regarding the quality of symptom control afforded to those in their last days of life, the Institute of Medicine (IOM) called for the implementation of palliative care measures even as curative measures were still ongoing (56). Despite the clear need for improved pain control in this patient group, palliative care remains problematic at the end of life.

Treatment Considerations

While ageist attitudes and age-related misconceptions about pain cannot be tackled directly through multidisciplinary approaches to care, such approaches are more likely to mitigate the harmful effects of ageism than are single discipline approaches. Of course, there are other attributes of multidisciplinary teams that also are likely to influence treatment positively: (1) their capacity to perform comprehensive assessments of medical, social, functional, and psychological elements of adaptation to pain; (2) the presence of specialized expertise in pain management and, possibly, geriatrics; and (3) multidisciplinary input into treatment decisions (57).

Multidisciplinary approaches to treatment are of particular value when patients have failed standard medical therapies and demonstrate multiple comorbidities that contribute to dysfunction. As noted earlier, pain-related disability in such patients can jeopardize their capacity for independent living. Because return of function is a critical goal of care for this patient group, input from physical and occupational therapists obviously is critical. Given the comorbidities that are likely to complicate rehabilitation, medical oversight also is crucial. Not only can physicians be helpful in deciding the safe limits within which functional restoration should operate, but their medication management can also greatly facilitate functional recovery (58).

The role of nurses, psychologists, and social workers is also critical in the care of these patients. Many of the patients described above also grapple with depression; indeed, both activity restriction and repeated exacerbations of pain can occasion major depressive episodes (59,60). Not only can counseling be of value in treating mood disorders, but nurses, psychologists, and social workers also can serve as coaches in the rehabilitation process.

There are reasonable data that support the value of multidisciplinary approaches to the treatment of pain in older adults. Some of these data are derived from specialized programs developed explicitly to treat older adults (61). For the most part, however, the data are derived from more general programs. Those data indicate that older adults do benefit from such treatment, although the measurable benefit may be less than that demonstrated by younger adults (62).

As mentioned earlier, older adults with moderate-to-severe cognitive deficits pose particular challenges to pain assessment and treatment. Unfortunately, multidisciplinary treatment, while a necessary condition to effective care, is no panacea for these difficult cases. Effective care hinges on careful observations of behavior, typically undertaken by nursing staff or aides, which reflect a sudden increase in agitation or a sudden decrease in activity, each of which can be occasioned by the onset of pain. While abrupt changes in behavior are sometimes obvious, more often the changes are insidious. Effective protocols for identifying patients who fall into the latter category are elusive. At present, the best approaches utilize a mix of professionals: (1) psychologists who identify/develop observational protocols, usually in conjunction with nursing; (2) nursing staff and nurse aides who implement the observational system; and (3) physicians who prescribe analgesics as indicated (63). Indeed, some promising approaches have melded these approaches, building an observational protocol around an analgesic intervention to ascertain whether the analgesic impacted behavior or not (55,64).

A final area in which the benefits of multidisciplinary care are clear occurs at the end of life, as exemplified by the hospice setting. Hospice teams often have representation from many disciplines: medical oncology and/or palliative medicine, nursing, social work, psychology, the chaplaincy, etc. (65). As noted earlier, the effectiveness of this approach to maintain comfort for dying patients is well-established (56). Nonetheless, hospice continues to be an underused service for dying patients, many of whom are not referred for hospice until shortly before their death (66). The reasons for resistance to hospice are many and are well-described in the IOM report; they must be overcome if this approach to care is to be used to an appropriate extent for these vulnerable patients.

CHILDREN

Sources of Vulnerability

While children are at the other end of the age continuum, they also are vulnerable to inadequate pain care. For years, inadequate care was provided to neonates because of a widely held belief that their nervous systems were not sufficiently developed to experience pain (67). While that belief has been debunked, children remain vulnerable to undertreatment.

While reasons for this vulnerability are multiple, a primary factor underlying their risk for undertreatment relates to their dependence upon others for care. Hence, their pain control hinges to a great degree on the assessment and attitudes of those upon whom they depend. Research has shown that parents tend to underestimate children's pain (68), pointing to a fundamental problem in pain assessment, especially in the context of home-based care. Similarly, research has shown that parental attitudes toward analgesics can impede adequate pain control, such that children are often undermedicated, even after a surgical procedure (69). Of course, dependency is not restricted to children's interactions with their parents. Children are also dependent on health-care providers. There, too, evidence suggests that health-care providers underestimate pain in children, such that pain also is poorly controlled after operative procedures in hospital settings (70).

Another issue that can complicate pain assessment in children involves the instruments used in the process. Secondary to a variety of developmental issues, children differ greatly in their capacity to report pain, even with validated measures (71). Hence, a variety of measures have been developed for children, ranging from standard self-report scales to behavioral measures to physiologic measures. Aside from the specifics of a measure, children's pain reports can be colored by the nature of the interaction with an examiner—unless children are made comfortable, they may not provide useful information (72).

Lack of pharmacologic research that explicitly targets children also contributes to inadequate treatment. Until recently, children were treated pharmacologically as though they were simply "little adults." Of course, evidence now shows substantial differences between adults and children in both pharmacodynamics and pharmacokinetics (72). Similarly, research has shown minors to be more vulnerable to serious adverse events associated with drugs in common use [e.g., increased risk of suicidality in response to the use of selected antidepressants (73)]. For these and other reasons, the Food and Drug Administration (FDA) now requires studies that specifically target minors before a compound can be labeled for use in that population.

While the need for such targeted research is clear, that requirement can also complicate treatment. For example, fentanyl patches were developed as a long-term, intradermal analgesic delivery system for severe chronic pain. Unfortunately, the dosages that were approved for adult use are poorly tolerated by children. Until research had documented the safety, tolerability, and effectiveness of lower dosages (74), children were deprived of the benefits of an analgesic with clear benefits when used in patients requiring long-term analgesia for pain.

Finally, children lack pain-related coping skills (75). Indeed, for most children, the experience of pain is frightening, especially when pain is persistent or recurrent. While pain-related coping skills can be taught, even to young children, the training often is left to parents who have little expertise in the area and, in fact, who may reinforce maladaptive responses to pain (76).

Treatment Considerations

Most common childhood pain conditions can be treated in a straightforward manner with the use of medication, physical therapy, etc. There are several classes of childhood pain, recurrent and/or chronic, however, that can require more intensive care: headache, abdominal pain, rheumatic disease, sickle cell disease, and pain secondary to catastrophic illness (e.g., cancer). For these conditions, specialty expertise in pediatric pain management is needed.

The management of medication in children, crucial in the successful treatment of all of the severe pain conditions described above, is increasingly recognized as a specialty area of importance in pain medicine (77,78). Relative to adults, analgesic pharmacology differs among infants and children for all of the major classes of analgesics, including nonsteroidal inflammatory agents, acetaminophen, adjuvant medications, and opioids. In addition, children can be candidates for other medical interventions, including neural blockade, conscious sedation, and other anesthesiologic procedures (79,80).

Of course, nursing also is central to the treatment of serious pediatric pain conditions. In many facilities, nursing is considered the backbone of pain treatment, as nurses perform extensive clinical evaluations and provide input to physicians and other health-care providers (81). Further, nurses are often involved in educational interventions for children, parents, and staff (82). Indeed, some facilities rely even more heavily on nursing for pediatric pain management: nurses not only play crucial consultative roles but also direct pediatric pain management teams (83).

Psychological counseling and coping skills training is another area of recognized value in treating pediatric pain. Psychological approaches, including relaxation training, hypnosis, and other cognitive-behavioral techniques, have been found useful in helping children to cope with repeated painful procedures (e.g., bone marrow aspirations) (84,85) and to manage chronic conditions (e.g., headache) (86). Interesting applications of cognitive-behavioral strategies also have been proposed for sickle cell disease, regarding which it has been suggested that early training in such techniques can reduce the frequency of crises (87) and the frequency of hospital admissions (88). Further, psychological counseling can be of great value to both children and families of children facing death from disease progression (89).

Finally, rehabilitative approaches to pain can be critical to the successful treatment of a number of pain conditions, including headache (90) and various rheumatologic conditions (91). Even when physical therapy is not directly curative of painful symptoms, its promotion of exercise can be generally beneficial in children who may become activity avoidant in the presence of unremitting pain (92).

Of course, children with catastrophic illnesses such as cancer need all of the above services. These children present numerous complexities: (1) most are chronically ill; (2) their clinical course is often erratic, with a poor long-term prognosis; (3) therapy is generally aggressive and associated with debilitating side effects; (4) there is a frequent need for repeated painful procedures; and (5) both the illness and its treatment produce severe disruptions to daily life. For patients undergoing major surgery or who have sustained major fractures (and who are likely to be in pediatric intensive care units), pain control challenges may be different, but difficult, nonetheless. These challenges are even greater when children are unable to communicate about their pain, not an uncommon occurrence in pediatric intensive care settings (93).

While the importance of pediatric pain expertise has been recognized in hospital settings, recognition of the effectiveness of multidisciplinary teams has been slower to come. There is, however, a growing literature that speaks to the effectiveness of multidisciplinary care (75). Although most studies are small (94), the results consistently support the value of rehabilitative and psychological interventions when combined with medical therapies (91). Nonetheless, there are still relatively few comprehensive clinics that specialize in the treatment of pediatric pain (75).

In those institutions in which multidisciplinary pediatric pain services are available, they can assume various forms. One form, described above, is strictly consultative, utilizing pain resource nurses who function as mentors for their colleagues involved in front-line treatment of pediatric patients (82,83). Another consultative model involves a larger team with representatives from medicine, nursing, and pharmacy (79). A still larger consultative model also has been described, comprised of several physicians, nurses, psychologists, pharmacists, and physical therapists (78). While the latter model is clearly more comprehensive, it is noteworthy that financial challenges affect the provision of such a range of services—in the latter case, multiple departments subsidized the service.

Of course, the most comprehensive form of a pediatric pain service involves the freestanding model that provides inpatient and outpatient services across a range of disciplines. As of this writing, there are only about a dozen such clinics in the country (75). As noted previously, the availability of such services is limited less by clinical need than by financial considerations.

PATIENTS WITH PSYCHIATRIC DISORDERS (WITH SPECIAL ATTENTION TO SUBSTANCE ABUSE)

Sources of Vulnerability

There is a high incidence of psychiatric disorders in the chronic pain population. It is estimated that over 75% of pain patients meet the criteria for a lifetime history of a DSM disorder, particularly depression, anxiety, and substance abuse; nearly 60% of patients meet criteria with current symptoms (95). Because of psychiatric comorbidities that complicate treatment, these patients can be "doomed to fail" if their physical symptoms are treated without attention to psychological factors (96). There are several reasons for a high failure rate: (1) both anxiety and depression can decrease pain tolerance, (2) both anxiety and depression are associated with an increased intensity of medical problems, (3) both anxiety and depression can complicate the assessment of pain symptoms and vice versa, and (4) both anxiety and depression can interfere with the high levels of patient self-management often required for successful treatment (97). Accordingly, it is well-accepted that attention to psychiatric disorders is a requisite for effective pain treatment (98).

There is less of a consensus regarding the management of substance abuse in patients with chronic pain. Indeed, a history of substance abuse, affecting an estimated 6–15% of people in the United States, is often associated with undertreatment of pain (99,100). Physician attitudes, patient behaviors (e.g., pseudoaddiction), and legal concerns contribute to undertreatment. "Opiophobia," the widely held fear among physicians of using opioids to manage pain, is particularly problematic when treating patients who have a history of substance abuse (101,102).

Of course, negative attitudes toward opioids can also assume more subtle forms in patients without histories of substance abuse. For example, physicians may overestimate the side effects associated with opioid treatment of chronic pain (e.g., respiratory depression) (103). Similarly, physicians may prescribe inadequate analgesic doses and/or fail to provide analgesics to cover breakthrough pain, especially if their pain control goals are not aggressive, as is often the case with cancer pain (5). This pattern of undertreatment is not only a problem for the "standard" patient with chronic pain, but it also increases the risk of relapse among patients with a history of substance abuse (104).

Patients with psuedoaddiction, an iatrogenic syndrome in which patients with inadequately treated pain exhibit behavioral symptoms that mimic psychological addiction (105), are often mistaken for those with bona fide substance abuse disorders. Typically, pseudoaddicted patients will start by asking for more medication. When that request is spurned, they exhibit pain behaviors that escalate in frequency and intensity, a response that usually elicits more physician concerns about addiction. Unless pain is properly treated, this escalating cycle of patient–provider mistrust can only end in mutually unsatisfactory outcomes.

Much of the misinformation regarding analgesic use and abuse can be traced to inadequate medical school training. Surveys show that little time is dedicated to teaching about either pain treatment or substance abuse, nor has this time increased in the past 3 years (106). Aside from inadequate training, another risk factor for inadequate analgesic treatment involves the community in which a physician practices. Physicians practicing in communities of 100,000 people or less are more likely than their counterparts in larger communities to fear iatrogenic addiction and are less willing to prescribe opioid treatment (103).

The fear of legal repercussions further heightens physician concerns about prescribing opioids (100). Indeed, state statutes regarding prescribing practices are often vague and/or inconsistent (107) such that they provide little direction or solace to the physician who prescribes opioids. While legislative progress has clarified statutory language in a number of states, considerable work remains if the statutes are to allow physicians to prescribe appropriate analgesics without fears of legal repercussions.

Of course, patient factors also contribute to undertreatment. Patients with a history of substance abuse (including many patients with pain secondary to HIV) may resist opioids out of fear of becoming readdicted (108). Similarly, patients may be reluctant to take opioids due to fears that the medicines will be ineffective later in the course of their illness, fear that they will lose custody of their children, and fear that the opioids will harm their immune system. Finally, as noted previously, some patients may not have access to controlled medicines in their neighborhood pharmacies (42).

Treatment Considerations

Multidisciplinary care is indicated in patients with complex treatment needs, such as those with psychiatric and/or substance abuse disorders (95,98). While there is no agreement about the optimal composition of a multidisciplinary team to care for chronic pain patients with psychiatric comorbidities, most agree that treatment should include a mental-health professional (108). While psychiatrists are experienced in working with patients with psychiatric disorders, including those with substance abuse, relatively few have received specialty training in pain management (109). Hence, specialty trained psychologists or other mental-health professionals are often incorporated into multidisciplinary teams (110,111).

Pharmacy is another specialty of value in treating patients with psychiatric disorders that is often represented on multidisciplinary pain management teams. A pharmacist can serve several useful functions: (1) consulting with physicians regarding the management of analgesic medications; (2) consulting with physicians regarding the use of psychotropic medications, including psychotropic medications with analgesic qualities; and (3) overseeing general pharmacotherapy to minimize the occurrence of adverse side effects and/or drug–drug interactions (110). Aside from these roles within the pain management team, pharmacists are ideally suited to patient education regarding medication management.

Clearly, the management of opioids in patients with histories of substance abuse requires more than pharmacy participation. Many pain services use opioid contracts with patients that are expected to receive long-term opioids (112). While the effectiveness of such contracts is not established, there is agreement as to their purposes: (1) to specify the terms and consequences for breaching the contract, (2) to clarify patient and physician responsibilities, (3) to stipulate the consensual (rather than obligatory) nature of the doctor–patient relationship, and (4) to outline conditions wherein the terms of the contract may be renegotiated. Of course, multidisciplinary pain services can expand on the standard contract. In one innovative approach, a committee, comprised of the director of the medical practice, two attending physicians, a nurse, and two resident physicians, was developed to handle substance misuse and to evaluate suspected misuse. Patients that committed serious substance misuse were referred for counseling, and candidacy for opioid treatment was reevaluated by the committee after 6 months. Thus, treatment was not permanently terminated, and patients could rejoin the treatment program if they could bring their substance abuse under control (110).

Several studies have supported the efficacy of multidisciplinary care for chronic pain patients with psychiatric disorders, including both past and current substance abuse. A study that followed up on multidisciplinary treatment showed that patients with comorbid depression, a history of substance abuse, and other psychiatric disorders demonstrated decreased pain and depression as well as an improved quality of life (110). A 10-week multidisciplinary treatment for addiction and pain management also supported benefits of multidisciplinary treatment, including decreased pain, decreased emotional distress, decreased reliance on pain medications, increased self-control, and improved coping skills (113). In one of the few comparative studies, a randomized controlled trial found that patients with a history of substance abuse had better responses to an integrated model of treatment than an independent treatment for addiction treatment and medical care (111). The latter study also demonstrated that the integrated treatment model was cost-effective.

OTHER VULNERABLE POPULATIONS

Prisoners

Nowhere is the lack of attention to the treatment needs of a vulnerable group more glaring than in the case of pain in prisons. Prisoners are more likely to experience pain and other health problems than like-aged adults in the general population, secondary to higher rates of physical injury, poor general health, high rates of substance use, etc. (114,115). Despite the relatively high prevalence of pain in prisons, the general treatment of pain in prisoners has received little formal study.

Indeed, the only systematic attention to pain treatment that these authors could find involved pain among the terminally ill prisoners. That population has been growing in recent years, secondary to the increased length of prison terms meted out to those convicted of criminal offenses, resulting in increased numbers of older inmates (116). While 55,000 state and federal prisoners were over 50 years of age in 1995, that number was estimated to have increased to at least 125,000 by 2000 (117). Moreover, the trend suggests that the latter figure will continue to grow.

The treatment of pain in terminally ill prisoners has proved problematic for a number of reasons. First, the opioid analgesics required to treat such pain successfully are tightly controlled, a requirement that poses logistical difficulties for prisoners who continue to reside within the general prison populace. Second, physicians who are charged with managing pain in prisoners describe concerns about misuse/diversion and question the credibility of prisoner self-reports (118). Third, the option of moving the terminally ill patient from the general populace to a specialty setting, while preferable from a purely health-care perspective, is problematic because the prisoners view being moved as tantamount to a death sentence (119). Further, such a move reduces their access to the support systems that they have developed in the prisons over time.

In light of the above complications, it is not surprising that different prison systems have evolved different approaches to the management of this prisoner group. Some approaches have left the prisoners in the general populace until their final days, while others have created hospice settings (called designated death units) in which to house them (117,119). While the solutions differ substantially, most involve some form of multidisciplinary care, typically including nurses, physicians, psychologists, psychiatrists, social workers, clergy, and security officials. A number of programs involve prisoners who provide hospice-type support, attending to the patient's medical and emotional needs, advocating for changes in care, and attending case conferences in which treatment options are discussed (116). This approach is thought to have multiple benefits, both to the dying prisoner who remains capable of accessing support from fellow prison mates with whom he or she may have developed a friendship, and to the prisoner-provider, who is given responsibilities and the latitude to discharge those responsibilities despite the otherwise-restrictive environment in which he or she lives.

While it is gratifying to see innovative approaches being taken to the care of this patient group, it is troublesome to see that pain management remains inadequate for these inmates (118). Even more troublesome, however, is the lack of attention to chronic pain conditions to such a degree that it is difficult to determine the incidence and prevalence of this condition in prisons. While the lack of information is diagnostic of this group's vulnerability, it also makes it difficult to assess the extent of the problem in this population.

Workers' Compensation

Some would argue against the inclusion of workers' compensation (WC) claimants in a listing of vulnerable populations. Unlike other vulnerable groups, they have access to care (WC insurance coverage is mandated by state and federal governments). Indeed, the argument has been made that WC patients are over- rather than undertreated.

On the other hand, WC claimants can stake a claim to their own share of negative stereotypes that impugn the validity of their symptoms, reflected in such terms as malingerer, compensation neurosis, greenback poultice, and others (19). Further, the rate of success for the treatment for WC claimants is lower than that of comparable patients whose pain did not originate in a work-related accident, such that the dynamics of the system have been cited as causing iatrogenic disability (120,121). Finally, within the WC system, there is evidence that vulnerable patient groups (e.g., Blacks) are subject to disparities in care at least equal to those found in other sectors of health care (10).

The point of this brief discussion is to argue that WC claimants represent a vulnerable class of patients because of *ineffective* treatment that largely ignores the unique vulnerabilities that characterize them. In making this argument, the principal focus will be on neither those workers who are injured but do not report their injuries (122) nor those workers who make the expected recovery from their injuries, but rather on the 5–10% of workers who fail to recover function and who account for an inordinate proportion of WC costs (123).

At present, the latter group receives largely the same care as that provided to patients who demonstrate good outcomes, although most nonresponders can be identified as such by 3 months postinjury (124). While this approach may be defensible, it fails to consider the multiple patient, provider, and system stresses outlined in Figure 1 that may be obstacles to good outcomes. Treatment approaches that address those obstacles are likely to yield superior outcomes to standard care. Indeed, a review of the literature indicates this to be so: multidisciplinary programs that integrate functional restoration, medical management, psychoeducational services, and vocational counseling have yielded good outcomes, despite their focus on workers who have failed multiple prior treatments, often including surgery (125). Moreover, these outcomes have been replicated across states with different WC administrative structures, as well as across countries (126–128). Nonetheless, with rare exceptions, patients for whom such programs may be appropriate are delayed or redirected to other, less successful approaches (123), a pattern that supports classification of WC patients as another vulnerable group.

CLOSING COMMENTS

This chapter has reviewed a variety of patient groups that are vulnerable to inadequate treatment. As noted earlier, these groups are drawn from the general population of patients with chronic pain, all of which are vulnerable to undertreatment. The groups reviewed in this chapter are distinguished by the complex, albeit different, factors that render each particularly vulnerable. While this review has been telegraphic (each group deserves its own chapter), we hope that it has shown that an array of factors can contribute to vulnerability.

Given the complex clinical and social problems presented by these vulnerable patient groups, a good case can be made that each would benefit from multidisciplinary treatment, as this approach was developed to address the complexities posed by patients with chronic pain. While the rationale for such treatment may be strong, there is a disappointing level of empirical research available that speaks to the effectiveness of multidisciplinary approaches of these groups. Especially lacking is research that examines the relative (i.e., incremental) effectiveness of multidisciplinary versus single-discipline or standard-care approaches to chronic pain in vulnerable populations.

There are several reasons why the multidisciplinary research cupboard is bare in relation to these patients. First, our attention to vulnerable populations is relatively recent, and therefore relatively little time has passed during which to accrue data relevant to their treatment. Second, attention was drawn to these groups because of profound disparities in the delivery of health-care services that they received. Those services reflect current standards of care, and standards of care are slow to change. Finally, these developments have occurred within an environment where insurance reimbursement for multidisciplinary pain treatment has eroded, occasioning a reduction in the number of multidisciplinary treatment programs available to patients in pain (129,130). Clearly, these trends have not been conducive to the conduct of the type of empirical research that is needed to evaluate the relative efficacy of multidisciplinary approaches to the care of vulnerable patients.

While none of the latter trends are propitious, awareness of disparities in the delivery of health-care services to minorities and other vulnerable populations is increasing (11). To some degree, that awareness has been accompanied by increased federal funding for research that might reduce disparities in treatment. Thus, there is potential support for studies that could test the effectiveness of multidisciplinary treatment programs in reducing disparate outcomes. Should such evidence support the value of multidisciplinary approaches to the treatment of vulnerable populations (as we would expect), it could have implications for all patients with chronic pain (a rising tide lifts all boats).

Of course, programmatic research such as that described above comes slowly and at a cost so that it offers no short-term solution. Indeed, there are no guarantees of federal funding for such projects. Thus, it is important that pain practitioners, especially those involved in the delivery of multidisciplinary pain treatment, pay particular attention to vulnerable populations while designing their treatments and conducting their own outcome evaluations. Not only is this approach the ethical thing to do, such work can only serve to strengthen the argument that multidisciplinary treatment deserves far greater levels of support than it has received.

REFERENCES

1. Merskey H, Teasell RW. The disparagement of pain: social influences on medical thinking. Pain Res Manage 2000; 5:259–270.
2. Taylor AG, Skelton JA, Butcher J. Duration of pain condition and physical pathology as determinants of nurses' assessments of patients in pain. Nurs Res 1984; 33:4–8.
3. Chibnall JT, Tait RC, Ross LR. The effects of medical evidence and pain intensity on medical student judgments of chronic pain patients. J Behav Med 2000; 38:529–538.
4. Desbiens NA, Wu AW, Broste SK, et al. Pain and satisfaction with pain control in seriously ill hospitalized adults: findings from the SUPPORT research investigations. Crit Care Med 1996; 24:1953–1961.
5. Green CR, Wheeler JRC. Physician variability in the management of acute postoperative and cancer pain: a quantitative analysis of the Michigan Experience. Pain Med 2003; 4:8–20.
6. Grossman SA, Sheidler VR, Swedeen K, et al. Correlation of patient and caregiver ratings of cancer pain. J Pain Symp Manage 1991; 6:53–57.
7. Todd KH, Samaroo N, Hoffman JR. Ethnicity as a risk factor for inadequate emergency department analgesia. JAMA 1993; 269:1537–1539.
8. Bernabei R, Gambassi G, Lapane K, et al. Management of pain in elderly patients with cancer. SAGE Study Group. JAMA 1998; 279:1877–1882.
9. Green CR, Anderson KO, Baker TA, et al. The unequal burden of pain: confronting racial and ethnic disparities in pain. Pain Med 2003; 4:277–294.
10. Tait RC, Chibnall JT, Andresen EM, et al. Management of occupational back injuries: differences among African Americans and Caucasians. Pain 2004; 112:389–396.
11. Institute of Medicine of the National Academies of Science. Unequal treatment: confronting racial and ethnic disparities in health care. Washington, DC: National Academies Press; 2002.
12. Rush SL, Harr J. Evidence-based pediatric nursing: does it have to hurt? AACN Clin Issues 2001; 12:597–605.
13. Schechter NL, Berde CB, Yaster M. Pain in infants, children, and adolescents: an overview. In: NL Schechter, CB Berde, M Yaster, eds. Pain in Infants, Children and Adolescents. Philadelphia, PA: Lippincott Williams & Wilkins; 2003:3–18.
14. Vincent CVH. Nurses' knowledge, attitudes, and practice regarding children's pain. Am J Matern Child Nurs 2005; 30:177–183.

15. Herr K. Pain assessment in the older adult with verbal communication skills. In: SJ Gibson, DK Weiner, eds. Pain in Older Persons. Seattle, WA: IASP Press; 2005:111–133.
16. Tait RC, Chibnall JT. Pain in older subacute care patients: associations with clinical status and treatment. Pain Med 2002; 3:231–239.
17. Sengstaken EA, King SA. The problems of pain and its detection among geriatric nursing home residents. J Am Geriatr Soc 1993; 41:541–544.
18. National Commission for the Protection of Human Subjects of Biomedical and Behavioral Research. The Belmont Report: Ethical Principles and Guidelines for the Protection of Human Subjects of Research. Washington, DC: DHEW Publication No. (OS) 78–0012; 1978.
19. Tait RC. Compensation claims for chronic pain: effects on evaluation and treatment. In: Dworkin RH, Breitbart WS, eds. Psychosocial Aspects of Pain: A Handbook for Health Care Providers. Seattle, WA: IASP Press; 2004:547–569.
20. Loeser JD. Multidisciplinary pain programs. In: Loeser JD, Butler SH, Chapman CR, et al., eds. Bonica's Management of Pain, 3rd edn. Philadelphia, PA: Lippincott Williams & Wilkins; 2001:255–266.
21. Picket JP, et al., eds. The American Heritage Dictionary of the English Language, 4th edn. Boston, MA: Houghton Mifflin Company; 2000.
22. Agency for Healthcare Research and Quality. AHRQ's Patient Safety Initiative: Building Foundations, Reducing Risk. Interim Report to the Senate Committee on Appropriations. Rockville, MD: AHRQ Publication No. 04-RG005; 2003.
23. Dworkin RH, Banks SM. A vulnerability-diathesis-stress model of chronic pain: herpes zoster and the development of postherpetic neuralgia. In: Gatchel RJ, Turk DC, eds. Psychosocial Factors in Pain: Critical Perspectives. New York: Guilford Press; 1999:247–269.
24. Chibnall JT, Tait RC, Andresen EM, et al. Race and socioeconomic differences in post-settlement outcomes for African American and Caucasian Workers' Compensation claimants with low back injuries. Pain 2005; 114:462–472.
25. McCracken LM, Matthews AK, Tang TS, et al. A comparison of Blacks and Whites seeking treatment for chronic pain. Clin J Pain 2001; 14:249–255.
26. Riley JL, III, Wade JB, Myers CD, et al. Racial/ethnic differences in the experience of chronic pain. Pain 2002; 100:291–298.
27. Gatchel RJ, Polatin PB, Mayer TG. The dominant role of psychosocial risk factors in the development of chronic low back pain disability. Spine 1995; 20:2402–2709.
28. Edwards RR, Doleys DM, Fillingim RB, et al. Ethnic differences in pain tolerance: clinical implications in a chronic pain population. Psychosom Med 2001; 63:316–323.
29. Edwards RR, Moric M, Husfeldt B, et al. Ethnic similarities and differences in the chronic pain experience: a comparison of African American, Hispanic, and White patients. Pain Med 2005; 6:88–98.
30. Jordan MS, Lumley MA, Leisen JCCC. The relationships of cognitive coping and pain control beliefs to pain and adjustment among African-American and Caucasian women with rheumatoid arthritis. Arthrit Care Res 1998; 11:80–88.
31. Ibrahim SA, Siominoff LA, Burant CJ, et al. Differences in expectations of outcome mediate African American/White patient differences in "willingness" to consider joint replacement. Arthrit Rheum 2002; 46:2429–2435.
32. LaVeist TA, Nickerson KJ, Bowie JV. Attitudes about racism, medical mistrust, and satisfaction with care among African American and White cardiac patients. Med Care Res Rev 2000; 57(Suppl 1):146–161.
33. Cooper-Patrick L, Gallo JJ, Gonzales JJ, et al. Race, gender and partnership in the patient-physician relationship. JAMA 1999; 282:583–589.
34. Frantsve LME, Kerns RD. Patient-provider interactions in the management of chronic pain: current findings within the context of shared medical decision making. Pain Med 2007; 8:25–35.
35. Tait RC, Chibnall JT. Racial and ethnic disparities in the evaluation and treatment of pain: psychological perspectives. Prof Psychol Res Pract 2005; 36:595–601.

36. Shutty MS, DeGood DE, Tuttle DH. Chronic pain patients' beliefs about their pain and treatment outcomes. Arch Phys Med Rehabil 1990; 71:128–132.
37. Brown KS, Folen RA. Psychologists as leaders of multidisciplinary chronic pain management teams: a model for health care delivery. Prof Psychol Res Pract 2005; 36:587–594.
38. Schulz A, Williams D, Israel B, et al. Unfair treatment, neighborhood effects, and mental health in the Detroit metropolitan area. J Health Sco Behav 2000; 41:314–332.
39. Williams DA, Keefe FJ. Pain beliefs and the use of cognitive-behavioral coping strategies. Pain 1991; 46:185–190.
40. Kalauokalani D, Franks P, Oliver JW, et al. Can patient coaching reduce racial/ethnic disparities in cancer pain control? Secondary analysis of a randomized controlled trial. Pain Med 2007; 8:17–24.
41. Davidson PM, Paull G, Introna K, et al. Integrated, collaborative palliative care in heart failure. J Cardiovasc Nurs 2004; 19:68–75.
42. Morrison RS, Wallenstein S, Natale DK, et al. "We don't carry that"—Failure of pharmacies in predominantly nonwhite neighborhoods to stock opioid analgesics. New Engl J Med 2000; 342:1023–1026.
43. Clark R, Anderson NB, Clark VR, et al. Racism as a stressor for African Americans. A biopsychosocial model. Am Psychol 1999; 54:853–866.
44. Brochet B, Michel P, Barberger-Gateau P, et al. Population-based study of pain in elderly people: a descriptive survey. Age Ageing 1998; 27:279–284.
45. Gibson SJ, Farrell MJ, Katz B, et al. Multidisciplinary management of chronic nonmalignant pain in older adults. In: Ferrell BR, Ferrell BA eds. Pain in the Elderly. Seattle, WA: IASP Press; 1996:91–99.
46. Pitkala KH, Strandberg TE, Tilvis RS. Management of nonmalignant pain in home-dwelling older people: a population-based survey. J Am Geriatr Soc 2002; 50:1861–1865.
47. Mantyselka P, Hartikainen S, Louhivuori-Laako K, et al. Effects of dementia on perceived daily pain in home-dwelling elderly people: a population-based study. Age Ageing 2004; 33:496–499.
48. Hall S, Gallagher R, Gracely E, et al. The terminal cancer patient: effects of age, gender, and primary site on opioid dose. Pain Med 2003; 4:125–134.
49. Butler RN. Age-ism: another form of bigotry. Gerontol 1969; 9:243–246.
50. Baltes M, Carstensen L. The process of successful aging. Ageing Soc 1996; 16:397–422.
51. Herr K, Garand L. Assessment and measurement of pain in older adults. Clinics Geriatr Med 2001; 17:457–478.
52. Backonja M- M. Painful neuropathies. In: Loeser JD, Butler SH, Chapman CR, et al., eds. Bonica's Management of Pain, 3rd edn. New York: Lippincott Williams & Wilkins; 2001:371–387.
53. Virani A, Mailis A, Shapiro LE, et al. Drug interactions in human neuropathic pain pharmacotherapy. Pain 1997; 73:3–13.
54. Chibnall JT, Tait RC. Pain assessment in cognitively impaired and unimpaired older adults: a comparison of four scales. Pain 2001; 92:173–186.
55. Chibnall JT, Tait RC, Harmon B, et al. Effect of acetaminophen on behavior, well-being, and psychotropic medication use in nursing home residents with moderate-to-severe dementia. J Am Geriatr Soc 2005; 53:1921–1929.
56. Foley KM, Gelband H, eds. Improving palliative care for cancer: summary and recommendations. Institute of Medicine and Commission on Life Sciences National Research Council. Washington, DC: National Academy Press; 2001.
57. Katz B, Scherer S, Gibson SJ. Multidisciplinary pain management clinics for older adults. In: Gibson SJ, Weiner DK, eds. Pain in Older Persons. Seattle, WA: IASP Press; 2005:309–326.
58. Hanlon JT, Guay DRP, Ives TJ. Oral analgesics: efficacy, mechanism of action, pharmacokinetics, adverse effects, drug interactions, and practical recommendations for use in older adults. In: Gibson SJ, Weiner DK, eds. Pain in Older Persons. Seattle, WA: IASP Press; 2005:205–222.

59. Erdal KJ, Zautra AJ. Psychological impact of illness downturns: a comparison of new and chronic conditions. Psychol Aging 1995; 10:570–577.
60. Williamson GM, Schulz R. Activity restriction mediates the association between pain and depressed affect: a study of younger and older adult cancer patients. Psychol Aging 1995; 10:369–378.
61. Helme RD, Katz B, Neufeld M, et al., The establishment of a geriatric pain clinic—a preliminary report of the first 100 patients. Aust J Ageing 1989; 8:27–30.
62. Gagliese L, Katz J, Melzack R. Pain in the elderly. In: Wall PD, Melzack R, eds. Textbook of Pain, 4th edn. London: Churchill Livingstone; 1999:991–1006.
63. Kovach CR, Weissman DE, Griffie J, et al. Assessment and treatment of discomfort for people with late-stage dementia. J Pain Symptom Manage 1999; 18:412–419.
64. Manfredi PL, Breuer B, Wallenstein S, et al. Opioid treatment for agitation in patients with advanced dementia. Int J Geriatr Psychiatry 2003; 18:700–705.
65. King LA, Arnold R. Cancer pain and end-of-life issues. In: Gibson SJ, Weiner DK, eds. Pain in Older Persons. Seattle, WA: IASP Press; 2005:403–420.
66. Field M, Cassel C, eds. Approaching death, improving care at the end of life. Committee on Care at the End of Life. Institute of Medicine. Washington, DC: National Academy Press; 1997.
67. McGrath PJ, Unruh AM. Pain in Children and Adolescents. New York: Elsevier Science Publishers; 1987.
68. Chambers CT, Reid GJ, Craig KD, et al. Agreement between child and parent reports of pain. Clin J Pain 1998; 14:336–342.
69. Finley GA, McGrath PJ, Forward SP, et al. Parents' management of children's pain following 'minor' surgery. Pain 1996; 64:83–87.
70. Gauthier JC, Finley GA, McGrath PJ. Children's self-report of postoperative pain intensity and treatment threshold: determining the adequacy of medication. Clin J Pain 1998; 14:116–120.
71. McGrath PA, Gillespie J. Pain assessment in children and adolescents. In: Turk DC, Melzack R, eds. Handbook of Pain Assessment, 2nd edn. New York: The Guilford Press; 2001:97–118.
72. Ross DM, Ross SA. The importance of type of question, psychological climate and subject set in interviewing children about pain. Pain 1984; 19:71–79.
73. Food and Drug Administration. FDA public health advisory: suicidality in children and adolescents being treated with antidepressant medications. Available on www.fda.gov/cder/drug/antidepressants/SSRIPHA200410.htm.
74. Finkel JC, Finley A, Greco C, et al. Transdermal fentanyl in the management of children with chronic severe pain: results from an international study. Cancer 2005; 104:2847–2857.
75. Zeltzer LK, Schlank CB. Conquering Your Child's Chronic Pain: A Pediatrician's Guide for Reclaiming a Normal Childhood. New York: HarperCollins; 2005.
76. Reid GJ, McGrath PJ, Lang BA. Parent-child interactions among children with juvenile fibromyalgia, arthritis, and healthy controls. Pain 2005; 113:201–210.
77. Greco C, Berde C. Pain management for the hospitalized pediatric patient. Pediatr Clin N Am 2005; 52:995–1027.
78. Shapiro BS, Cohen DE, Covelman KW, et al. Experience of an interdisciplinary pediatric pain service. Pediatrics 1991; 88:1226–1232.
79. Alexander M, Richtsmeier AJ, Broome ME, et al. A multidisciplinary approach to pediatric pain: an empirical analysis. Child Health Care 1993; 22:81–91.
80. Reeves ST, Havidich JE, Tobin DP. Conscious sedation of children with propofol is anything but conscious. Pediatrics 2004; 114:74–76.
81. Gordon DB, Pellino TA, Enloe MG, et al. A nurse-run inpatient pain consultation service. Pain Manage Nurs 2000; 1:29–33.
82. Turner HN. Complex pain consultations in the pediatric intensive care unit. AACN Clin Issues 2005; 16:388–395.
83. McCleary L, Ellis JA, Rowley B. Evaluation of the pain resource nurse role: a resource for improving pediatric pain management. Pain Manage Nurs 2004; 5:29–36.

84. Jay S, Elliott CH, Fitzgibbons I, et al. A comparative study of cognitive behavior therapy versus general anesthesia for painful medical procedures in children. Pain 1995; 62:3–9.
85. Liossi C, Hatira P. Clinical hypnosis versus cognitive behavioral training for pain management with pediatric cancer patients undergoing bone marrow aspirations. Int J Clin Exper Hypnosis 1999; 47:104–116.
86. Engel JM. Relaxation training: a self-help approach for children with headaches. Am J Occupat Ther 1992; 46:591–596.
87. Gil K, Wilson J, Edens J. The stability of pain coping strategies in young children, adolescents, and adults with sickle cell disease over an 18-month period. Clin J Pain 1997; 13:110–115.
88. Dumaplan CA. Avoiding admission for afebrile pediatric sickle cell pain: pain management methods. J Pediatr Health Care 2006; 20:115–122.
89. Postovsky S, Ben Arush MW. Care of a child dying of cancer: the role of the palliative care team in pediatric oncology. Pediatr Hematol Oncol 2004; 21:67–76.
90. Jay GW, Brunson J, Branson SJ. The effectiveness of physical therapy in the treatment of chronic daily headaches. Headache 1989; 29:156–162.
91. Anthony KK, Schanberg LE. Pediatric pain syndromes and management of pain in children and adolescents with rheumatic disease. Pediatr Clin N Am 2005; 52:611–639.
92. Goldschneider KR, Mancuso TJ, Berde CB. Pain and its management in children. In: Loeser JD, Butler SH, Chapman CR, et al., eds. Bonica's Management of Pain, 3rd edn. New York: Lippincott Williams & Wilkins; 2001:797–812.
93. Breau LM, Camfield CS, McGrath PJ, et al. Risk factors for pain in children with severe cognitive impairments. Develop Med Child Neurol 2004; 46:364–371.
94. Bursch B, Walco GA, Zeltzer L. Clinical assessment and management of chronic pain and pain-associated disability syndrome. J Dev Behav Pediatr 1998; 19:45–53.
95. Gatchel RJ. Comorbidity of chronic pain and mental health disorders: the biopsychosocial perspective. American Psychologist 2004; 59:795–805.
96. Dersh J, Gatchel RJ, Polatin P, et al. Prevalence of psychiatric disorders in patients with chronic work-related musculoskeletal pain disability. J Occup Environ Med 2002; 44:459–468.
97. Glajchen M. Chronic pain: treatment barriers and strategies for clinical practice. J Am Board Fam Pract 2001; 14:211–218.
98. Sullivan MD, Turk DC. Psychiatric illness, depression, and psychogenic pain. In: JD Loeser, SH Butler, CR Chapman, et al., eds. Bonica's Management of Pain, 3rd edn. Philadelphia, PA: Lippincott Williams & Wilkins; 2001:483–500.
99. Kirsh KL, Passik SD. Palliative care of the terminally ill drug addict. Cancer Invest 2006; 24:425–431.
100. Prater CD, Zylstra RG, Miller KE. Successful pain management for the recovering addicted patient. Primary care companion. J Clin Psychiatry 2002; 4:125–131.
101. Breitbart W. Pain management and psychosocial issues in HIV and AIDS. CARING Magazine 1996; 15:26–35.
102. Kowal N. What is the issue? Pseudoaddiction or undertreatment of pain. Nurs Econ 1999; 17:348–349.
103. Weinstein SM, Laux LF, Thornby JI, et al. Physician's attitudes toward pain and the use of opioid analgesics: results of a survey from the Texas Cancer Pain Initiative. South Med J 2000; 93:479–487.
104. Weaver MF, Schnoll SH. Opioid treatment of chronic pain in patients with addiction. J Pain Palliat Care Pharmacother 2002; 16:5–26.
105. Weissman DE, Haddox JD. Opioid pseudoaddiction—an iatragenic syndrome. Pain 1989; 36:363–366.
106. Miller NS, Sheppard LM, Colenda CC, et al. Why physicians are unprepared to treat patients who have alcohol- and drug-related disorders. Acad Med 2001; 76:410–418.
107. Pain and Policy Studies Group. Achieving Balance in Federal and State Pain Policy: A Guide to Evaluation, 3rd edn. University of Wisconsin Paul P. Carbone Comprehensive Cancer Center, Madison, Wisconsin, 2006.

108. Kemp C. Managing chronic pain in patients with advanced disease and substance-related disorders. Home Healthc Nurs 1996; 14:255–261.
109. Leo RJ, Pristach CA, Streltzer J. Incorporating pain management training into the psychiatry residency curriculum. Acad Psychiatry 2002; 27:1–11.
110. Chelminski PR, Ives TJ, Felix KM, et al. A primary care, multi-disciplinary disease management program for opioid-treated patients with chronic non-cancer pain and a high burden of psychiatric comorbidity. BMC Health Serv Res 2005; 5:1–13.
111. Weisner C, Mertens J, Parthasarathy S, et al. Integrating Primary Medical Care with addiction treatment: A randomized controlled trial. JAMA 2001; 286:1715–1723.
112. Fishman SM, Kreis PG. The opioid contract. Clin J Pain 2002; 18:S70–S75.
113. Currie SR, Hodgins DC, Crabtree A, et al. Outcome from integrated pain management treatment for recovering substance abusers. J Pain 2003; 2:91–100.
114. Kjelsberg E, Hartvig P. Can morbidity be inferred from prescription drug use? Results from a nation-wide prison population study. Eur J Epidemiol 2005; 20:587–592.
115. Mara CM, McKenna C. "Aging in place" in prison: health and long-term care needs of older inmates. Pub Policy Aging Rep 2000; 10:1–8.
116. Yampolskaya S, Winston N. Hospice care in prison: general principles and outcomes. Am J Hospice Palliat Care 2003; 20:290–296.
117. Maull FW. Issues in prison hospice: toward a model for the delivery of hospice care in a correctional setting. Hospice J 1998; 13:57–82.
118. Lin JT, Mathew P. Cancer pain management in prisons: a survey of primary care practitioners and inmates. J Pain Sympt Manage 2005; 29:466–473.
119. Dubler NN. The collision of confinement and care: end-of-life care in prisons and jails. J Law Med Ethics 1998; 26:149–156.
120. Gallagher RM, Myers P. Referral delay in back pain patients on workers' compensation: costs and policy implications. Psychosomatics 1996; 37:270–284.
121. Hadler NM, Carey TS, Garrett J. The influence of indemnification by Workers' Compensation insurance on recovery from acute backache. North Carolina Back Pain Project. Spine 1995; 20:2710–2715.
122. Biddle J, Roberts K, Rosenman KD, et al. What percentage of workers with work-related illnesses receive workers' compensation benefits? J Occup Environ Med 1998; 40:325–331.
123. Frymoyer JW. Cost and control of industrial musculoskeletal injuries. In: Nordin M, Andersson GBJ, Pope MH, eds. Musculoskeletal disorders in the workplace: principles and practice. St. Louis, MO: Mosby-Year Book; 1997:62–71.
124. Frank JW, Brooker A-S, DeMaio SE, et al. Disability resulting from occupational low back pain. Part II: What do we know about secondary prevention? A review of the scientific evidence on prevention after disability begins. Spine 1996; 21:2918–2929.
125. Mayer T, McMahon MJ, Gatchel RF, et al. Socioeconomic outcomes of combined spine surgery and functional restoration in workers' compensation spinal disorders with matched controls. Spine 1998; 23:598–606.
126. Cutler RB, Fishbain DA, Rosomoff HL, et al. Does nonsurgical pain center treatment of chronic pain return patients to work? A review and meta-analysis of the literature. Spine 1994; 19:643–652.
127. Guzman J, Esmail R, Karjalainen K, et al. Multidisciplinary rehabilitation for chronic low back pain: a systematic review. BMJ 2001; 322:1511–1516.
128. Turk DC. Clinical effectiveness and cost-effectiveness of treatments for patients with chronic pain. Clin J Pain 2002; 18:355–365.
129. Schatman ME. The demise of multidisciplinary pain management clinics? Pract Pain Manage 2006; Jan/Feb:30–35.
130. Schatman ME. The demise of the multidisciplinary chronic pain management clinic: bioethical perspectives on providing optimal treatment when ethical principles collide. In: Schatman ME, ed. Ethical Issues in Chronic Pain Management. New York: Informa Healthcare; 2007:43–62.

10 Developing an Interdisciplinary Multidisciplinary Chronic Pain Management Program: Nuts and Bolts

Steven P. Stanos
Chronic Pain Care Center, Rehabilitation Institute of Chicago, and Department of Physical Medicine and Rehabilitation, Northwestern University Medical School, Feinberg School of Medicine, Chicago, Illinois, U.S.A.

The way a team plays as a whole determines its success. You may have the greatest bunch of individual stars in the world, but if they don't play together, the club won't be worth a dime.

Babe Ruth

MULTIDISCIPLINARY AND INTERDISCIPLINARY TREATMENT

Developing a multidisciplinary (MPC) and/or interdisciplinary (IPC) pain treatment program involves a thorough understanding of coordinating well-supported individual treatment approaches for chronic pain (physical and occupational therapy, pain psychology, relaxation training, therapeutic recreation, medical management, and vocational therapy) into an integrative program. In doing so, the program must have the flexibility to meet the needs of a heterogeneous patient population, third-party payers, and numerous stakeholders to a patient's chronic pain condition such as employers, case managers, insurance adjustors, referring physicians, and family members. Goals of treatment shift the focus to patients as active participants, helping to educate and empower them to take more active roles in treatment and enabling them to self-manage pain-related difficulties, pacing, limit setting, stress management, and problem solving. Less attention is paid to reducing pain versus improving overall function.

This chapter will discuss the "nuts and bolts" of the interdisciplinary pain program at the Rehabilitation Institute of Chicago's Chronic Pain Care Center (CPCC) as an example of an interdisciplinary functional restoration program. It is understood that this type of comprehensive treatment can be delivered in a number of ways. Variations in program structure are based on regional variability in practice scope, reimbursement patterns, referral practices, and the type of facility in which they are housed. The chapter will examine (1) general program content, (2) individual team member goals and responsibilities, (3) concepts important to successful team building and communication, (4) general financial aspects related to program survival, and (5) referral development, marketing, and networking in the community.

Introduction

The terms "multidisciplinary" and "interdisciplinary" approaches, although sometimes used interchangeably, represent two distinct models along a continuum of more collaborative approaches. Although interdisciplinary is an extension of a more general multidisciplinary approach, both the models use the biopsychosocial model to address the multifactorial causes of pain, pain-related suffering, and loss of function.

Multidisciplinary and interdisciplinary treatment models are part of a continuum of medical care which ranges from a unimodal model of patient care to a completely integrative one. These models include, in order of increasing comprehensiveness and philosophical complexities, parallel, collaborative, coordinated, multidisciplinary, interdisciplinary, and finally, integrative approaches (1). Parallel practice is commonly seen in acute medical conditions such as acute cardiac chest pain management. In an emergency-room cardiac unit, a number of physicians and ancillary staff provide care independently. Often, in the early management of work-related injuries, collaborative and coordinated models may include practitioners acting independently and sharing patient records, with facilitation by a case manager. Acute pain and musculoskeletal injuries may also be managed by a more simple collaborative or coordinated approach. Chronic pain, however, necessitates a more comprehensive and collaborative treatment model.

Interdisciplinary and Multidisciplinary Pain Treatment Programs

The history and evolution of multidisciplinary and interdisciplinary treatment programs is reviewed in chapter 1 in this volume. These programs evolved following the establishment of mainstream integration of cognitive and behavioral approaches to the field of pain management in the 1970s and 1980s. In this chapter, "multidisciplinary" treatment will refer to those programs that generally involve one or two specialists (e.g., a surgeon, pain interventionalist, and nurse) directing services of a number of team members, often having independent goals, with treatment components delivered at different facilities. "Interdisciplinary" pain programs provide outcome-focused, coordinated, and goal-oriented services usually delivered at one setting. The inter- and multidisciplinary models have been used effectively in a number of other medical specialties (e.g., internal medicine, palliative care, and rehabilitation medicine) to more effectively and efficiently treat complex conditions such as diabetes mellitus, asthma, poststroke, and spinal cord disorders. The "interdisciplinary" model is characterized by team members working together for a common goal, making collective therapeutic decisions, and having face-to-face meetings and patient team conferences to facilitate communication as a means of improving patient outcomes. Interdisciplinary teams are typically led by a physician, psychologist, or nurse.

Initial patient assessment in an IPC may include a coordinated pain medicine examination, pain psychology and physical therapy assessment, and, in the case of an injured worker, vocational rehabilitation. Patients may then be placed into a number of different treatment programs based on the initial team assessment. Programs may vary in intensities and content, usually involving 3–8 weeks of 4–8 hour per day treatment, with both individual (one-on one) and group therapies provided in an outpatient-based setting. A small number of hospital-based inpatient programs remain active and are often integrated with a substance abuse or detoxification program. A similar biopsychosocial treatment approach is used with work hardening and early intervention programs, although the focus on psychological issues and patient education may differ.

CHRONIC PAIN CARE CENTER TEAM

History of the CPCC

Program content has evolved over the center's 25-year history. Initially set up in an inpatient setting, patients received physical, occupational, nursing, and psychological services at the RIC flagship inpatient acute rehabilitation hospital. The inpatient setting exposed patients to other disabled patients, many of whom evidenced significantly more overt physical impairments and limits in function (acute post-stroke, spinal cord injury, and trauma). Some team members felt that this helped to encourage the pain patients to succeed and return to more normal function. Due to changes in reimbursement, the inpatient model was abandoned in the 1980s, and the program was converted into an outpatient day program with the addition of less-intense modified treatment programs. The CPCC moved to a non–hospital-based setting in a downtown Chicago high-rise in 2000. The approximately 5000 square foot facility is located adjacent to a private full service health club which includes free weights, exercise machines, a basketball court, pool, and group studio rooms. The center has an ongoing formal relationship with the gym, at which approximately 15 full memberships are maintained and available on a rotating basis to patients in our formal pain program. Most importantly, the use of a community-based exercise facility helps to encourage community reentry for patients and ongoing use of a gym for long-term management. Membership fees offset any additional clinical costs that would have to be paid to cover building expenses, rent, equipment, and additional staff needed to manage an exercise facility or gym. Physical and occupational therapists are encouraged to use the gym facility when necessary for individual and group treatments. The gym is an integral part of the formal program and is used for various group activities, including scheduled open gym time (in which patients use aerobic equipment, exercise machines, and strengthening machines), pool therapy, and relaxation classes held in more private gym studios. Group exercise sessions include dedicated gym time (strengthening and aerobic exercises under the supervision of a physical therapist) and Feldenkrais classes (a deep breathing and flexibility class) 2–3 days per week.

CPCC Staff

The clinic employs three full-time equivalent board certified physicians [physical medicine and rehabilitation (PM&R) and pain subspecialty], three full-time physical and occupational therapists, three full-time pain psychologists, two biofeedback/relaxation therapists, and part-time vocational and therapeutic recreation specialists. A dedicated business support manager and a clinic manager are responsible for coordinating scheduling of evaluations, obtaining insurance precertification, and managing program flow (scheduling, discharge, and organizing and communicating to case managers and referring physicians appropriate progress notes and team conference documents). The clinic manager [0.5 full-time equivalents (FTE) administrative, 0.5 FTE occupational therapy) is responsible for weekly scheduling for the formal pain program (4 weeks) and modified programs (once, weekly, and biweekly programs). Daily and weekly modification and rearranging of schedules is necessary due to the ever-changing total number of patients in the respective programs. Approximately 15–20% of patients are "discharged early" from the formal program due to poor compliance, tolerance, and limited progress. Approximately

9–10 new patients start in the formal program every other week. Group and individual treatments each constitute approximately 50% of the program.

Pain Program Evaluation

The CPCC clinic evaluates approximately 16–17 new patients per week. All patients undergo a physical medicine evaluation (1.5 hours), pain psychology assessment (1 hour), and, if a workers' compensation case, vocational assessment (1 hour) as part of the comprehensive evaluation. At the conclusion of the evaluation, recommendations are reviewed with the patient, and if possible, with the assigned or dedicated case manager of the workers' compensation patient. Yearly clinic volumes include approximately 4700 physician visits and 75,000 therapy units (physical and occupational therapy, psychology, relaxation training, therapeutic recreation). The CPCC has approximately 1200 active patients in the practice. Patients represent a wide range of payers (approximately 40% commercial, 25% Blue Cross/Blue Shield, 30% Medicare, and 10% Medicaid). Free funding is available for patients and potential program candidates meeting hospital financial need requirements.

Treatment Programs

Level of treatment is determined following completion of an interdisciplinary assessment, which includes physiatric evaluation, pain psychology evaluation, and with work-related cases, vocational assessment. Patients are placed in one of a number of treatment programs depending on physical and psychological impairment and level of disability. Treatment programs include, in order of increasing scope of treatment intensity, unimodal physical medicine management (i.e., medication management, interventional procedures, and physical therapy) to more interdisciplinary programs which include weekly, and biweekly interdisciplinary programs 5 hours per day (medical management, physical and occupational therapy, relaxation training, pain psychology, aerobic conditioning) and a 4-week, 8 hour per day "formal" treatment program (see figures with schedules for weekly and modified programs). The formal treatment program additionally incorporates recreational and vocational training. The interdisciplinary model involves ongoing communication between all members of the treatment team, helping to facilitate patient progress while they participate in the behavioral, cognitive, and active therapy treatments. Patients are discussed individually in a team-conference format on a weekly basis, enabling ongoing communication of progress and adjustment of treatment goals. Medical follow-ups with the physiatrist are provided weekly in the modified programs and two to three times per week in the formal program.

Each "group" is reviewed by the team on a weekly basis. Team conferences are scheduled, during which each patient is reviewed individually, typically for 10–15 minutes. When possible, case managers are present in order to observe the conference, monitor progress, and answer questions that staff may have regarding the involved patient. This also helps facilitate vocational recommendations and coordinate scheduling for functional capacity evaluations (FCEs), which are usually performed during the final week of the pain program or within 1 week from discharge, and clarify job status and restrictions.

Early in the program, there is a focus on restoring lost function related to leisure pursuits, which is the primary focus of group and individual therapeutic recreation counseling. Program focus later turns to vocational issues in which parallels between loss of function at home and the workplace are made, thus preventing the patient's development of the misconception that "return to work" (RTW) is in itself the only focus of the comprehensive rehabilitation program.

Comprehensive Treatment Programs

The CPCC also offers less-intense programs based on a similar biopsychosocial model of the full program and include

1. Monday and Wednesday half-day program (4 p.m.–7:30 p.m.)—4 weeks
2. Tuesday half day (12 noon to 5 p.m.)—6 weeks
3. Thursday half day (12 noon to 5 p.m.)— 6 weeks

These programs include 45-minute round-robin type schedules which include medical management, physical therapy, occupational therapy, relaxation training, nurse education, and Feldenkrais therapy.

More modified treatment programs have developed over the past 5 years as a means of meeting the demands of patients' schedules (i.e., working, care giving of family member responsibilities), insurance coverage, and level of program needs. These programs may also serve as a trial program for patients who are too impaired, whether due to poor sitting, standing, or walking tolerance, and/or questionable motivation, for more comprehensive treatment. Those patients demonstrating progress are then transferred to the formal 4-week program.

ASSESSMENT AND TREATMENT FOCUS

Chronic pain patients are typically subject to a number of failed interventions and therapies. As a result, the pain patient is often demoralized and turns from an active participant in his or her care to a more passive individual, often with great affective distress. This reaction serves only to perpetuate subjective disability and learned helplessness. Successful treatment of these individuals relies on an appreciation of the multiple psychosocial and physical issues that shape their presentation.

Medical Assessment

The physiatrist may serve as the team leader, assessing patients at the initial evaluation through a comprehensive musculoskeletal examination that includes assessment of compensatory postural and muscular imbalances that may perpetuate ongoing pain and dysfunction. The physiatrist must also assess and document observed pain behavior and level of affective distress, motivation, readiness, and expectancies for treatment, and discuss issues related to RTW and previous levels of functioning.

Factors Related to Disability and the "Sick Role"

In many cases, disability behaviors are thought to be perpetuated by financial, vocational, and psychological rewards related to not working or "being sick." This concept of "secondary gain" is often erroneously equated with malingering. In fact, it is more appropriate to relate secondary gain to a number of more complex psychosocial issues. The works of Gatchel, Fishbain, and Kwan (2–5) have described these important related and evolving concepts of "secondary gain and loss" and "tertiary gain and loss." In this regard, "losses" or "gains" associated with illness

TABLE 1 Common Secondary Gains and Losses Related to Chronic Disease

Gains	Losses
Gratification of preexisting and unresolved dependency/revengeful strivings	Economic
Attempt to illicit care or sympathy	Community/family/personal approval
Entitlement for years of struggling	Social stigma/guilt of disability
Ability to withdraw from responsibility or unsatisfactory life role	Quality of life
Adoption of sick and needy role	Respect
Drug availability and use	

and disability may impact both the patient and the patient's family or work colleagues (see Table 1 for examples).

Abandoning the Patient as a "Victim"

Although it is not expected that all patients will quickly grasp a rehabilitation approach, motivation for even considering changing maladaptive thoughts and beliefs must be assessed by the physician along with the evaluating psychologist and vocational counselor. Beardwood and colleagues (6) recently examined perceptions and experiences of injured workers in Ontario, Canada. Upon reviewing a number of structured interviews, important themes emerged (Table 2). Many believed that they were "victimized" by their experiences, rendering them powerless and dependent on others. Health professionals and "bureaucrats" in turn impeded their rehabilitation and quests for pain relief and a return to preinjury function. The impact of injury often includes financial, functional, social, and emotional domains. Although this may not be the case with every patient, understanding similar concepts and misconceptions is important for the rehabilitation team as a first step in helping chronic pain patients change maladaptive thoughts and behaviors, and facilitate a successful rehabilitation program.

The treating pain clinician must develop trust and rapport with the patient in order to understand barriers to recovery (i.e., contentious relationships involving family, employer, case manager, and the legal system) that may potentially lead to delay of clinical improvement and case resolution. Many times, the success of developing that relationship begins at the initial evaluation. Understandably, patients in MPC treatment are asked to make significant changes in the ways they cope with pain and function. Readiness to make such important changes has been found to be associated with treatment success (7,8) and readiness to self-manage pain increases from pre- to post-MPC treatment (9). Based on the transtheoretical model of behavior change, individuals are seen as progressing through a number of stages involving decisions about change and include precontemplation, *contemplation, action, maintenance* phases (10). These basic concepts are important for the physician to explore during the evaluation and often becomes a focus of discussion between the evaluating team (i.e., pain psychologist, physician, and vocational counselor) when deciding whether the patient is an appropriate candidate for interdisciplinary treatment. Unfortunately, like many psychosocial and operant issues, the patient's own "story" and representation of these issues may vary between the evaluating individuals.

TABLE 2 Understanding the Injured Worker

Pathways to becoming injured	Seeking treatment	Seeking return to adequate work	Living as an injured worker
Work, workplace, and degree of unsafe practices lead to injury	Desperate for a diagnosis, difficulty accessing appropriate and timely treatment	Returned to modified work yet disillusioned to find accommodations short-lived or nonexistent	Financial hardships, loss of marriages, change in family structure
Fear of unemployment, continued hazardous job	Negative attitudes by doctors and other health practitioners toward the injured worker	Lack of choice and control over vocational issues	Legal action with compensation system drained of financial resources, adding to distress
Lack of knowledge about reporting injuries	Medical uncertainty led to different diagnoses from different specialists; uncertainty led to more doctor shopping and inconsistent message regarding level of activity, restrictions	Workers believed employer-based actions on the need of company rather than the workers	Psychological deterioration; limitation in self-care activities led to feelings of dependency and social isolation

Source: From Ref. 6.

Patients not Determined to be Candidates for Interdisciplinary Treatment

As many patients may still be resistant to change or have other operant factors that seem to be acting as an overwhelming force that prevents them from abandoning the "sick role," expecting them to take a more active role in their treatment will only lead to additional treatment "failures." These same patients, if involved in a comprehensive program, will only limit the progress of other patients and add unnecessary burden to the treating team. Many of these patients suffer from serious characterological disturbances, and the inclusion of these patients in a multidisciplinary or interdisciplinary chronic pain management program can serve as a serious perturbation to the system (11). Although there is presently no psychometric instrument available to screen out this type of patient, close attention to potential yellow flags for treatment failure should not be ignored. Many times, formal treatment is not offered, and patients are told that overwhelming operant factors need to be addressed first (e.g., closing a personal injury or workers' compensation claim).

MAKING AN INTERDISCIPLINARY APPROACH WORK

Interdisciplinary treatment requires a comprehensive assessment of potential treatment targets. The following section reviews key disciplines in interdisciplinary chronic pain management. Unique to interdisciplinary treatment is a common set of treatment goals and commonalities of treatment that need to be assessed at evaluation to determine patient candidacy for treatment and during the program, as a means of conveying a unified message to patients.

Goals to Pain Management Success

Clear, focused, and manageable short- and long-term goals are the hallmark of successful outcomes for interdisciplinary chronic pain management programs. Unrealistic goals will only lead to patient disappointment. Short- and long-term goals are discussed at the initial evaluation and frequently during the formal program with the patient, family members, and clinicians (physician, pain psychologist, and vocational therapist), and include

- pain reduction
- increased activity and function
- resolution of disability claims, RTW
- reduction of reliance on opioid analgesia; more appropriate opioid use
- reduction of emotional distress; mastery of coping techniques
- decreased medical resource utilization

Commonalities of treatment across all disciplines include

- reconceptualization of the patient's pain
- fostering optimism; combating demoralization
- encouragement of proactive patient participation and responsibility
- focusing training for a specific effect
- encouragement of feelings of success, self-control, and self-efficacy

Medical Management

Medical management is focused on helping patients progress through their individualized treatment programs, supporting treatment goals across all disciplines (physical and occupational therapy, relaxation training, therapeutic recreation, and vocational counseling), providing feedback on progress, facilitating final RTW, and other discharge planning. Pharmacologic trials target improving mood, restoring sleep, and improving analgesia with a rational polypharmacy approach, often including decreasing or eliminating the use of opioid or other dependency-producing medications. The question of high-dose opioid use remains a dilemma in considering patient candidacy. Many times, referral for opioid detoxification or significant preprogram reduction in dose along with initiation of a rational polypharmacy approach by the physician may be necessary prior to initiating the formal pain program. Although this may require additional time, it may be the greatest means to ensuring better outcomes for the patient and other stakeholders involved. Otherwise, starting a patient in the program while concomitantly reducing opioids may be too much of a distraction to the functional restoration approach. It is imperative, when possible, that patients begin the formal program when they are the most "ready." A recent study demonstrated that patients on stable opioid therapy can benefit from MPC or interdisciplinary treatment with no difference in functional or RTW outcomes as compared to those patients not on opioids (12). If a reduction of opioids is a treatment goal, success can be achieved with close medical monitoring, which is provided two to three times per week. The CPCC also has the ability to perform frequent urine toxicology screens for more objective evidence of compliance.

- Dysfunctional attitudes, beliefs, and expectations about pain and disability
- Inappropriate attitudes, beliefs, and expectations about health care
- Uncertainty, anxiety, fear avoidance
- Depression, distress, low mood, negative emotions
- Passive or negative coping strategies (e.g., catastrophizing)
- Lack of motivation and readiness to change, failure to take personal responsibility for rehabilitation, awaiting a "fix," lack of effort
- Illness or pain behavior

FIGURE 1 Yellow flags for developing prolonged disability (17).

Pain Psychology

Pain psychology assessment and therapeutic interventions focus on both cognitive and behavioral factors related to pain. Operant treatments, based on Fordyce's model (13,14), are designed to eliminate pain behaviors and promote well behaviors. The primary goal of treatment is not to reduce an individual's subjective experience of pain, but to restore functioning by modifying overt pain behaviors that can interfere with functioning and quality of life. The pain psychologist initially helps the patient understand and identify these maladaptive behaviors. The focus of treatment includes targeting (1) pain behaviors or lack of well behaviors; (2) the discriminative stimuli that precede and influence these behaviors; and (3) the reinforcers and punishments for these behaviors. The pain psychologists help the patient integrate the understanding of his or her own behavior with the pathophysiology involved in order to set realistic expectations for physical functioning. The patient is made aware of how learning and behavior play in one's functioning and how his or her cognitions (e.g., attributions, fears, beliefs) can either enhance or interfere with effective coping and function.

Psychological treatment is also focused on identifying and treating cognitive factors related to chronic pain. The cognitive-behavioral model takes into account the complex interactions between the cognitive, behavioral, affective, and social aspects of the pain experience. Maladaptive cognitive factors involved in the development of and perpetuation of chronic pain include anxiety, fear–avoidance behavior, pain catastrophizing, and learned helplessness. A number of these factors are considered "yellow flags" for increased risk for prolonged disability (15,16). Interestingly, these yellow flags for disability are targets of the psychological assessment and subsequent treatment program (17) (Fig. 1). The reader is directed to chapter 4 in this volume for a more detailed discussion of the role of psychological assessment in multidisciplinary chronic pain management. Factors identified with improvement in adjustment to chronic pain include self-efficacy, pain-coping strategies, readiness to change, and acceptance. Psychological intervention focuses on unlearning maladaptive responses and reactions to pain, while fostering feelings of improved self-efficacy, wellness, perceived control, decreased catastrophizing, and acceptance, thereby improving coping. Our psychologists highlight decreasing catastrophic thoughts as a crucial aspect of treatment, as catastrophizing has empirically been more strongly associated with quality of life than is pain intensity (18). Phases of individual and group-based treatment include education, skills training and application, and relapse prevention.

Insurance coverage and reimbursement for pain psychology services remain a challenge, despite a number of randomized controlled studies and meta-analytic evidence supporting efficacy for improving psychosocial functioning and reduced

TABLE 3 Health and Behavioral Codes for Pain Management

CPT codes	Intervention
96150	Initial assessment
96151	Reassessment
96152	Intervention to modify psychological, behavioral, cognitive, and social factors
96513	Group intervention
96514/96155	Family intervention with/without patient present

subjective reports of pain (19–21). Patients often do not have coverage through their private insurers for "psychological" services, which may be "carved out" from multidisciplinary or interdisciplinary treatment program, thereby affecting overall treatment efficacy. Please refer to chapter 3 in this volume for an in-depth analysis of the detrimental effects of the "carving out" phenomenon. Many patients are unwilling or unable to pay "out of pocket" for psychological services.

Abandoning the use of traditional mental-health codes, the CPCC has more recently shifted to using "Health and Behavioral" Current Procedural Terminology (CPT) codes in its billing. Health and Behavioral CPT codes for pain psychology services may be used for patients with an established illness (pain) or symptoms who are not diagnosed with mental illness. In general, Health and Behavioral Assessment codes (CPT 96150–96154) are used to bill for services intended to assess factors that may affect the recovery or progression of a diagnosed physical health problem or illness. In addition to the standard diagnosis of a Pain Disorder Associated with Both Psychological Factors and a General Medical Condition (CPT code 307.89), billing should also include a diagnosis of the physical cause of pain (e.g., LBP/724). The initial assessment is billed according to the Health and Behavioral Assessment (96150) guidelines, which includes a health-focused interview, behavioral psychophysiological observation and monitoring, and assessment of health-oriented questionnaires. These services are usually billed in 15-minute face-to-face increments. Documentation must include clear rationale regarding why assessment is required, assessment of mental status and ability to understand and respond meaningfully, and expected treatment goals. Evidence of referral by a medical provider managing the patient's case, evidence of coordination of care, time of treatment spent (in minutes), and a medical diagnosis (ICD-9-CM) reflecting the condition should be included (Table 3).

Psychology groups meet for two to three sessions per week over the 4-week treatment period. Each Monday, the program starts with "weekend review," in which patients discuss what transpired over the weekend. Topics usually include patients' levels of success in being able to incorporate self-management techniques (pacing, relaxation exercises, and home occupational/physical therapy exercises) into their normal routines. Other psychology groups are structured around topics from a well-known pain management patient resource, *Managing Pain Before It Manages You* (22).

Psychology groups focus on education related to

- understanding relationships between chronic pain and psychological functioning

- self-management versus medical management
- acute versus chronic pain
- role of biofeedback in relaxation training
- gait control theory of pain, fight-or-flight syndrome, and chronic pain experience
- operant factors affecting pain
- problem solving, catastrophizing, attention, diversion, imagery, and distraction
- family issues, role of reinforcement and other solicitous reactions, alternative and adaptive reactions
- cognitive factors affecting pain, patients' own distorted thinking that may contribute to maladaptive responding to pain and stress
- cognitive-behavioral techniques: challenging assumptions, reality checking, thought stopping to alter negative attitudes
- identification of sources of anger and role in pain and anger management strategies
- distinguishing passive–aggressive from assertive behavior, learning and practicing active listening, developing appropriate communication strategies to improve coping with pain
- weekend review: emphasis on improving functional activity levels while maintaining or reducing subjective levels of pain, or attributing increased levels of pain as expected, or temporarily, as a result of normal or increased physical activity
- problem-solving skills, realistic solutions, dealing with stressful situations involving pain
- identifying negative and dysfunctional thoughts leading to negative affective arousal, increased stress, and increased pain
- discharge management, relapse prevention

Relaxation Training and Biofeedback

Relaxation training focuses on acquiring self-management tools for reducing tension and decreasing pain. Patients are seen individually and in groups. Initial work involves basic education explaining how biofeedback works, as patients become able to control their own bodies by "seeing" or "hearing" their own physiologic function (i.e., breathing, limb temperature, and perspiration). Skill training includes the use of basic biofeedback technology such as respiratory biofeedback, surface electromyography, and thermal biofeedback. Techniques include diaphragmatic breathing (DB), progressive muscle relaxation (PMR), and autogenic techniques (AT). Patients are encouraged to log their practice sessions in their relaxation practice logs.

Patients in the full program are seen 2–3 hours per week for individual relaxation training sessions and three group relaxation sessions. Trained biofeedback specialists are responsible for individual therapy, and groups are primarily run by a team psychologist. Billing is done in 15-minute intervals with a standard biofeedback code (90901). Billing requires the continuous presence of a physician or qualified nonphysician practitioner. Documentation includes plan of care (goals of therapy, exercise prescription, and measurable objectives), along with evidence of necessity for biofeedback therapy. Relaxation training remains one of the highest ranked disciplines by patients who successfully complete any of the interdisciplinary treatment programs at CPCC.

Physical and Occupational Therapies

Physical and occupational therapists involved in interdisciplinary chronic pain treatment programs must be adept in their ability to assess initial levels of functional ability, and then monitor and progressively increase the level and complexity of therapeutic exercises. Most patients report limited results or "failing" previous physical or occupational therapy. The majority of chronic pain patients have secondary impairments in addition to their primary pain–related diagnoses (i.e., general inflexibility, deconditioning, regional myofascial pain and dysfunction, and other related postural abnormalities), which expands the area of treatment focus. Physical and occupational therapists apply a more functional cognitive and behaviorally mediated therapeutic approach to help the patient slowly integrate other aspects of the program (e.g., pacing, breathing) into his or her home program. This approach may help foster patient optimism, decrease the fear of reinjury, and maximize patient compliance.

Physical and occupational therapists use active therapy techniques, and, less often, passive therapeutic techniques (e.g., manual treatments, passive physical modalities). Active treatment focuses on reducing deficits in flexibility, strength, balance, neuromuscular control, posture, functional mobility, locomotion, and endurance. While there is some crossover between the skill sets of physical and occupational therapists, they possess established core competencies that are unique.

The pain physicians and treating physical and occupational therapists are in general agreement regarding not using any modalities while patients are actively enrolled in treatment. Instruction regarding self-application of ice or heat preparations is sometimes provided, often to be used during off-clinic or program time (i.e., at home or over the weekend). Modality use may be appropriate during flare-ups only. The team is in general agreement that the chronic use of most modalities has limited benefit and may only serve to encourage pain behavior. The use of outside chiropractic or manipulative techniques, massage therapy, and other passive techniques or modalities is rarely supported. Weaning patients from assistive gait devices, braces, and splints is an early priority of treatment. Discontinuation and/or weaning from such devices is usually coordinated and managed by both the occupational and physical therapist, only after significant discussion and agreement with the patient and treatment team. Written logs and a short- and long-term schedule supported by the entire staff are often necessary to ensure successful weaning from these devices.

Physical Therapy

Physical therapists specialize in gait training, locomotion, core stability, upper- and lower-extremity biomechanics, and judicious use of manual therapy. Manual therapy includes techniques based on the Maitland and McKenzie schools (23,24). Group treatments directed by the physical therapist also include Feldenkrais sessions, gym participation (free weights and aerobic conditioning), and creative movement class. The creative movement class emphasizes body mobility and awareness while decreasing patients' fear of movement (kinesophobia) and facilitating improved coordination and confidence in movement.

Occupational Therapy

Occupational therapy focuses primarily on functional mobility and activities of daily living (ADLs), as well as activity tolerance and ergonomic retraining.

Occupational therapists typically concentrate on educating patients regarding proper posture and ergonomics related to upper limb functional activities such as lifting and computer usage as well as proper standing, sitting, carrying, and lifting postures. Occupational therapists address upper extremity–related ADLs including feeding, hygiene, grooming, bathing, and dressing. Physical and occupational therapists also play a primary role in the education of patients, family, and other caregivers.

A valuable part of the formal treatment program involves the occupational therapist videotaping patients early in the program and at its conclusion. This group activity involves recording an individual patient walking, bending, and performing basic functional tasks. Pain behavior, posture, and positioning are identified, discussed, and reviewed as a group. At the conclusion of the program (usually week 4), the same activity is re-recorded, giving visual feedback of improvement to the patient and other members of the group. Patients are also given a hard copy of their session that they may share with family members.

The occupational therapist also works individually with patients on their own "pie of life" exercise. Here, patients reflect on how they spend different parts of their day engaged in various types of activities (work, sleep, self-care, and leisure) before and after their injury or onset of pain. The therapist is then able to work with the patients in improving their daily routines, incorporating pacing, taking appropriate breaks, and prioritizing activities while incorporating self-management skills learned in the program.

The occupational therapist is also responsible for directing group tolerance activities. "Tolerance" may include scheduled extended periods of time during the week (1–3 hours) during which a patient is engaged in a planned activity (e.g., a craft or wood project) in which sitting, standing, and pacing are observed and increased in a graded fashion. The therapist is also a facilitator of a planned and group-coordinated meal preparation. In the meal preparation exercise, patients develop a menu, purchase the food, and prepare a lunch (usually organized during the final week of the program) while using the techniques learned in the program, thereby reinforcing the importance of incorporating these techniques into daily activities.

Therapeutic Recreation

Therapeutic recreation specialists evaluate and plan leisure activities for the promotion of mental and physical health. The therapeutic recreation groups are meant to supplement the individual's general pain program goals and facilitate carry-over of strategies patients have learned in the program. The therapeutic recreation specialist helps the patient analyze habitual leisure patterns and potential realistic alternatives for change. An individualized recreational assessment includes many of the important leisure activities that had been abandoned or neglected by the patient after developing their pain (e.g., sports, recreational, community outings). Short- and long-term goal setting may be followed by individual and group projects and supervised outings. The groups act as a forum to discuss past and future activity participation. Additional group sessions focus on developing new leisure skills with exposure to new activities. During sessions, tolerance, pacing, proper body mechanics, and posture adjustments are practiced.

Weekly group outings involve 2–3 hour activities in the Chicago area including various museum outings, grocery shopping excursions, and other seasonal activities. During the community outings, the therapeutic recreation therapist is also able to document individual compliance and inconsistencies. Other goals include increasing social interaction, walking tolerance, and practicing problem solving for community situations. Successful therapeutic recreation may segue into similar issues related to vocational disabilities. Therapeutic recreation activities are billed as a group and supervised by the therapeutic recreation specialist and physical therapist.

Nursing Educators

The program nurse or nursing staff members play an essential role in coordinating patient progress and care during evaluation, treatment, and ongoing follow-up. Nurses play a critical role in educational aspects of treatment, including basic instruction on pain pathways, pharmacology, nutrition, and sleep hygiene. They can also serve as patient advocates in ongoing communication with team members and help facilitate changes in schedules or other personal requests by patients that may occur throughout the program.

Nurse educators conduct weekly lectures to individuals in all program groups and include topics such as

- basic pharmacology for pain management
- sleep: sleep hygiene, relationship between insomnia and chronic pain
- nutrition: basic concepts related to proper diet, weight loss, nutrition, and stress
- laughter and humor as a pain management tool
- sexuality and back pain: communication between patient and loved one, positioning, physiologic benefits

Vocational Therapy

Vocational counselors participate in the analysis of current or prior job descriptions, provide suggestions for work accommodation or modification, and if necessary, facilitate vocational testing and targeted retraining. RTW is conceptualized as part of an evolving process, with four key phases: "off work," "work reentry," "retention," and "advancement" (25). This conceptualization helps the vocational counselor and the treatment team better understand, focus, and develop individually based goals and areas of treatment. An RTW "goal" can be viewed as a mutually acceptable RTW target.

At the end of the rehabilitation process, vocational counselors can help coordinate FCE testing and finalize RTW issues (e.g., restrictions, level of work). Information is also acquired from the physical therapists, occupational therapists, and physician to address instructions regarding any limitation of duty (full or limited), and functional restrictions or modifications that might be required. These restrictions or modifications include sitting or standing tolerance, walking, and lifting. All patients with work-related injuries undergo an FCE at the conclusion of the formal program. Data from the FCE as well as clinical information from the treatment program help determine a final RTW assessment, which is forwarded to the employer and case manager. Most patients are released at maximum medical improvement (MMI) at the conclusion of the program.

A number of studies have demonstrated significant evidence to acknowledge chronic pain conditions and their disability-related sequelae as a multifactorial problem, with physical, medical, psychological, social, economic, and legal factors each contributing to its natural history (26,27). Psychosocial factors are thought to influence disability duration (28,29) and are an important focus for the vocational counselors in their interactions with the injured worker. Prolonged work disability may be directly correlated with the following risks for poor RTW rates: (1) heavy physical work, (2) high psychological job demands, (3) low job control, (4) high job strain, (5) low peer support, and (6) lack of work schedule flexibility (30). Krause and colleagues found duration of work disability to be independent of injury severity and level of physical work. High physical and psychological demands were associated with 20% lower RTW rates in a retrospective study of 433 LBP workers' compensation claimants (30). The vocational counselor can help facilitate dialogue in one-on-one and group meetings, helping patients to identify, problem solve, and manage job stressors with incorporation of techniques learned in the program. All patients are included in the group discussion, regardless of whether they are working. Patients who are retired as well as those who are actively employed may serve as role models for other patients in the group, contributing valuable insight in group discussions.

Vocational counseling also focuses on preparing patients for potential, modified work positions. Unfortunately, this is not always feasible due to barriers beyond control of the program, such as a union position that will not accept the return of a patient to any job level with restrictions, or the termination of a previous work position.

Final Recommendations for Treatment

Most workers' compensation patients undergo a formal FCE during the final week of their treatment program or immediately following completion. Results of the FCE are used to develop a final RTW assessment which includes a level of RTW, possible time frame for adjusting level of work, and a general statement regarding how self-management techniques and other strategies learned in the program may be incorporated into the workplace. Although in many instances FCEs provide definitive answers in a variety of situations involving physical work, practical limitations need to be realized. Unfortunately, a patient's job requirement is often based on a somewhat vague job "title," and standard job descriptions can be inaccurate. Evaluation of sincerity of effort, ability to perform complex or variable jobs, and prediction of injury based on FCE data is problematic (31). FCE outcomes are used as part of the decision process for the final RTW assessment. In some instances, the FCE is completed while the patient is in the process of improving physical strength and tolerances. Adjustment of level of work determined by the FCE is done at the 4-week recheck or shortly thereafter. Reliability may be limited or poor due to variations in pain, position, self-limitation to avoid injury, equipment function or testing protocol, or subject comprehension (32). Poor performance may be due to failure to understand effort required, test anxiety, depression, fear–avoidance, illness behavior, or malingering (33).

Follow-up for Formal Interdisciplinary (4 Week) Program

Patients are seen 4 weeks after completion of the program by key disciplines including physical and occupational therapy, pain psychology, relaxation training, and medical management. A formal summary of the 4-week recheck is forwarded to the case manager and referring physician. Compliance with treatment, adjustment of home exercise program, and updates on functional status (i.e., at home, work, and in the community) are the focus of most disciplines. Rarely is any further individual treatment recommended. Patients are occasionally referred to the physical therapist for a small number of visits in order to upgrade their home exercise programs. After the comprehensive 1-month "team" follow-up, patients are seen by the physician at 3 months, 6 months, and 1 year following completion of the program. Over this time frame, depending on the referring provider and patient needs, most patients are returned to the care of their primary-care physician or initial referring pain practitioner. Those patients completing modified programs are referred back to the initial evaluating physician 4–6 weeks after completing the program for ongoing maintenance. At that visit, the treatment team physician reviews the self-management program (physical therapy, occupational therapy, relaxation therapy) for compliance, as well as making any necessary medication adjustment. With further medical follow-ups, additional individualized therapy (usually physical therapy or occupational therapy) may be prescribed in order to progress patients' home programs or to manage any severe flare-ups of pain.

NAVIGATING DIFFICULT ISSUES AND POOR PATIENT OUTCOMES

"Noncompleters"

The CPCC discharges an average of 20% of its patients prior to completion of the program, primarily due to reasons including treatment noncompliance, inconsistencies, treatment plateau, and severe pain and lack of progress despite the application of all conservative measures and techniques. A small number of patients are found to be candidates for the treatment program, despite having a poor prognosis for RTW, having poor or unrealistic goals for treatment, or significant secondary gain for remaining disabled. These patients may be provided with a "trial" in the treatment program as a last effort for gaining improvement in function or reduction in pain. These same patients are more likely to fail the trial period, and are usually discharged from the program based on a team decision 1–2 weeks into treatment. Those discharged patients who are sponsored by workers' compensation will undergo functional capacity testing, the results of which will serve as the basis of an RTW assessment. Patients in this category are more likely to be found at MMI, and it is more likely that it will be recommended that they pursue case closure. A recent prospective study found many of the "noncompleters" of a comprehensive multidisciplinary treatment program to have more comorbid health problems, greater rates of smoking, unresolved financial disputes, negative relationships with their employers, lengthier periods of prereferral disability, and utilized more health-care services following discharge than completers (34). Surely, helping even a small number of the noncompleters reach some type of closure (e.g., with their insurance carrier or workers' compensation provider, despite poor progress in the program) in itself can be a useful endpoint for all stakeholders and help patients move on with their lives. Additionally, documentation of function, tolerance, and inconsistencies may provide a valuable service to referral sources.

Malingering/MMI

Regarding a number of chronic pain patients, questions relating to possible "malingering" need to be addressed to the best of the treatment team's abilities. Malingering can be defined as "the willful, deliberate, and fraudulent feigning or exaggeration of the symptoms of illness or injury done for the purpose of a consciously desired end" (35). Blatant malingering is rarely seen, and if so, those patients would most likely be screened out for comprehensive treatment at the initial evaluation. Much more difficult to determine is the significance of high levels of somatic focus, more dramatized complaints, lower or decreased interest in treatment, and poor treatment compliance across one or a number of disciplines. Again, monitoring more closely for inconsistencies and changes in maladaptive thoughts and behaviors may be critical early in the treatment program. It is important to realize that in a small number of patients, these behaviors may quickly resolve in response to improvements in mood or sleep early in the program and/or increase in patient trust of the treatment team. We have found that a number of these "difficult patients" can make relatively significant gains in treatment. The treating physician's core responsibility is to help monitor these issues and discuss these topics in order to create an open dialogue with the patient during the two or three weekly medical follow-ups. Concise, consistent, and coherent feedback from the team through review of weekly team conference notes with the patient is essential. The patients who are unable to demonstrate any progress, despite these team efforts, are discharged from treatment as early as possible. Many times, discharge of a patient may help to encourage other patients in the group to improve their compliance or efforts in the treatment program. Difficult interpatient group conflicts are managed primarily by the treating team psychologist or vocational counselor.

ADMINISTRATIVE AND REFERRAL DEVELOPMENT ISSUES

Referral Process and Demographics

Patients are referred to our tertiary-based pain treatment center primarily from the greater Chicago area. Additionally, a growing referral source includes out-of-state referrals generated from case managers via a number of catastrophic and reinsurance companies. The CPCC is presently a "preferred provider" for two national insurance companies, serving as a regional pain management provider for their respective networks. These relationships, although presently evolving, are facilitated by a more comprehensive case management process, including on-line scheduling, evaluation, team conference, and therapy reports. This virtual networking capability should facilitate a more streamlined and efficient scheduling process, decreased time for obtaining treatment approval, shorter wait times for initiating program treatment, and case closure. Referrals are generated from exposure gained from physician and staff member lectures and presentations on chronic pain, delivered at a number of venues and multidisciplinary pain scientific and clinical organizations [i.e., American Pain Society (APS), Midwest Pain Society, American Academy of Pain Medicine (AAPM), American Society of Pain Management Nurses (ASPMN), American Society of Regional Anesthesiologists (ASRA), and American Academy of Physical Medicine and Rehabilitation (APM&R)], and regional and national news features on our clinic, which are facilitated by the Rehabilitation Institute of Chicago's public relations office. Recent exposure has also been made through presentations by pain clinician team members at regional primary-care review meetings (PRIMED, and MedEx) in the Chicago area, which enable physicians to present to a number of health-care providers (200–500 physicians per lecture). Additionally, the CPCC is a training center for a combined university medical

TABLE 4 Team-Related Values for IPC

Team-related values	Comments
1. Team unity and credibility	Key factors in taking appropriate action and enhancing worker trust
2. Collaboration with stakeholders	Effective for coordination of care, constraining if hindered team decisions
3. Worker's internal motivation	Demonstrated by autonomy and assertiveness
4. Worker's adherence to the program	Worker and team acting as "allies"
5. Worker's reactivation	Overcome fear of movement and reinjury
6. Single message	Regarding patient condition, goals, and actions of the team
7. Patient and team member reassurance	While playing down distressing, less helpful information
8. Graded intervention	Psychological and physical progression in order for patient to restore confidence
9. Pain is multidimensional	Must also be actively controlled
10. Work is therapeutic	Expose patient/worker to workplace obstacles, positive relationship between worker and employer, and preparing for work hardening and conditioning

Source: From Ref. 37.

center (Northwestern University Medical School) anesthesiology, PM&R, neurology and psychiatry departments (ACGME) accredited multidisciplinary pain fellowship. The clinic is also an outpatient training sight for medical students and PM&R residents, many of whom will presumably practice in the area and serve as potential future referral sources for the program. Continuing medical education activities, including grand round presentations at local hospitals by pain team staff, are also organized by the university medical center and help highlight our programs.

Building a Successful Rehabilitation Team

The interdisciplinary team must learn to have a broader view of the disability problem than is typically evidenced in the medical community. Communication between team members and other patient stakeholders (i.e., case managers, adjustors, family members, referring physicians) may have some similar, as well as divergent or conflicting, goals. Success of the team may be determined by team values and the decision-making process. Curtis (36) has identified four values important to the rehabilitation team, which include altruism, choice, empowerment, and equality and individualism. Important values underlying any team decision-making process have more recently been identified (37). Ten common decision values were identified in an observational study of an interdisciplinary team treating injured workers. The identified ten values were divided into four categories: (1) team-related values, (2) stakeholder-related values, (3) worker-related values, and (4) general values influencing the intervention (Table 4).

Financial Issues: Refusal for Treatment

Unfortunately, insurance providers are all too frequently reluctant to approve interdisciplinary treatment despite the number of reports supporting the model's efficacy and cost-effectiveness (38–41). Schatman (42,43) has identified possible inappropriate reasons for stakeholder denial of treatment approval including

(1) "sticker shock" of a 4–6-week comprehensive treatment program (while ignoring the more critical costs of ongoing disability payments and routine medication and medical follow-up and procedure costs);
(2) third-party payers maintaining somewhat unreasonable expectations that all patients entering treatment will have a successful vocational and pain reduction outcomes, ignoring the multidimensional nature of the injured workers pain problem (e.g., limitations in job retraining and placement, operant factors, complicated psychological issues) that may continue to act as barriers to improved function and return to previous level of work;
(3) MPCs compete with pharmaceutical and device companies whose primary service is to produce products, despite being based on a more biomedical model that ignores important psychosocial factors;
(4) a trend toward decreasing reimbursement for noninterventional services (follow-up appointments, physical and occupational therapy, and medication management).

SUMMARY

Developing an interdisciplinary pain treatment program involves a thorough understanding of coordinated, well-supported individual treatment approaches for chronic pain (physical and occupational therapy, pain psychology, relaxation training, therapeutic recreation, medical management, and vocational therapy). Flexibility in administrative and team management is necessary to meet the needs of a heterogeneous patient population, insurance referral sources, and other stakeholders to a patient's chronic pain condition. Goals of treatment shift the focus to the patient as an active participant, educating and empowering patients to take more active roles in treatment that enables them to self-manage pain-related difficulties, pacing, limit setting, stress management, and problem solving.

After a comprehensive assessment (medical, pain psychology, and vocational therapy), patients found to be appropriate candidates are placed in one of a number of treatment program types varying from daily to weekly programs. While in treatment, regular communication between team members is crucial to developing treatment goals and to delivering a consistent message to the patient, as the patient develops his or her own self-management life skills.

Occupational therapist and physical therapist work to help the patient improve aerobic capacity, decrease fear of movement and activity, and improve strength and activity tolerance. Relaxation therapy provides the patient with a number of tools (e.g., deep breathing, PMR, imagery and distraction, etc.) that are helpful in terms of decreasing levels of muscle tension, decreasing daily pain, and managing flare-ups more independently. Vocational, recreational, and occupational therapy goal settings are based on improving function, increasing activity tolerances, and learning techniques to manage ongoing work and life stressors. Pain psychology focuses on helping patients identify, understand, and unlearn complex maladaptive behavioral and cognitive patterns, helping patients improve psychosocial functioning and return to an improved quality of life. The team physician, who is often the program leader, guides patient progress through appropriate counseling and improving medication regimens focusing on decreasing pain and improving mood and sleep quality. The physician, as the team leader, helps facilitate team unity, team communication, and community and referral education. The interdisciplinary approach is a true team endeavor and serves as an invaluable tool to help chronic pain patients reclaim their lives by decreasing their pain and improving psychosocial functioning.

REFERENCES

1. Boon H, Verhoef M, O'Hara D, et al. From parallel practice to integrative health care: a conceptual framework. BMC Health Serv Res 2004; 4:15.
2. Dersh J, Polatin PB, Leeman G, et al. The management of secondary gain and loss in medicolegal settings: strengths and weaknesses. J Occup Rehabil 2004; 14:267–279.
3. Fishbain D. Secondary gain concept: definition problems and its abuse in medical practice. Am Pain Soc J 1994; 3:264–273.
4. Gatchel RJ. Psychosocial factors that can influence the self-assessment of function. J Occup Rehabil 2004; 14:197–206.
5. Kwan O, Ferrari R, Friel J. Tertiary gain and disability syndromes. Med Hypotheses 2001; 57:459–464.
6. Beardwood BA, Kirsh B, Clark NJ. Victims twice over: perceptions and experiences of injured workers. Qual Health Res 2005; 15:30–48.
7. Jensen MP. Enhancing motivation to change in pain treatment. In: Turk DC, Gatchel RJ, eds. Psychological approaches to pain management: a practitioner's handbook. New York: Guilford Press; 1996:78–111.
8. Kearns RD, Rosenberg R, Jamison RN, et al. Readiness to adopt a self-management approach to chronic pain: the Pain Stages of Change Questionnaire (PSCOQ). Pain 1997; 72:227–234.
9. Jensen MP, Nielson WR, Turner JA, et al. Changes in readiness to self-manage pain are associated with improvement in multidisciplinary pain treatment and pain coping. Pain 2004; 111:84–95.
10. Prochaska J, DiClemente C. The transtheoretical approach: crossing traditional boundaries of therapy. Homewood, IL: Dow Jones Irwin; 1984.
11. Schatman ME. Dramatically disturbed patients in interdisciplinary pain programs. Pract Pain Manage 2004:4,24–29.
12. MacLaran JE, Gross RT, Sperry Jam Boggess JT. Impact of opioid use on outcomes of functional restoration. Clin J Pain 2006; 22:392–398.
13. Fordyce WE. Behavioral methods for chronic pain and illness. St. Louis, MO: Mosby Year Book; 1976.
14. Fordyce WE, Fowler RS, DeLateur B. An application of behavior modification technique to a problem of chronic pain. Behav Res Ther 1968; 6:105–107.
15. Kendall N, Linton S, Main C. Guide to assessing psychosocial yellow flags in acute low back pain. Risk Factors for Long-term Disability and Work Loss. Wellington, NZ: Accident Rehabilitation and Compensation Insurance Corporation of New Zealand and the National Health Committee; 1997.
16. Main CJ, Burton AK. Economic and occupational influences on pain and disability. In: Main CJ, Spanswick CC, eds. Pain Management. An Interdisciplinary Approach. Edinburgh: Churchill Livingstone; 2000:63–87.
17. Waddell G, Burton AK. Concepts of rehabilitation for the management of low back pain. Best Pract Res Clin Rheumatol 2005; 19:655–670.

18. Lame I, Peters M, Vlaeyen J, et al. Quality of life in chronic pain is more associated with beliefs about pain, than with pain intensity. Eur J Pain 2005; 9:15–24.
19. Morley S, Eccleston C, Williams A. Systematic review and meta-analysis of randomized trials of cognitive behavior therapy and behavior therapy for chronic pain in adults, excluding headache. Pain 1999; 80:1–13.
20. McCracken LM, Turk D. Behavioral and cognitive-behavioral treatment for chronic pain: outcome, predictors of outcome, and treatment process. Spine 2002; 27:2564–2573.
21. Hoffman BM, Papas RK, Chatkoff DK, et al. Meta-analysis of psychological interventions for chronic low back pain. Health Psychol 2007; 26:1–9.
22. Caudill M. Managing Pain Before it Manages You, revised edn. New York: Guilford Press; 2002.
23. Maitland GD. Vertebral Manipulation, 4th edn. Boston, MA: Butterworths; 1977.
24. McKenzie R. The Lumbar Spine: Mechanical Diagnosis and Therapy. Waikenae, New Zealand: Spinal Publications; 1981.
25. Young AE, Roessler RT, Wasiak R, et al. A developmental conceptualization of return to work. J Occup Rehabil 2005; 15:557–568.
26. Frank J, Sinclair S, Hogg-Johnson S, et al. Preventing disability from work-related low back pain. New evidence gives new hope—if we can just get all the players onside. J Can Med Assoc 1998; 158:1625–1631.
27. Krause N, Frank JW, Sullivan T, et al. Determinants of duration of disability and return to work after work-related injury and illness: challenges for future research. Am J Ind Med 2001; 40:464–484.
28. Deyo RA, Diehl AK. Psychosocial predictors of disability in patients with low back pain. J Rheumatol 1988; 15:1557–1564.
29. Feuerstein M, Berkowitz SM, Huang GD. Predictors of occupational low back disability: implications for secondary prevention. J Occup Environ Med 1999; 41:1024–1031.
30. Krause N, Dasinger LK, Geegan LJ, et al. Psychosocial job factors and return-to-work after compensated low back injury: a disability phase-specific analysis. Am J Ind Med 2001; 40:374–392.
31. Pransky GS, Dempsey PG. Practical aspects of functional capacity evaluations. J Occup Rehabil 2004; 14:217–229.
32. Innes E, Tuckwell N, Straker L, et al. Test-retest reliability on nine tasks of the physical work performance evaluation. Work 2002; 19:243–253.
33. Hirsch G, Beach G, Cookde C, et al. Relationship between performance on lumbar dynamometry and Waddell score in a population with low-back pain. Spine 1991; 16:1039–1043.
34. Proctor TD, Mayer TG, Theodore B, et al. Failure to complete a functional restoration program for chronic musculoskeletal disorders: a prospective 1-year outcome study. Arch Phys Med Rehabil 2005; 86:1509–1515.
35. Dorland's Illustrated Medical Dictionary, 25th edn. Philadelphia, PA: W.B. Saunders; 1974.
36. Curtis RS. Values and valuing in rehabilitation. J Rehabil 1998; 64:42–47.
37. Loisel P, Falardeau M, Baril R, et al. The values underlying team decision-making in work rehabilitation for musculoskeletal disorders. Disabil Rehabil 2005; 27:561–569.
38. Turk DC, Okifuji A. Treatment of chronic pain patients: clinical outcomes, cost-effectiveness, and cost-benefits of multidisciplinary pain centers. Crit Rev Physiol Rehabil Med 1998; 10:181–208.
39. Guzman J, Esmail R, Karjalainen K, et al. Multidisciplinary rehabilitation for chronic low back pain: a systematic review. BMJ 2001; 322:1511–1516.
40. Turk DC. Clinical effectiveness and cost-effectiveness of treatments for patients with chronic pain. Clin J Pain 2002; 18:355–365.

41. Kitahara M, Kojima KK, Ohmura A. Efficacy of interdisciplinary treatment for chronic nonmalignant pain patients in Japan. Clin J Pain 2006; 22:647–655.
42. Schatman ME. The demise of multidisciplinary pain management clinics? Pract Pain Manage 2006; 6:30–41.
43. Schatman ME. The demise of the multidisciplinary chronic pain management clinic: bioethical perspectives on providing optimal treatment when ethical principles collide. In: Schatman ME, ed. Ethical Issues in Chronic Pain Management. New York: Informa Healthcare; 2007:43–62.

11 Approaches to Psychological Assessment Prior to Multidisciplinary Chronic Pain Management

Allen H. Lebovits
Neurology and Integrative Pain Medicine ProHealth Care Associates, LLP, Lake Success, New York, U.S.A.

One of the controversial issues in chronic pain management today is whether every chronic pain patient who is being treated should first receive a psychological evaluation. The arguments against this are practical in nature—there are increased costs associated with this as well as limited resources (access to mental-health professionals with pain expertise may be quite limited). Additionally, the fear of communicating to the patient that their "pain is in their head," as well as resistance on the part of referring doctors (particularly in settings where referrals are made for specific procedures to be done) are all very practical and significant considerations. Some patients with chronic pain react negatively to being referred to a psychologist, most often believing that the purpose of the psychological evaluation is to determine whether their pain is "real."

The other side of the argument, however, is based on clinical experience as well as research. Almost all practicing pain management specialists today would agree that there is a high incidence of comorbid psychopathology associated with chronic pain, such as depression and posttraumatic stress disorder (PTSD). Treating the emotional disorder often helps the pain disorder quite significantly, while not treating the psychiatric disorder can hamper improvement of the physical pain regardless of any medical intervention. Additionally, there is a growing body of literature showing that most predictors of both treatment success and failure with interventional procedures are psychological. A careful explanation from the referring physician about the mind–body relationship and the usefulness of techniques, such as biofeedback with chronic pain, very often will allay any fears patients might have about why they are being referred to a mental-health professional.

As the practice of chronic pain management has moved toward the use of increasingly invasive "high-tech" procedures, partly as a response to economic pressures on pain management centers, the psychological evaluation of every chronic pain patient has become increasingly essential so that (1) patients are carefully screened to determine (or predict) their suitability for such procedures, and (2) more conservative, less costly treatments, such as cognitive-behavioral methods, can first be implemented within a multidisciplinary approach.

While there are many excellent psychological assessment tools to choose from to assist the clinician in diagnosing and treating the patient with chronic pain, there is no substitute for listening to the patient and his or her story. Patients appreciate being listened to, rather than being dismissed as having imaginary pain. One important question to keep in mind when listening to their stories is how their lives have changed as a result of their pain. Invariably, the more their lives have changed, the greater the suffering and emotional distress. One needs to read between the lines, however, in evaluating the pain patient. One needs to be the "Lieutenant Columbo" of clinicians, rather than always sticking to the facts, as "Sergeant Joe Friday" did. The experienced clinician can thus take his or her pain questionnaire, clinical interview, and psychological assessment measures, and apply them together with sound clinical judgment in formulating a diagnosis and treatment plan that is individually tailored to that patient.

TRANSITION FROM ASSESSMENT TO TREATMENT

Although the treatment of a patient with chronic pain mandates a comprehensive evaluation of the medical as well as psychological contributors to the etiology, maintenance, and exacerbation of pain, evaluating and treating chronic pain patients with a unimodal, strictly medical approach still occurs. Evaluating chronic pain patients with a unimodal, strictly medical approach is not in the patient's best interests. Radiological findings are not reliable indices of pain; significant spinal abnormalities are often found in patients who do not experience pain (1). The unimodal medical pain evaluation without a psychological evaluation can lead to iatrogenic effects such as failed surgical interventions and pharmacologic disasters with attendant side-effects and exacerbation of pain. Not appreciating the psychopathology of some pain patients, such as somatization, often results in repeated medical interventions that lead, in turn, to medical and psychological morbidity.

The interdisciplinary evaluation of these patients, requiring collaboration among health-care professionals, is essential (2–4). The well-meaning clinician who has not done a thorough psychological evaluation can soon find himself or herself with an increasingly difficult to manage patient on increasingly high doses of opioids with unremitting pain. Therefore, the Commission on Accreditation of Rehabilitation Facilities (CARF) only accredits chronic pain programs that are interdisciplinary in both their evaluation and treatment of patients and that require a psychologist or psychiatrist as part of the core pain team. The American Academy of Pain Management's accreditation service, while less prescriptive in its staffing requirements, also requires that the needs of the whole patient, including any psychological needs, be assessed and treated as part of a comprehensive treatment approach.

The multidisciplinary evaluation and treatment approach is widely practiced today and considered to be the standard of care (2). The psychological evaluation and assessment of chronic pain patients has evolved from one-dimensional to multidimensional models, and the utility of these approaches has increased exponentially (5). As its sophistication has increased so has its distance from the standard mental-health intake assessment.

The inadequate assessment of the pain patient is based on a surprising lack of knowledge and misunderstanding about chronic pain issues. In a survey of pain knowledge and attitudes of nearly 700 health-care providers in three hospitals, Lebovits et al. (6) found a correct response rate of only 56%, with the addiction knowledge–related items responded to least correctly. Seventy-two percent of providers agreed incorrectly with the item "25% of patients receiving narcotics around the clock become addicted," when, in fact, the prevalence rate of opioid addiction in patients with chronic pain is much lower than the prevalence of substance use disorders in the population at large. The unwarranted fear of addiction is a misunderstood concept in pain management that can lead to the undertreatment of pain, a problem that has been well documented in AIDS and cancer patients (7–10).

Treatment in a multidisciplinary pain center must be based on both the medical and psychological evaluations. Direct communication between specialists as well as with the patient is essential in deciding treatment direction. Every patient with chronic pain is unique; one cannot apply a "cookie cutter" approach. Rather, treatment must be individualized, with only the most appropriate psychological and medical interventions uniquely suited for that particular patient applied.

OBJECTIVES OF THE PSYCHOLOGICAL EVALUATION

The objective of the psychological evaluation of the patient with chronic pain is *not* to determine whether the patient's pain is real or imagined (all pain is "real") but rather to:

1. determine the degree of psychological adaptation to chronic pain, which includes mood state, coping skills, effect on family, and level of physical functioning,
2. evaluate the patient's premorbid psychological state, personality factors, and their influence on the onset and etiology of pain,
3. establish the role of psychological factors in the maintenance and exacerbation of pain,
4. formulate a DSM-IV diagnosis,
5. determine which psychological and medical interventions would be most appropriate for the patient,
6. identify environmental reinforcers of chronic pain and illness behaviors such as family, litigation status, and disability insurance status,
7. devise a treatment plan in conjunction with the patient and the rest of the multidisciplinary team,
8. predict a likely outcome of invasive medical procedures such as surgical implantation of spinal cord stimulators (SCSs) or intrathecal pumps, and
9. evaluate the likelihood of the development of chronic pain–related disability.

STANDARD PAIN CENTER EVALUATION PROTOCOL

The standard procedure in many multidisciplinary pain centers is to mail a background and demographic questionnaire before the patient's first visit to either send back prior to the visit or bring along at the first visit. This allows for review of data, which can save valuable time for the clinician who can begin to frame the clinical interview. It also serves as a very valuable educational lesson for the patient, structuring their thoughts in a certain direction such as relating pain to various factors, and most significantly, introducing the concept of the relationship between psychological factors and pain. This is an important therapeutic principle that many patients have a great deal of defensiveness about. Unless this can be overcome, psychological interventions will not succeed. The standard evaluation protocol of most pain centers is the pain questionnaire, the clinical interview, pain assessment measures, and a psychological evaluation. Many patients perceive the careful, detailed analysis of their pain and related factors as an understanding and willingness to listen to them, something prior health-care personnel may have been reluctant to do.

Pain center pain questionnaire—a structured questionnaire, with open-ended questions kept at a minimum, which facilitates data entry and speeds up the time it takes to complete it. The questionnaire should be designed to yield objective clinical outcome measures for accreditation, as per the criteria of the CARF and the American Academy of Pain Management. Most questionnaires include the following information: demographic characteristics (age, marital status, ethnicity, occupation, and educational level), pain location, intensity (typically evaluated on a 0 to 10 rating scale regarding least, average, and worst severity), duration, sensory and affective descriptors, factors that make the pain better and worse, pain interference with sleep, and date and circumstances of onset of pain. Also included typically is a review of prior interventions and their efficacy, prior hospitalizations for pain, current and past medication use, litigation and compensation status, job status and enjoyment, interference of pain with various psychosocial factors such as general activity, mood, work ability, relationships, sexual activity, and social/recreational activities (rated on a 0 to 10 rating scale of degree of interference due to pain), health perception, and functional status (number of hours spent resting during the day because of the pain, number of blocks able to walk, ability to perform household chores such as laundry, meal preparation, cleaning, shopping, child care, and financial management).

Structured clinical interview—a structured clinical interview is typically performed as part of any comprehensive psychological evaluation and assessment of chronic pain patients. It represents a good opportunity to review the data obtained on the pain questionnaire with the patient, which often may be incomplete or inconsistent. It is an even better opportunity to observe the patient and his or her subjective experience of pain, as well as any illness behavior (facial expressions, frequent posture change, aids used in ambulation, and guarding/bracing). It is an excellent idea to evaluate the patient together with their significant other, which facilitates evaluation of the response of the partner to the patient's pain—whether it is a solicitous, punishing, or distracting response (11). Family relationships are often disrupted when there is an individual in the family suffering with chronic pain. The significant other should be asked about how he or she views the patient's pain and what they would recommend for treatment (12). The evaluating mental-health professional should also pay attention to the words that are used to describe pain. Patients who describe their pain in very "affective" terms such as "horrible" may be communicating a strong emotional component to their pain perception.

The clinical interview is ideally suited to review the patient's pain complaints. This initial focus on pain helps establish rapport by focusing the agenda of the interview on pain and may allay the fears and defensiveness that pain patients have about seeing a mental-health professional. Additional areas of evaluation that should also be covered include onset of pain and relationship to trauma, prior medical and psychiatric history (including patient's family, medical, and psychiatric history), prior alcohol and drug usage, current marital and family environment, current functional level, disability status, motivation to return to work, secondary gain issues, and ability to sleep and utilization of coping skills.

Inquiring about previous experiences with mind–body interventions such as relaxation training and biofeedback is extremely important as it gives the psychologist insight into the patient's knowledge and receptivity to these methods and also enables the proper introduction to potential interventions. An additional area of investigation of the clinical interview, particularly with women presenting with chronic pelvic pain, is a history of childhood physical, emotional, or sexual abuse. Studies have shown a high rate of incidence of childhood abuse appearing later in adulthood as physical pain (13).

Patients with chronic pain often have a traumatic onset etiology. A significant number of patients seen by chronic pain specialists may therefore experience considerable amounts of psychological distress and some may have PTSD. PTSD has been estimated to occur in about 10% of chronic pain patients (14,15). When patients with pain resulting from an accident are referred for psychological treatment, the reported PTSD rate increases from 50% to 100%. The failure to diagnose and treat PTSD properly in chronic pain patients can lead to minimal or inadequate pain relief. A useful assessment measure for patients with chronic pain and trauma is the posttraumatic chronic pain test (PCPT) (16). The PCPT contains six true–false items that evaluate the presence of PTSD related to the accident that caused the pain. General levels of stress need to be monitored as well. Many patients report stress as a result of pain such as significant financial hardships, litigation concerns, anger at the employer, and fears about the future.

The clinical interview also affords the opportunity to evaluate the patient's beliefs and cognitions about their pain. The primary utility, however, of the clinical interview is to formulate a diagnosis in conjunction with the standardized questionnaires. Particular diagnostic areas that need to be carefully evaluated include levels of depression and anxiety, PTSD, and somatization disorders. This facilitates the design of a comprehensive treatment plan, devised together with the patient, as well as the rest of the multidisciplinary team.

Pain assessment measures—the third important aspect of all pain evaluation protocols is the assessment of the intensity and quality of pain.

1. Verbal, numerical, and visual analogue scales are commonly used to assess the intensity of pain.
   (a) Verbal rating scales consist of a list of adjectives that describe different levels of pain intensity. The patient is asked to choose the adjective from as few as 4 to over 10, depending on the scale used, that best describes his or her pain. Verbal rating scales are easy to administer, score, and understand but are less sensitive than visual analogue scales because of fewer response categories which may miss small changes in pain intensity (17).
   (b) Numerical rating scales are based on asking pain patients to rate their pain from 0 to 10 or 0 to 100, with the anchor descriptors of "no pain" and "worst imaginable pain." Numerical rating scales are easy to administer, score, and understand and have demonstrated their validity as pain intensity measures (18).
   (c) Visual analogue scales usually are 10 cm lines, with defined anchors at the ends of the line ranging from "no pain" to "worst pain imaginable." The patient is required to make a mark along the line on a spot that best reflects their pain intensity. Scoring is accomplished by measuring the distance from

the left end of the scale ("no pain") to the mark. Although there is demonstrated validity with this technique, older patients have difficulty with this method (18), and photocopied versions change the length of the line (17). Visual analogue scales are effective, however, with a pediatric population (19).

2. In the pediatric setting, age-appropriate pain intensity measures have been devised for the different developmental stages of the child. The Poker Chip Tool (20) requires the 4–8 year old to choose one to four poker chips, representing the "pieces of hurt" experienced. Various faces scales have also been devised for young children, with each face being assigned a numerical value reflecting its order within a series of facial expressions. Excellent psychometric properties have been demonstrated for these pediatric pain measures (21).
3. One of the most commonly used pain assessment tools is the McGill Pain Questionnaire (MPQ) (22). When it first appeared, the MPQ differed significantly from standard pain intensity measures in that it offered for the first time a multidimensional assessment of pain, evaluating the sensory, affective, and evaluative dimensions of pain. Patients are asked to choose an adjective from each of 20 subclasses of adjective groupings. Each word is associated with a specific numerical score. Pain-rating indices are calculated for the total score as well as for each dimension. The MPQ is useful in differentiating psychiatric patients from those who do not have a psychiatric disturbance, and particularly in its ability to discriminate between patients who have different kinds of pain. For example, postherpetic neuralgia (PHN) is often described using the adjectives "tender, burning, throbbing, stabbing, shooting, sharp" which correlate with the three different types of pain experienced with PHN:

   (a) steady throbbing or burning pain
   (b) an intermittent sharp or shooting pain
   (c) allodynia (tender) (pain in response to a stimulus that does not normally provoke pain)

Confirmatory factor analyses of the MPQ have shed some doubt on the original three subscales of the test (23). Holroyd et al. (24) conducting a multicenter evaluation of the MPQ with 1700 chronic pain patients showed that a factor analysis revealed a four-factor model instead of three factors: one affective, one evaluative, and two sensory factors. Furthermore, examination of the relationships between the MPQ and the Minnesota Multiphasic Personality Inventory (MMPI) failed to provide evidence of the discriminant validity of the MPQ subscales. They concluded that the utility of the three scale scores in clinical decision making remains unstandardized and their value in diagnosis or forming useful subgroups of patients remains unclear.

Administration of the test needs to be carefully monitored to make sure that no more than one word is selected from each subclass and to ensure that the patient understands each word. Patients for whom English is not their first language have particular difficulty with this test, although foreign language versions are available. The short form of the MPQ (SF-MPQ) has gained popularity due to its brevity and good reliability (25). The SF-MPQ consists of 15 representative words from the sensory and affective categories of the original MPQ as well as an additional word "splitting" because it is a discriminant word for dental pain. The SF-MPQ is sensitive to clinical changes from therapeutic interventions (26).

MEASURES OF PSYCHOLOGICAL STATUS

Because of the close interplay of psychological factors, stress, and emotional reactions with the etiology, maintenance, and exacerbation of pain, measures of psychological status have become part of the standard pain center evaluation protocol. Measures of psychological symptomatology as well as specific pain-coping measures are widely used.

Depression

The Beck Depression Inventory (BDI) (27) is one of the most widely used tests with chronic pain patients because it is a relatively quick measure of depression, a mood state closely interlinked with chronic pain (28). The most prevalent psychological characteristic of chronic pain patients is depression. Depression and chronic pain occur together so frequently that it is often difficult to determine whether the depression is a precipitant of the pain or a consequence of living with intractable pain. Levels of depression can range from minor mood state disturbances to major clinical depressions with active suicidal ideation. In an unpublished study, the author has found that 25% of 821 chronic pain patients score in the moderate to severe range of depression on the BDI (see Fig. 1). The BDI is a 21-item questionnaire requiring the patient to endorse various symptoms of depression that produce a total score ranging from 0 to 63. Scores above 10 reflect minor depressive states, while those above 17 are indicative of a moderate to severe state. The BDI is easy to administer and score. The item on suicidal ideation is helpful in assessing suicidality in chronic pain patients, which always needs to be carefully monitored. The BDI is able to distinguish between depressed and nondepressed chronic pain patients (29). Comparing the BDI to another measure of depression, the Center for Epidemiologic Studies Depression (CES-D), Geisser et al. found that both the BDI and the CES-D discriminated significantly between chronic pain patients who were depressed and those who were not (30). One of the criticisms of the use of an instrument such as the BDI is that some of the physical "vegetative" items such as sleeplessness, which can be endorsed because of pain, can artificially elevate BDI scores for pain patients. Geisser et al found, however, that removal of these somatic items did not improve its accuracy (30).

Anxiety

The Spielberger State-Trait Anxiety Inventory (STAI) (31) is the most widely used measure of anxiety, a construct that is not used as extensively as depression is, but nevertheless a very important one with pain patients. The STAI is a 40-item inventory that assesses "trait" anxiety—a characterological, stable dimension of anxiety that is relatively consistent over time—as well as "state" anxiety—transitory feelings of anxiety usually in response to specific situations. Patients are asked to rate statements on a 4-point scale regarding how they feel right now (state anxiety) and how they feel generally (trait anxiety).

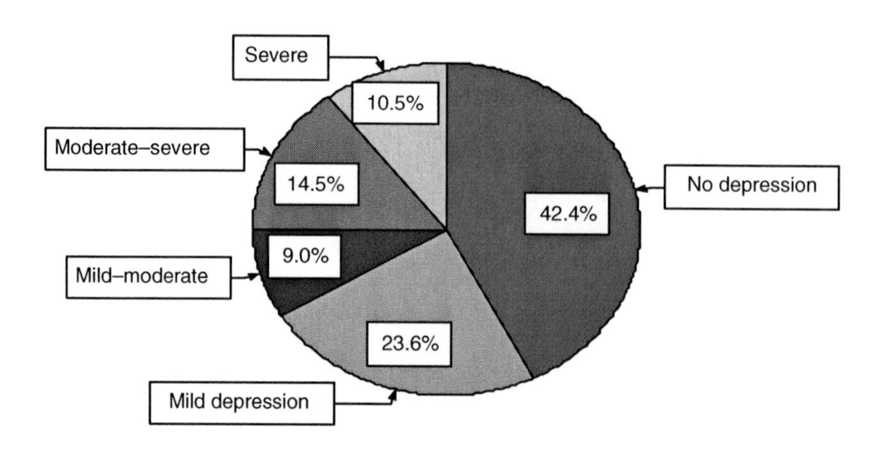

FIGURE 1 Level of depression at first visit.

Comprehensive Personality/Psychiatric Measures

The MMPI (32), one of the most widely used and researched tests of all time, is used quite extensively with chronic pain patients. For the decade of 1990–1999, 12% of all MMPI citations in the literature are pain related. The MMPI is a 566-question true–false test that evaluates the presence of psychopathology by taking into account scores on three validity scales (which assess the degree to which respondents may be trying to distort their true persona). The 10 most commonly used clinical scales are *hypochondriasis, depression, hysteria, psychopathic deviance* (history of antisocial behavior and nonconformance), *paranoia, psychasthenia* (obsessive–compulsive tendencies as well as anxiety), *schizophrenia, hypomania, masculinity–femininity,* and *social introversion.* Two additional scales used with chronic pain patients are the *low back pain scale* and the *dorsal scale.* Careful examination of the pattern or "profile" of scale scores, particularly those above a normative percentile *T* score of 70, enables the experienced clinician to evaluate the degree of psychological distress experienced by the patient as well as treatment compliance and responsiveness.

The most common profile seen in chronic pain patients is the "conversion V" with elevations on the hypochondriasis, depression, and hysteria scales. Individuals whose profiles reflect greater psychopathology tend to display more severe pain symptoms (17). Problems utilizing the MMPI with chronic pain patients include its length (over 2 hours to complete) and its strong orientation to psychopathology (which suggests to pain patients that they are being perceived as "crazy" and their pain is in their head). A criticism that has been directed at the use of the MMPI with chronic pain patients is that there is an overlap of symptoms of chronic pain with MMPI items, which can lead to erroneous estimates of psychopathology (33). For example, five items on the MMPI reflect the presence and severity of rheumatoid arthritis. Each of these items code on both scales 1 and 3 (hypochondriasis and hysteria). Three items also code on scale 2 (depression).

The MMPI-2, the recent revision of the MMPI, has reduced some of the psychiatric bias and has also updated the normative samples. While some pain centers administer the MMPI or MMPI-2 as part of the standard evaluation protocol, others reserve its use for patients with suspected major psychopathology or for the treatment of refractory patients.

The Symptom Checklist-90-Revised (SCL-90-R) (34) is a commonly used assessment of psychological symptom patterns that is also used, on a more limited basis, with chronic pain patients. Patients indicate the degree to which they are bothered by 90 symptoms on a 5-point scale ranging from "not at all" to "extremely," which yield nine "symptom dimensions": *somatization, obsessive–compulsive, interpersonal sensitivity, depression, anxiety, hostility, phobic anxiety, paranoid ideation*, and *psychoticism*. There are also three general measures of distress: *global severity index, positive symptom distress index*, and *positive symptom total*. The SCL-90-R is shorter and easier to administer than the MMPI and is considered to be a state-oriented measure sensitive to treatment changes (35).

The Brief Symptom Inventory (BSI) is the short version of the SCL-90-R that consists of only 53 items utilizing the same rating scale and yielding the same symptom patterns and global indices as the SCL-90-R. Correlations between the BSI and the SCL-90-R are 0.92 and higher for each of the scales. If testing time is an issue with the patient, as is often the case in a multidisciplinary pain center, then the BSI may be a more suitable instrument to use than the SCL-90-R.

Specific Pain Questionnaires

The Multidimensional Pain Inventory (MPI) (11), originally derived from the West Haven-Yale Multidimensional Pain Inventory (WHYMPI) (36), is a specific self-report pain measure, based on a cognitive-behavioral approach that evaluates subjective, behavioral, and psychophysiological indices. The first section assesses

1. perceived interference of pain with daily activities,
2. support experienced from significant others,
3. pain severity and level of suffering,
4. perceived self-control over life and life's problems, and
5. affective distress.

The second section is unique in that it evaluates the patient's perception regarding the responses of his or her significant other to the patient's pain:

1. the degree to which the patient's pain behavior is reacted to with irritation, frustration, or anger by the significant other (punishing responses)
2. the frequency with which the significant other responds to pain behavior with encouragement (soliciting responses)
3. the level of distracting responses that the significant other uses in response to pain behavior (distracting responses)

The third section assesses the frequency with which the patient participates in five categories of activity:

1. household chores
2. outdoor work
3. activities away from home

4. social activities
5. general activity level

The MPI is easily administered, has face validity for the patient (the relationship to pain is obvious), and is a multidimensional tool that is unique in its assessment of environmental contingencies.

Pain-Coping Measures

The Coping Strategies Questionnaire (CSQ) (37) is a specific pain measure, designed to evaluate how pain patients cope with their pain. Based on patients' responses to 48 items on a seven-point Likert type scale, six cognitive coping strategies (diverting attention, reinterpreting pain sensations, calming self statements, ignoring pain sensations, praying and hoping, and catastrophizing) and two behavioral coping strategies (increasing behavioral activity and increasing pain behaviors) are combined into three general coping measures: cognitive coping and suppression, helplessness, and diverting attention and praying. The three general measures are predictive of other pain-related variables as well as mood state (17). The CSQ has recently been revised, retaining only 27 of the original items (38). The original *catastrophizing* and *diverting attention* subscales were most robust, and although the original six cognitive factors were retained, the behavioral factors were not replicated.

Generally speaking, the literature has identified the adaptive coping strategies associated with less pain as the active coping strategies of staying busy, ignoring pain, and distraction. Maladaptive coping strategies, associated with increased pain, include catastrophizing as well as the passive coping strategies such as restricting activities, wishful thinking, and depending on others. A particularly "bad" coping strategy that has been identified in the literature as being associated with poor outcomes is "catastrophizing" (interpreting events in a negative light). The objective of pain management is to improve the functional status of the patient. One approach to doing this is to improve the patient's coping skills, to get individuals who have been dealt a "bad" hand to "stay in the game":

> So we accept it as it is. It is a day to day thing, sometimes hour to hour. But this is what they call life. Sometimes it does deal you cards you weren't ready to play, but the cards have been dealt. You either play them and try to make a winning hand, or you fold the sons of bitches and walk away. I think I will stay to play. (39)

PREDICTORS OF OUTCOME OF INVASIVE PROCEDURES AND OF DISABILITY

As pain management has become more technologically sophisticated and aggressive in its approach, one of the more common uses of the psychological evaluation has been to determine the appropriateness of a potential candidate for implantation of an SCS or implantable pump, based on a set of predetermined psychosocial characteristics. The purpose of such evaluations is to optimize the outcome of these interventions (40). Nelson and colleagues (41) conducted a meta-analysis of the literature on this topic and concluded that patients should be excluded from receiving implantable SCSs if they had active psychosis, suicidality, untreated major depression, somatization disorder, alcohol or drug dependency, compensation/litigation disincentive to recovery, lack of social supports, or cognitive deficits. Additional considerations for exclusion include unusual pain ratings, personality disorders, physical incongruence, a high elevation on the depression scale of the MMPI, or elevations on four or more MMPI scales. Doleys et al. (42), however, were not as optimistic about the predictability of these factors. They concluded that there were no definitive multicenter studies that could identify a statistically significant psychological factor that predicts outcome. The authors did feel that the psychological evaluation is useful if not necessary, but advised caution in interpreting test data. One of the limiting factors in evaluating data in these studies is that the definition of success of SCS is not standard, although one predictive factor identified was that seriously personality disordered patients are not likely to improve.

In clinical practice, the mental-health specialist needs to evaluate for these factors and use them together with his or her own judgment in deciding whether to allow or exclude a patient from treatment. Sometimes the recommendation might be to delay implantation until a severe depression can be better controlled. Other times, a patient's level of motivation to return to work might be so impressively high that it would mitigate the presence of some of the above-delineated exclusion criteria. Patient expectations about the success of the device is a very important area of evaluation (40). An unrealistically high expectation, such as complete "cure" of their pain, is a red flag for problems. Additionally, patients who are very concerned about body image, such as commonly found in young women, need to be assessed regarding their willingness to accept the body protrusion brought about by the stimulator implantation.

Similarly, surgical success has also been "predicted" on the basis of psychological factors: the MMPI has been shown to be a very powerful predictor of the success of lumbar surgery. In one study, six MMPI scales administered preoperatively were predictive of surgical outcome in a herniation but not in a stenosis group (43). In another study, 84 patients, evaluated before lumbar discectomy with an objective evaluation system (neurological signs, sciatic-tension signs, MMPI, and lumbar myelography), accurately predicted treatment outcome 1 year later (accounting for 40% of the variance) (44). The MMPI was the most powerful predictor of treatment outcome. Block and Callewart (45) have developed a presurgical scoring card that predicts surgical success based on three groups of factors that might impede optimal outcome: *medical* (chronicity of condition, previous spine surgery, smoking, and/or obesity); *psychological interview* (litigation, workers' compensation, job dissatisfaction, heavy lifting job, substance abuse, family reinforcers of pain, marital dissatisfaction, abuse, and/or a preinjury psychiatric history); and *psychological testing* (elevations on five MMPI scales, Hypochondriasis, Depression, Hysteria, Psychopathic Deviance, and Psychasthenia, as well as choosing poor coping strategies on the CSQ). Psychological interventions such as biofeedback, smoking cessation, or weight loss strategies, either pre- or postsurgically, may be recommended based on the evaluation.

Unresolved traumatic stress can help maintain chronic pain for many years or actually activate physical pain many years later. In a study of 100 spinal surgery patients, 95% of patients who recalled no developmental traumas (physical, sexual, or emotional abuse, or alcohol/drug abuse in caregiver, or abandonment) had a successful postsurgical outcome (13). Only 15% of patients who recalled three or more of these traumas/risk factors had a successful postsurgical outcome. Thus, childhood traumas were significantly predictive of surgical success many years later.

The authors of this study theorized that for those patients with a history of abuse, surgery is another traumatic event that reactivates the childhood template of abuse. Patients who can be consoled are likely to improve; those who have been psychologically traumatized and are not readily consolable may not improve.

As disability claims are increasing in alarming rapidity, another purpose of the psychological evaluation has arisen: the prediction of the development of disability. Gatchel et al. conducted a prospective study of 504 acute low back pain patients to identify work status 1 year later (46). A logistic regression analysis identified 91% of patients' work status 1 year later. Patients were more likely not to be at work if they were female, had workers compensation injuries, scored high on self-reported pain and disability, and scored high on the *hysteria* scale of the MMPI.

Another use of the psychological evaluation is to assess patients with noncancer pain before initiating opioid treatment to determine which patients might be susceptible to substance abuse. Patients with a significant and or recent history of substance abuse or dependence need to be evaluated very carefully before initiation of opioids.

THE PAIN PATIENT WITH A SUSPECTED SUBSTANCE ABUSE PROBLEM

Among the most difficult to manage and treat populations of chronic pain patients are the patients who present with a current or past history of addiction to illicit substances, alcohol, or prescription drugs (47). Pain patients who are perceived to have addictive disorders are often undertreated. The unwarranted fear of addiction is a misunderstood concept in pain management that can lead to the undertreatment of pain. The increasingly accepted management of chronic nonmalignant pain with opioid therapy underscores the importance of understanding the nature of opioid addiction. As important as the psychological assessment of the chronic pain patient is in general, it takes on added significance with the patient who presents with a history of past or present substance abuse. Observation, history, monitoring, and being aware of the "red flags" are very important in the specific assessment of the chronic pain patient with suspected abuse.

Specific substance abuse/addiction measures that can be of help include the Drug Abuse Screening Test (DAST-20) (48), Cage Questions Adapted to Include Drugs (CAGE-AID) (49), and the Cyr-Wartman Screen (50). The CAGE questionnaire is increasingly popular in clinical settings because of its ease of use. Patients who screen positively on the CAGE also reported a higher opioid intake (51). Patients who screen positively on one of these questionnaires should be referred to a mental-health professional with experience in evaluating addiction. Passik et al. have recently developed the Pain Assessment and Documentation Tool (PADT) (52), a 41-item tool that assesses four domains: analgesia, activities of daily living, adverse events, and potential aberrant drug-related behavior. The PADT has been formatted for use as a chart note designed to assist clinicians in assessing and documenting these four main outcome domains during long-term opioid use. Pain specialists need to educate themselves about standards of care in addictive disease and substance abuse disorders as well as be knowledgeable about the prescribing and practice laws in their state.

CONCLUSIONS

There is an ethical imperative for all pain specialists to assess the pain patient as a whole person, including all their biological, social, and psychological dimensions (53). Although the evaluation and management of the patient with unremitting pain is very complex, it needs to be done in a sensitive and nonjudgmental manner, with comprehensive knowledge of the relevant issues. Nowhere is this more essential than with the chronic pain patient. Better, more individualized assessment of pain patients, particularly those with comorbid psychiatric issues, can only lead to more effective treatment of this very difficult-to-treat population. To paraphrase Sir William Osler, it is not the type of disease that a patient has that is as important as the type of patient that has the disease. Nowhere in medicine is this truer than with the patient suffering from chronic pain.

REFERENCES

1. Jensen MC, Brant-Zawadzki MN, Obuchowski N, et al. Magnetic resonance imaging of the lumbar spine in people without back pain. N Engl J Med 1994; 331:69–73.
2. Lebovits AH. Chronic pain: the multidisciplinary approach. Int Anesthesiol Clin 1991; 29:1–7.
3. Okifuji A. Interdisciplinary pain management with pain patients: Evidence for its effectiveness. Semin Pain Med 2003; 1:110–119.
4. Turk DC, Stieg RL. Chronic pain: the necessity of interdisciplinary communication. Clin J Pain 1987; 3:163–167.
5. Lebovits AH. The psychological assessment of chronic pain patients. Curr Rev Pain 2000; 4:122–126.
6. Lebovits AH, Florence I, Bathina R, et al. Pain knowledge and attitudes of health care providers: practice characteristic differences. Clin J Pain 1997; 13:237–243.
7. Lebovits AH, Lefkowitz M, McCarthy D, et al. The prevalence and management of pain in patients with AIDS: a review of 134 cases. Clin J Pain 1989; 5:245–248.
8. Lebovits AH, Smith G, Maignan M, et al. Pain in hospitalized patients with AIDS: analgesic and psychotropic medications. Clin J Pain 1994; 10:156–161.
9. Breitbart W, Rosenfeld BD, Passik SD, et al. The undertreatment of pain in ambulatory AIDS patients. Pain 1996; 65:239.
10. Cleeland C, Gonin R, Hatfield A, et al. Pain and its treatment in outpatients with metastatic cancer. N Engl J Med 1994; 330:592–596.
11. Turk DC, Rudy TE. Toward an empirically derived taxonomy of chronic pain patients: integration of psychological assessment data. J Consult Clin Psychol 1988; 56:233–238.
12. Turner JA, Romano JM. Psychological and psychosocial evaluation. In: Loeser JD, Chapman CR, Turk DC, eds. Bonica's Management of Pain. 3rd edn. Philadelphia: Lippincott, Williams & Wilkins; 2001.
13. Schofferman J, Anderson D, Hines R, et al. Childhood psychological trauma correlates with unsuccessful lumbar spines surgery. Spine 1992; 17:S138–S144.
14. Benedikt RA, Kolb LC. Preliminary findings on chronic pain and posttraumatic stress disorder. Am J Psychiatry 1986; 143:908–910.
15. Muse M. Stress-related posttraumatic chronic pain syndrome: criteria for diagnosis, and preliminary report on prevalence. Pain 1985; 23:295–300.
16. Muse M, Frigola G. Development of a quick screening instrument for detecting posttraumatic stress disorder in the chronic pain patient: construction of the Posttraumatic Chronic Pain Test (PCPT). Clin J Pain 1986; 2:151–153.

17. Karoly P, Jensen MP. Multimethod Assessment of Chronic Pain. London: Pergamon Press; 1987:152.
18. Jensen MP, Karoly P, Braver S. The measurement of clinical pain intensity. Pain 1986; 27:117–126.
19. Varni JW, Jay SM, Masek BJ, et al. Cognitive-behavioral assessment and management of pediatric pain. In: Holzman AD, Turk DC, eds. Pain Management: A Handbook of Psychological Treatment Approaches. New York: Pergamon Press; 1986:168–192.
20. Hester NK, Foster R, Kristensen K. Measurement of pain in children: generalizability and validity of the pain ladder and the poker chip tool. In: Tyler DC, Krane EJ, eds. Advances in Pain Research and Therapy: Pediatric Pain. New York: Raven Press; 1990:79–84.
21. Bieri D, Reeve RA, Champion GD, et al. The faces pain scale for the self-assessment of the severity of pain experienced by children: development, initial validation, and preliminary investigation for ratio scale properties. Pain 1990; 41:139–150.
22. Melzack R. The McGill Pain Questionnaire: Major properties and scoring methods. Pain 1975; 1:277–299.
23. Turk DC, Rudy TE, Salovey P. The McGill Pain Questionnaire reconsidered: confirming the factor structure and examining appropriate uses. Pain 1985; 21:385–397.
24. Holroyd KA, Holm JE, Keefe FJ, et al. A multi-center evaluation of the McGill Pain Questionnaire: results from more than 1700 chronic pain patients. Pain 1992; 48:301–311.
25. Melzack R. The short-form McGill Pain Questionnaire. Pain 1987; 30:191–197.
26. Backonja M, Beydoun A, Edwards KR, et al. Gabapentin for the symptomatic treatment of painful peripheral neuropathy in patients with diabetes mellitus: a randomized controlled trial. J Am Med Association 1998; 280:1831–1836.
27. Beck AT, Rush AJ, Shaw BF, et al. Cognitive Therapy of Depression. New York: Guilford; 1979.
28. Romano JM, Turner JA. Chronic pain and depression: does the evidence support a relationship? Psychol Bull 1985; 97:18–34.
29. Turner JA, Romano JM. Self-report screening measures for depression in chronic pain patients. J Clin Psychology 1984; 40:909–913.
30. Geisser ME, Roth RS, Robinson ME. Assessing depression among persons with chronic pain using the Center for Epidemiological Studies-Depression Scale and the Beck Depression Inventory: a comparative analysis. Clin J Pain 1997; 13:163–170.
31. Spielberger CD. Manual for the State-Trait Anxiety Inventory Palo Alto, CA: Consulting Psychologists Press; 1983.
32. Butcher NB, Dahlstrom WG, Graham JR, et al. MMPI-2, Manual for Administration and Scoring. Minneapolis: University of Minnesota Press; 1989.
33. Pincus T, Callahan LF, Bradley LA, et al. Elevated MMPI scores for hypochondriasis, depression, and hysteria in patients with rheumatoid arthritis reflect disease rather than psychological status. Arthritis Rheum 1986; 29:1456–1466.
34. Derogatis LR. The SCL-90R: administration scoring and procedures manual I. Baltimore: Clinical Psychometrics Research, 1977.
35. Lynch NT, Lyman DR. Psychological assessment in chronic pain syndrome. In: Lefkowitz M, Lebovits AH, Wlody D, et al., eds. A Practical Approach to Pain Management. Boston: Little Brown and Co.; 1996:115–123.
36. Kerns RD, Turk DC, Rudy TE. The West Haven-Yale Multidimensional Pain Inventory (WHYMPI). Pain 1985; 23:345–356.
37. Rosenstiel AK, Keefe FJ. The use of coping strategies in chronic low back pain patients: relationship to patient characteristics and current adjustment. Pain 1983; 17:33–44.
38. Riley JL, Robinson ME. CSQ: five factors or fiction? Clin J Pain 1997; 13:156–162.
39. Letter to the Editor. Clin J Pain 1997; 13:178–179.
40. Menefee LA. Psychological evaluation of the patient with chronic pain. In: Pappagallo M, ed. The Neurological Basis of Pain. New York: McGraw-Hill; 2005:219–223.

41. Nelson DV, Kennington M, Novy DM, et al. Psychological selection criteria for implantable spinal cord stimulators. Pain Forum 1996; 5:93–103.
42. Doleys DM, Klapow JC, Hammer M. Psychological evaluation in spinal cord stimulation therapy. Pain Rev 1997; 4:189–207.
43. Herron LD, Turner J, Clancy S, et al. The differential utility of the Minnesota Multiphasic Personality Inventory. A predictor of outcome in lumbar laminectomy for disc herniation versus spinal stenosis. Spine 1986; 11:847–849.
44. Spengler DM, Tillete EA, Battie M, et al. Elective discectomy for herniation of a lumbar disc. Additional experience with an objective method. J Bone Joint Surg 1990; 72:230–237.
45. Block AR, Callewart C. Surgery for chronic spine pain: procedures for patient selection and outcome enhancement. In: Block AR, Kremer EF, Fernandez E, eds. Handbook of Pain Syndromes. Mahwah, NJ: Erlbaum; 1999:191–212.
46. Gatchel RJ, Polatin PB, Mayer TG. The dominant role of psychosocial risk factors in the development of chronic low back pain disability. Spine 1995; 20:2702–2709.
47. Lebovits AH. The psychological assessment of the chronic pain patient with a suspected substance abuse disorder. Tech Reg Anesth Pain Manage 2005; 9:195–199.
48. Skinner HA. The drug abuse screening test. Addict Behav 1982; 4:363–371.
49. Brown RL, Leonard T, Saunders LA. The prevalence and detection of substance use disorders among inpatients ages 18–49: an opportunity for prevention. Prev Med 1998; 27:101–110.
50. Cyr M, Wartman A. The effectiveness of routine screening questions in the detection of alcoholism. J Am Med Association 1984; 259:51–54.
51. Bruera E, Moyano J, Seifert L, et al. The frequency of alcoholism among patients with pain due to terminal cancer. J Pain Symptom Manage 1995; 10:599.
52. Passik S, Kirsh K, Whitcomb L, et al. A new tool to assess and document pain outcomes in chronic pain patients receiving opioid therapy. Clin Ther 2004; 26:552–561.
53. AAPM Council on Ethics. Ethics charter from American Academy of Pain Medicine. Pain Med 2005; 6:203–212.

12 Development of Policies and Procedures: Assurance of Consistent Chronic Pain Management Practice

Paula Spoonhour
Pinnacle Health Rehab Options, Harrisburg, Pennsylvania, U.S.A.

Michael E. Schatman
Consulting Clinical Psychologist, Bellevue, Washington, U.S.A.

INTRODUCTION

Chronic pain is a disorder of *the person*, and a number of authors (1–9) have called for a more phenomenological approach to treating the individual who suffers from chronic pain and its sequelae. While multidisciplinary chronic pain management programs should respect the individuality of each patient, a need for consistency in treatment still exists. Accordingly, effective multidisciplinary programs strive for consistency through the development and implementation of policies and procedures. This chapter will focus on the distinction between policies and procedures, the purpose and components of each, and the integral role they play in the day-to-day operation of a multidisciplinary chronic pain management program. Additionally, strategies for striking the delicate balance between consistency in treatment and respect for the individuality of each patient will be outlined. Examples of specific policies and procedures that guide the day-to-day operations of a program developed by the second author will be provided, along with the rationale behind their development. Finally, the important role of uniform policies and procedures in the process of gaining reimbursement from the health insurance industry for multidisciplinary chronic pain management will be discussed.

DEFINITIONS

The terms "policy" and "procedure" are often used interchangeably, resulting in confusion and inefficiency. A policy is a written guide for a course of action that is used to determine present and future decisions. A procedure, on the other hand, describes the specific steps that are to be used to carry out a given policy. Bruder and Mahan (10) state, "Procedures go hand-in-hand with policies. They articulate the detailed protocols or algorithms describing the who, what, where, when, and why of a given policy" (p. 25).

A policy has many purposes within an organization such as a multidisciplinary chronic pain clinic. First and foremost, it helps the treatment team members understand the program's vision and the activities expected of them in carrying out the daily operations of the clinic. This understanding is crucial if the numerous disciplines comprising a multidisciplinary treatment team are to function consistently and cohesively. As other chapters in this book cite the overwhelming empirical evidence of the clinical efficacy and cost-efficiency of multidisciplinary chronic pain management programs, there is no need to do so here. Yet, it is important to emphasize that without consistency and cohesion, treatment teams providing care to this challenging group of patients are likely to fail. Baszanger (11) describes the professionals who treat chronic pain from a team approach as "pluridisciplinary"; each of the disciplines has its own unique training methods and clinical experiences, and accordingly approaches the same patient with different assumptions and treatment methods. For example, a physical therapist may consider a patient's unwillingness to exercise as representative of conscious noncompliance, while a psychologist may view the same behavior as unconsciously motivated and at least temporarily out of the patient's control. In such a situation, there is the need for a policy that specifies how disagreements between treating team members will be handled in order to assure continued cohesion. Numerous studies (12–18) have indicated that patients with *antisocial, histrionic, narcissistic,* and *borderline personality disorders* are significantly represented in the chronic pain population. As these patients are often manipulative and prone to "splitting" team members, cohesion becomes even more important.

A policy theoretically may be a simple statement of fact (e.g., "Any patient who engages in physical violence in the clinic will be immediately discharged"), although it is likely to consist of multiple procedures. The actual number of procedures needed within the context of a policy is dependent upon the intricacy of the process required to outline the program's vision and expectations. Procedures should be directly stated and kept simple, presenting one idea, or action step, at a time. Each procedure should provide specific direction, and they should be written in a logical sequence that allows team members to understand the "big picture" as well as the individual steps that make up a policy.

DEVELOPMENT OF POLICIES AND PROCEDURES: PROCESS

There are a number of schools of thought regarding who should be responsible for the development of a program's policies and procedures. When a multidisciplinary chronic pain management program is housed within a larger organization (typically a hospital), it is crucial that the program has its *own* policy and procedure manual in addition to the institutional documents, as relying only upon the policies and procedures of the larger organization can be problematic. Typically, a hospital's general policies and procedures lack the specificity necessary to contribute to effective management of a chronic pain program. Virani (19) astutely notes, "There is frequently less 'buy-in' with centrally generated policies and procedures because few if any grassroots members are involved in their development" (p. 46). Multidisciplinary chronic pain management is certainly a complex undertaking, and the bureaucrats who develop general policies for hospitals generally lack the expertise to develop policies and procedures that will serve a pain treatment program well. It is important to note, however, that a policy and procedure manual specific to a pain program cannot be in conflict with the broader policies of the hospital, as this type of inconsistency can lead to confusion and potential legal issues.

What member or members of a treatment team should be responsible for and participate in the development of policies and procedures? Traditionally, it has been assumed that the manager of a business or department is the most logical individual to develop policies and procedures, as he or she will be using them to manage employees and carry out the general operations of the organization (20). However, multidisciplinary chronic pain management teams are unique entities, generally composed entirely of highly educated professionals. Virani (19) argues against centrally controlled development and review of policies and procedures, noting that such a process will potentially result in overload for those involved. Additionally, she states that when the process of development and review is overly centralized, "the policies and procedures are frequently incongruent with the current knowledge base in the content area" and that "this again reflects the lack of involvement of the organization members who have the most current practice, theory and research knowledge on a specific subject" (p. 46). The greatest strength of the multidisciplinary chronic pain management team is its diversity, and the manager who fails to take advantage of the breadth of knowledge and skills that each practitioner possesses does not manage effectively. Accordingly, we are recommending that while the program manager should have editorial privilege in the development of policies and procedures, their actual development and review should be conducted primarily by the professional to whom the specific policies and procedures most closely apply. For example, biofeedback policies and procedures should not be written by a program manager if he or she is a nurse; rather, the biofeedback therapist should be responsible for writing and reviewing the biofeedback policies and procedures (although that therapist should consider consultation with the psychologist or physical therapist from whom he or she receives clinical supervision). Likewise, administrative policies pertaining to the day-to-day operation of the "business" of a pain management clinic should be written and reviewed by the program manager/administrator rather than by the medical director. *All* highly effective multidisciplinary chronic pain management team members must be *selfless* to a degree, recognizing that "rank" on a team is far less important than is one's contribution to the team and patient welfare. Accordingly, the most effective program managers and medical directors are those who are willing to allow the team member with expertise to function in a manner maximizing the benefit of that expertise. Policies and procedures should ideally be developed with respect to this philosophy.

Regardless of how effectively a multidisciplinary chronic pain management program's policies and procedures are developed, it is important to recognize that they constitute a constantly evolving document that should reflect the changing reality of the specific program and of the state of chronic pain management as a discipline. For example, given the increased publicity and awareness associated with abuse and diversion of opioid analgesics over the past several years, it is likely that many programs have changed some of their policies and procedures regarding medications (e.g., more frequent urine toxicology screens). Even the most effective and cost-efficient chronic pain management program cannot rest on its laurels. The evidence base for treatment is continually evolving, and therefore changes in practice are inevitable. The program's policies and procedures should serve as a record of improvements that are found in the pain treatment and health-care delivery system literatures. According to the standards listed in the Pain Program Accreditation manual of the American Academy of Pain Management (AAPM) (21), policies and procedures should be reviewed by all treatment team members on an annual basis, with the review documented. We agree with this AAPM standard for review.

DEVELOPMENT OF POLICIES AND PROCEDURES: CONTENT

Pinnacle Health System Rehab Options is a comprehensive multidisciplinary chronic pain management program that was developed by Schatman in 1994 and is currently under the management of Spoonhour. This section of the chapter will focus on crucial elements of a policy and procedure manual for a multidisciplinary chronic pain management program, and will refer to specific policies and procedures developed by Rehab Options in order to provide concrete examples.

Rehab Options developed and adheres to policies and procedures covering five broad areas consistent with the standards for pain program accreditation set forth by the AAPM (21): organizational purpose and structure, business practices, personnel management, physical plant and safety, and clinical operations.

Policies and procedures for organizational purpose and structure pertain to, for example, mission statement, types of patients served, inclusion and exclusion criteria, program marketing, and appropriateness of training and experience of the program leadership. An example of such a policy and the procedures necessary to implement it can be found in Appendix 1. This policy is a crucial one for a number of reasons. First, it is disrespectful to bring patients into a challenging program when they are likely to fail. Patients suffering from chronic pain have, by definition, experienced multiple failures within the medical system. If this were not the case, they would not be presenting for comprehensive pain management. A policy stipulating that patients meet *empirically based* admission criteria enhances the likelihood that they will finally experience success in their efforts to become more functional across a wide variety of domains and improve their overall quality of life. Second, multidisciplinary chronic pain management programs are often accused by the health insurance industry of being willing to accept *anyone*, provided that the person has fee sponsorship. Clearly, well-defined policies and procedures regarding admission criteria will result in appropriately discerning selection practices, which should help third-party payers recognize that multidisciplinary programs are interested in facilitating success rather than in perpetuating failure.

Business practices are another important area for which clear policies and procedures are needed. Despite strong arguments against the commodification of chronic pain management (22,23), few would disagree with the notion that multidisciplinary chronic pain management programs need to be run, to a certain degree, like businesses if they are to become and remain financially viable. Policies and procedures relating to business practices include those pertaining to the administrative operation of the facility, maintenance of appropriate legal documents (including licenses, certificates, and permits) required for facility operation, general liability insurance for the facility, and appropriate professional liability for each licensed clinician who provides treatment to patients. An example of a business practice policy and procedures can be found in Appendix 2. The importance of current licensure is certainly obvious. A strong policy regarding the maintenance of licensure serves multidisciplinary chronic pain management programs by adding to their professional credibility, as well as assuring that they function within the letter of the law. While biofeedback therapists are not licensable in the state of Pennsylvania, Rehab Options insists that its biofeedback therapist obtain certification from the Biofeedback Certification Institute of America, ensuring maintenance of the highest professional standards in that field. Similarly, the program's vocational counselor, who is also unlicensed, is asked to obtain official recognition from the Commission on Rehabilitation Counselor Certification.

The management of personnel working in multidisciplinary chronic pain management demands well-founded policies and procedures, especially in light of the professional diversity necessary to treat chronic pain patients most effectively. As mentioned earlier in this chapter, the "pluridisciplinary" nature of effective pain management treatment teams translates to potential variance in the manners in which different health-care professionals approach the workplace. For example, research has suggested that physicians' attitudes regarding clinical safety have been found to be significantly less stringent than those of nurses (24). Accordingly, well-developed policies and procedures regarding personnel management are critical not only to patient well-being, but potentially to team cohesiveness as well. Personnel management policies and procedures should cover topics such as job descriptions, performance evaluations, personnel policies, personnel files, assurance of licensure, and CEU certification. An example of a relatively general personnel policy and procedures can be found in Appendix 3. The assessment of the competency of members of a multidisciplinary chronic pain management team may be more important than the assessment of providers in other health-care settings, simply because chronic pain sufferers are particularly complex. Since good multidisciplinary chronic pain management is based on a biopsychosocial model as opposed to the relatively simplistic traditional biomedical model (25), it is imperative that *all team members* possess a strong understanding of the psychosocial issues that their patients face. For example, a physical therapist on a multidisciplinary treatment team cannot afford to simply go through the motions of "shake-and-bake" that is typical of many physical therapists working in traditional acute care settings. Physical therapists working with chronic pain patients should be "full-time physical therapists and part-time psychologists," as they are often the team members who most commonly observe the maladaptive behavioral patterns that have developed during the metamorphosis into chronicity. As a multidisciplinary chronic pain management treatment team's members must all be able to implement behavioral interventions, it follows that competency assessments should include evaluation of the extent that providers are able to recognize and deal with maladaptive psychosocial phenomenon as well as being competent within the relatively narrow parameters of their specific disciplines. Rehab Options team members evaluate each other on an annual basis, with this "peer review" component of their competency assessment considered an integral aspect of the process.

Given the documented increase in litigation relating to pain management services (26), the importance of policies and procedures regarding physical plant and safety of multidisciplinary chronic pain management clinics cannot be overstated. These policies should cover issues including the physical accessibility and cleanliness of the facility, compliance with ADA and OSHA requirements, the handling of infectious waste, soiled linen, and "sharps," safety and maintenance of electrical and therapeutic equipment, fire detection, warning and suppression, emergency exits, and compliance with fire and other disaster codes. An example of a physical plant and safety policy and procedures is provided in Appendix 4. Such a policy is crucial to any ambulatory facility, as deficiencies in organizational structure and processes have been cited as a cause of safety failure (27,28). In addition to addressing the obvious legal and regulatory concerns, policies and procedures ensuring the physical safety of patients receiving multidisciplinary chronic pain management are important for their *psychological* well-being. With the experience of chronic pain may come a loss of one's sense of safety in the world, with this tendency toward fearfulness among chronic pain patients empirically supported by Asmundson et al. (29). By providing the patient with an environment that is safe, a multidisciplinary chronic pain clinic can ideally reduce some of its patients' anxieties, thereby resulting in enhanced clinical outcomes (30,31).

The largest group of policies and procedures for the operation of a multidisciplinary chronic pain management program is likely to pertain to clinical operations. Policies in this area pertain to appropriate documentation, multimodal pretreatment assessment of patients, development and tracking of treatment goals, outcomes assessment, discharge planning, follow-up and after-care of patients, external consultations, consents for treatment, releases of information, billing of patients, medical record maintenance and storage, and assurance of appropriate training of treatment team members to use therapeutic equipment. An example of a clinical operations policy and procedures can be found in Appendix 5. Documentation standards are of great importance in multidisciplinary chronic pain management programs for the same reasons that they are essential in any area of health care. Certainly, inadequate or poor documentation may result in the appearance of malpractice, negligence, fraud, and abuse. Additionally, while treatment team members will ideally engage in regular verbal interchange regarding patients, doing so is not always practical. In such instances, the availability of written information regarding patient goals and progress is essential. As third-party payers are often suspicious about the clinical efficacy and cost-effectiveness of multidisciplinary chronic pain management programs (despite the plethora of research supporting them, which is covered in chap. 2 in this volume), clear and detailed documentation serves the function of educating health insurers regarding the benefit of this type of treatment. If it is not documented, it did not happen. If it did not happen, treatment providers will not be paid. Despite their prejudices, third-party payers will find it difficult to argue against paying for treatment that is legitimated by well-documented progress.

RESPECT FOR THE INDIVIDUALITY OF THE PATIENT

The existence of detailed policies and procedures relating to patient care does not, nor should it, necessarily translate to a completely homogenized mode of treatment within multidisciplinary chronic pain management programs. Zaza and colleagues (32) calls for an individualized approach to treatment planning and outcomes measurement in multidisciplinary chronic pain management programs. In Chapter 14 in this book, Dr. Campbell calls for the use of the Pain Outcomes Profile (POP) for treatment planning and outcome measurement, and the Rehab Options program has developed a policy and procedures for the routine use of this measure. While the POP measures six dimensions of the chronic pain experience, the goals and condition *of the individual patient* should dictate which of these dimensions are emphasized. Chronic pain sufferers cannot be considered a homogeneous group, and overly rigid policies and procedures will not serve them well. For example, a policy that dictates that every patient receives two sessions of individual psychological counseling each week of the program is nonsensical, as the emotional and behavioral sequelae of the chronic pain experience vary from patient to patient.

Some patients with chronic pain are not particularly amenable to psychological counseling, and forcing them to spend a considerable proportion of their time in the clinic with a psychologist can potentially alienate them, thereby negatively influencing their motivation for treatment and consequently their ultimate success in the program. This is particularly true for members of certain racial and ethnic minority groups (33,34). Conversely, some patients in multidisciplinary chronic pain management programs experience high levels of emotional distress necessitating daily sessions with a psychologist in order to gain and maintain the emotional stability needed to benefit from treatment. A "one size fits all" approach to chronic pain management is doomed to failure, and policies and procedures should accordingly allow the flexibility to meet each individual patient's specific needs.

CONCLUSIONS

Numerous chapters in this volume address the uneasy relationship between the health insurance industry and multidisciplinary chronic pain management programs in the United States. Apparently, the copious body of research supporting the clinical efficacy and cost-efficiency of these programs has not been sufficient to convince third-party payers to consistently fund the treatment which often represents the only hope that chronic pain sufferers have of regaining a reasonable quality of life. While a robust and coherent set of policies and procedures that contribute to the consistency of treatment is not, in itself, likely to convince the insurance industry to fund treatment, their development contributes to an overall sense of professionalism of multidisciplinary chronic pain management clinics. In a number of states, chronic pain practitioners are actively lobbying third-party payers in an effort to help them understand that it is in the best interest of the insurance industry to support multidisciplinary chronic pain management. When policies and procedures "tell the story" of the rehabilitation of people who suffer from chronic pain, they can be used as a marketing tool in efforts to convince insurers of the benefit that we offer to *them* as well as to our patients. Of greater importance, practitioners of chronic pain management owe our patients the opportunity to be treated in facilities that function smoothly, as chronic pain brings a sense of chaos to many lives. Policies and procedures, if written in a thoughtful manner, can significantly contribute to the coherence of multidisciplinary chronic pain management programs, thereby enhancing their efficacy.

APPENDIX 1: REHAB OPTIONS ADMISSION CRITERIA

Policy No. 24.1B

Subject: Admission Criteria

Policy Statement: Patients admitted to Rehab Options will meet criteria as listed below:

Procedure Guidelines:

1. The patient has experienced unresolved pain that has persisted for at least 6 months.

2. The patient has demonstrated through psychological evaluation that he or she requires behavioral medicine intervention in order to improve his or her pain/disability status.
3. The patient has demonstrated through physical therapy evaluation that he or she demonstrates physical deficits in one or more of the following areas:

   A. range of motion
   B. strength
   C. material handling capacity
   D. posture
   E. aerobic capacity
   F. endurance

4. The patient is capable of independent ambulation.
5. The patient is willing to accept the philosophy of the Rehab Options program, and signs the behavioral contract signifying agreement with the philosophy.
6. The patient has fee sponsorship or is willing to self-fund the program.

Supersedes Policy No. 24.1A
Effective 4/1/05

Authored by: ______________________
Paula Spoonhour, BSN, RN, CDMS, Program Manager

Approved by: ______________________
Hospital Administrator

Review Dates:

4/1/06________
4/1/07________
____
____

APPENDIX 2: ENSURING CURRENT LICENSURE TO PRACTICE IN THE COMMONWEALTH OF PENNSYLVANIA

Policy No. 18.1A

Subject: Ensuring Current Licensure

Policy Statement: Rehab Options will ensure that all health-care providers on its treatment team that require licensure or other authorization to practice in the Commonwealth of Pennsylvania are currently licensed or authorized to practice at the time of employment, and that licenses or other authorizations are renewed at the officially designated intervals.

Procedure Guidelines:

1. The program manager is responsible for informing all applicants that they must be currently licensed or must have authorization to practice from the

Board of Examiners of their appropriate field by the first day of orientation.

2. On the first day of employment, the treatment team member will present proof of licensure or authorization to practice to the program manager.
3. A copy of a valid license or authorization to practice will be maintained in the team member's personnel file.
4. It is the responsibility of each treatment team member to assure that license or authorization renewal applications are filed with the Bureau of Professional and Occupational Affairs in a timely manner.
5. It is the responsibility of each treatment team member to provide a copy of the renewed license or authorization to the program manager within 30 days of its receipt.
6. Failure to comply with this policy will result in immediate suspension from employment without pay and will be subject to disciplinary action, until such time that proof of current licensure or authorization is presented to the program manager.

Effective 4/1/02

Authored by: ______________________________
Paula Spoonhour, BSN, RN, CDMS, Program Manager

Approved by: ______________________________
Hospital Administrator

Review Dates:
4/1/03__________
4/1/04__________
4/1/05__________
4/1/07__________

APPENDIX 3: REHAB OPTIONS STAFF COMPETENCY ASSESSMENT

Policy No. 58.1A

Subject: Competency Assessment

Policy Statement: Rehab Option recognizes its responsibility to ensure the competency of all staff members. "Competency" is defined as the skill, knowledge, and attitude necessary to fulfill performance requirements in a designated role and/or setting. Competency assessment ensures that all staff members are able to perform in a desired manner and fulfill the role expectations of their positions. Rehab Options provides an appropriate orientation to new staff members and ongoing education and training to support them in meeting competencies.

Procedure Guidelines:

1. Competency will be documented annually for staff members using any or all of the following criteria:

   A. licensure
   B. certification

C. duties as stated in position description
D. standards of practice
E. Rehab Options performance requirements for specific positions (see Policy No. 59.1B)

2. Competency assessment begins during the preemployment phase and continues into the orientation phase and ongoing assessment. The preemployment phase will consist of interviewing by the Rehab Options staff as appropriate (i.e., skills inventories, case studies, interpersonal assessment and peer interviews, etc.). The orientation phase will consist of educational meetings with treatment team members and others as seenappropriate by the program manager. Prior to the completion of orientation, the treatment team will reach consensus regarding the new staff member's ability to meet the requirements of his or her job description.
3. Competency assessment will be provided on an ongoing basis through a specific and consistent method of documenting clinical and nonclinical performance proficiency and by facilitating the achievement of individual learning needs. Methods of measurement include, but are not limited to, the following:

   A. inspection
   B. peer review
   C. case study
   D. customer evaluation
   E. testing
   F. continuing education units

4. When reviewing the need for a competency assessment, the following issues will be considered:

   A. age-specific needs of the population served
   B. psychosocial and physical needs of the population served
   C. cultural needs of the population served

5. Generally recognized types of competency as relevant to each position include the following:

   A. knowledge competency
   B. psychomotor skills
   C. critical thinking skills
   D. interpersonal skills

6. The program manager will oversee and be responsible for the competency assessment of the Rehab Options treatment team and support staff. Assessment records and of each staff member and supporting documentation will be maintained by the program manager.
7. Identified deficiencies in competency will necessitate a joint effort by the employee and his or her supervisor(s) to identify steps for remediation and develop an appropriate action plan. If remediation is unsuccessful, the staff member will be subject to disciplinary action (see Policy No. 59.4A).

Effective 4/1/02

Authored by: ______________________
Paula Spoonhour, BSN, RN, CDMS, Program Manager

Approved by: ______________________
Hospital Administrator

Review Dates:

4/1/03__________
4/1/04__________
4/1/05__________
4/1/07__________

APPENDIX 4: REHAB OPTIONS SAFETY PROGRAM

Policy No. 10.1B

Subject: Safety Program

Policy Statement: In carrying out its responsibility to provide a safe work environment for staff member, patients, and visitors, Rehab Options recognizes the necessity of aggressively managing the prevention of injuries. It is the philosophy of Rehab Options that *every* staff member has an obligation to make a positive contribution to the success of the facility's efforts to work in a safe manner and to report unsafe conditions to the compliance/safety manager, recognizing that every loss has a detrimental effect on the ability of the program to meet its objectives.

Procedure Guidelines:

1. The program compliance/safety manager and staff (as designated by the program manager) will design, implement, and evaluate programs and procedures to maintain a workplace that provides the highest quality of care under the safest possible conditions.
2. The safety staff will perform quarterly safety inspections and audits of the facility and make recommendations regarding potentially unsafe situations. The goal of these inspections and audits is compliance with JCAHO and other regulatory standards and to assure safe working conditions.
3. When an area of the clinic, equipment, or procedure is found to be noncompliant, written reports will be provided to the treatment team member responsible for that area, as well as to the compliance/safety manager and program manager.
4. The compliance/safety manager will provide feedback to the program manager regarding action plans to alleviate the identified concern(s) and compliance with the reported deficiencies.
5. Any reported deficiencies will be remedied within 30 days, with resolution documented in a written memorandum to the program manager.
6. The safety staff will meet on a quarterly basis in order to review any reports and actions that have been taken during the previous quarter. The staff will also identify concerns that may necessitate changes to policies

and procedures, orientation or education, or expenditure of funds to meet compliance standards.

7. As required by the law and accreditation authorities, safety staff will have the authority to immediately suspend any activity that is determined to put any staff member, patient, or visitor at risk of injury.

Supersedes Policy 10.1A
Effective 4/1/04

Authored by: ________________________
Paula Spoonhour, BSN, RN, CDMS, Program Manager

Approved by: ________________________
Hospital Administrator

Review dates:

4/1/05__________
4/1/06__________
4/1/07__________
____

APPENDIX 5: REHAB OPTIONS PROGRAM DOCUMENTATION

Policy No. 24.6A

Subject: Program Documentation

Policy Statement: The Rehab Options treatment team will document patient status through initial evaluation reports, daily and weekly progress notes, and discharge summary.

Procedure Guidelines:

1. Medical, physical therapy, behavioral medicine, biofeedback, and vocational evaluations will be typed and filed in the patient record according to discipline.
2. The referring physician will be sent a copy of the evaluation reports, accompanied by a cover letter. Others involved in the patient's treatment (e.g., primary-care physician, attorney) will be sent a copy of the reports with the patient's written request/consent.
3. Daily progress notes by the various disciplines will be handwritten in the patient's record on the day on which the service is provided.
4. Weekly progress will be documented by each discipline in a team conference report.
5. The team conference report will be sent to the referring physician and others designated to receive the report within 48 hours of the team conference.
6. The discharge summary and final team conference report will be sent to the referring physician and others designated to receive the report within 48 hours of the final team conference.

Effective 4/1/05

Authored by: ______________________
Paula Spoonhour, BSN, RN, CDMS, Program Manager

Approved by: ______________________
Hospital Administrator

Review Dates:

4/1/06__________
4/1/07__________
____
____

REFERENCES

1. Osborne M, Smith JA. The personal experience of chronic benign lower back pain: an interpretative phenomenological analysis. Br J Health Psychol 1998; 3:65–83.
2. Kugelmann R. Complaining about chronic pain. Soc Sci Med 1999; 49:1663–1676.
3. Honkasolo ML. Chronic pain as a posture towards the world. Scand J Psychol 2000; 41:197–208.
4. Steen E, Haugli L. Generalised chronic musculoskeletal pain as a rational reaction to a life situation? Theor Med 2000; 21:581–599.
5. Steen E, Haugli L. The body has a history: an educational intervention programme for people with generalised chronic musculoskeletal pain. Patient Educ Couns 2000; 41:181–195.
6. Dysvik E, Natvig GK, Eikeland OJ, et al. Coping with chronic pain. Int J Nurs Stud 2005; 42:297–305.
7. Steihaug S. Can chronic muscular pain be understood? Scand J Public Health 2005; 33(Suppl 66):36–40.
8. Engebretson J, Monsivais D, Mahoney JS. The meaning behind the words: ethical considerations in pain management. Am J Pain Manage 2006; 16:21–27.
9. Schatman ME. Psychological assessment of maldynic pain: the need for a phenomenological approach. In: Giordano J, ed. Maldynia: Inter-disciplinary Perspectives on the Illness of Chronic Pain. New York: Informa Healthcare; in press.
10. Bruder PT, Mahan D. Viable policies and procedures: building blocks to saving dollars and increasing effectiveness. Hosp Top 1989; 67:24–26.
11. Baszanger I. Definition of chronic pain and the organization of pain centers. Cah Sociol Demogr Med 1990; 30:75–83.
12. Reich J, Rosenblatt RM, Tupin J. DSM-III: a new nomenclature for classifying patients with chronic pain. Pain 1983; 16:201–206.
13. Fishbain DA, Goldberg M, Meagher BR, et al. Male and female chronic pain patients categorized by DSM-III psychiatric diagnostic criteria. Pain 1986; 26:181–197.
14. Polatin PB, Kinney RK, Gatchel RJ, et al. Psychiatric illness and chronic low-back pain. The mind and the spine–which goes first? Spine 1993; 18:66–71.
15. Gatchel RJ, Garofalo JP, Ellis E, et al. Major psychological disorders in acute and chronic TMD: an initial examination. J Am Dent Assoc 1996; 127:1365–1370, 1372, 1374.
16. Weisberg JN, Gallagher RM, Gorin A. Personality disorder in chronic pain: a longitudinal approach to validation of diagnosis. Paper presented at the 15th Annual Meeting of the American Pain Society, Washington, DC, 1996.

17. Burton K, Polatin PB, Gatchel RJ. Psychosocial factors and the rehabilitation of patients with chronic work-related upper extremity disorders. J Occup Rehabil 1997; 7:139–153.
18. Sansone RA, Whitecar P, Meier BP, et al. The prevalence of borderline personality among primary care patients with chronic pain. Gen Hosp Psychiatry 2001; 23:193–197.
19. Virani T. Making policy and procedure systems work effectively. Can J Nurs Adm 1996; 9:45–56.
20. Page SB. Establishing a System of Policies and Procedures. Westerville, OH: Process Improvement Publishing; 2002.
21. American Academy of Pain Management. Pain Program Accreditation On-site Surveyor's Worksheet. Sonora, CA: American Academy of Pain Management; 1999.
22. Schatman ME. The demise of multidisciplinary pain management clinics? Pract Pain Manage 2006; 6:30–41.
23. Schatman ME. The demise of the multidisciplinary chronic pain management clinic: bioethical perspectives on providing optimal treatment when ethical principles collide. In: Schatman ME, ed. Ethical Issues in Chronic Pain Management. New York: Informa Healthcare; 2007:43–62.
24. McDonald R, Waring J, Harrison S, et al. Rules and guidelines in clinical practice: a qualitative study in operating theatres of doctors' and nurses' views. Qual Saf Health Care 2005; 14:290–294.
25. Engel GL. The need for a new medical model: a challenge for biomedicine. Science 1977; 196(8):129–136.
26. Fitzgibbon DR, Posner KL, Domino KB, et al. American Society of Anesthesiologists. Chronic pain management: American Society of Anesthesiologists Closed Claims Project. Anesthesiology 2004; 100:98–105.
27. Leape LL. Error in medicine. JAMA 1994; 272:1851–1857.
28. Berwick DM, Leape LL. Reducing errors in medicine. Br Med J 1999; 319:136–137.
29. Asmundson GJ, Bonin MF, Frombach IK, et al. Evidence of a disposition toward fearfulness and vulnerability to posttraumatic stress in dysfunctional pain patients. Behav Res Ther 2000; 38, 801–812.
30. Tota-Faucette ME, Gil KM, Williams DA, et al. Predictors of response to pain management treatment. The role of family environment and changes in cognitive processes. Clin J Pain 1993; 9:115–123.
31. Watson PJ, Booker CK, Moores L, et al. Returning the chronically unemployed with low back pain to employment. Eur J Pain 2004; 8:359–369.
32. Zaza C, Stolee P, Prkachin K. The application of goal attainment scaling in chronic pain settings. J Pain Symptom Manage 1999; 17:55–64.
33. Schatman ME. Racial and ethnic issues in chronic pain management: challenges and perspectives. In: Boswell M, Cole BE, eds. Weiner's Pain Management: A Practical Guide for Clinicians. Boca Raton, FL: CRC Press; 2006:83–97.
34. Schatman ME. Racial and ethnic disparities in chronic pain management: recognizing the primacy of socioeconomic and cultural factors. In: Giordano J, Boswell MV, eds. Perspectives on Pain. New York: Informa Healthcare; in press.

13 Evaluating Outcomes in the Interdisciplinary Treatment of Chronic Pain: A Guide for Practicing Clinicians

Kevin E. Vowles
Pain Management Unit, Royal National Hospital for Rheumatic Diseases and University of Bath, Bath, U.K.

Richard T. Gross
Columbia Health Centre, Dartmouth, Nova Scotia, Canada

Lance M. McCracken
Pain Management Unit, Royal National Hospital for Rheumatic Diseases and University of Bath, Bath, U.K.

INTRODUCTION

Intensive, interdisciplinary treatments have been termed the "gold standard" of care for chronic, intractable pain that has not responded to other unimodal interventions (1–3). These treatments are usually rehabilitative, rather than curative, and biopsychosocial, rather than biomedical, in orientation. They capitalize on the expertise of multiple specialized providers, generally including some combination of physical therapy, occupational therapy, psychology, nursing, and medicine (4,5). Two recent reviews (1,3) suggest that such treatments are more cost-effective than many alternative interventions (including implantable devices, surgery, and "conservative" care), while achieving equal or greater success in outcomes [see also (6–8) and chap. 2 in this volume].

In spite of these documented successes, the number of treatment programs in the United States has declined, likely due to the increasing difficulties with reimbursement, poor understanding of treatment rationale and delivery methods, a general focus on cost containment in health care, and requirements for specialist training of providers (9,10). In order to begin to address these problems, it is imperative that treatment providers work toward educating third-party payers, medical personnel, patients, and the general public on the specifics of interdisciplinary treatment, with an emphasis on its benefits. For these purposes, there is a requirement for treatment providers to be empirically oriented toward their own interventions, as one method for meeting local concerns about appropriateness, treatment outcomes, and cost-effectiveness of intensive interdisciplinary treatment programs.

The present chapter is intended to serve as a "user's manual" in treatment outcome evaluation and is targeted at practicing clinicians, who may not have the time, training, interest, or resources to conduct funded clinical trials as a way of evaluating treatment effectiveness. The approach we outline emphasizes careful consideration of the targets and purposes of assessment, as well as issues of measure selection and data analysis on small samples of patients completing treatment. We will put forward a model based on a contemporary behavioral account of assessment. We hope that the chapter can be used to guide the collection and analysis of outcome data in order to support the continuation of this clearly efficacious set of treatments.

The chapter is broken up into two major sections. The first provides a conceptual background regarding the purposes and goals of assessment, in addition to potential targets to assess in determining outcomes. The second is concerned with issues of measurement and details specific domains to consider when evaluating treatment outcomes.

CONCEPTUAL AND THEORETICAL CONSIDERATIONS

So, why have a section on conceptual and theoretical issues in what is supposed to be a "hands-on" guide? Broadly speaking, assessment involves the gathering of data to form an opinion, diagnosis, or to formulate treatment objectives (11). Such a framework provides a guide within which the relevant issues can be identified and subsequently measured. Accurate and appropriate assessment is necessary in all facets of clinical decision making and treatment provision. We believe that performing assessment of treatment outcomes without a firm grasp of why the outcomes being assessed have been chosen and how those outcomes map on to theoretically derived treatment targets risks mistaken conclusions at best and ineffectual treatment at worst. Therefore, the first step in assessing treatment outcomes is deciding what will be assessed and why.

Purposes of Assessment

In a formal analysis of the purposes of individual assessment, Nelson and Hayes (12) suggest three primary areas of concern: (a) case conceptualization (which we would argue also includes selection for, or exclusion from, treatment), (b) routine symptom monitoring, and (c) determining the degree of treatment-related change. In one form or another, each of these three purposes is relevant to chronic pain treatment outcome evaluation. When all three purposes are addressed in assessment, the probability of providing a clear description of what a patient is like and an accurate description of why the patient is like that is increased (13). Considered in the context of treatment outcome specifically, the information gathered can also allow one to comment on what a patient was like before and how treatment has contributed to any observed change. These three purposes can be viewed as "guiding principles" in the assessment process and map directly onto the goals of assessment, detailed next.

Desirable Goals Following Assessment

One of the primary goals of assessment was detailed by Galton (14) over a century ago, which is to collect information that allows the comparison of an individual to a larger, presumably representative, group of individuals. This goal presumes that there is an inherent distinction between the individual presenting for some service and the population at large; documenting any observed similarities or differences is a key focus of assessment. Following assessment, it is common to provide information about the emotional, physical, cognitive, and social functioning of an individual, in comparison to other individuals with chronic pain (and perhaps those without chronic pain, as well). This commentary can include the specific identification of key issues that are particularly indicative of adaptive or maladaptive functioning, referred to as "target" behaviors in the applied behavior analysis field, as these behaviors are often targeted for change by intervention (15). In the case of the maladaptive functioning, these target behaviors are the important areas in need of clinical attention. In the case of adaptive functioning, these behaviors may be important areas of "strength" from which to begin treatment efforts.

A second purpose of assessment is to determine how a single individual's behavior varies across time and situation (16). For example, are there areas where functioning is more or less limited by pain and distress? How has functioning changed over time in response to previous treatment? These issues can be addressed through the repeated measurement of selected variables. In addition, if initial assessments identify relevant target behaviors, these behaviors can be specifically tracked over time as one additional way of evaluating treatment outcomes. Most interdisciplinary treatment programs assess at pre- and posttreatment time points, although it can also be useful to assess progress at various points during treatment, as well as several months or more after treatment has concluded. For example, repeating assessment in the middle of a treatment course can allow changes to be made in the content of the interventions if need be, whereas assessment made some time after treatment has concluded allows an evaluation of maintenance of treatment effects and longer term functioning.

Finally, outcomes assessment should not only attend to treatment outcome, but to the theorized process by which treatment is assumed to work. This last issue pertains to those key variables that are specifically targeted for change and is one way of supporting the validity of a treatment approach. Such analyses, variously referred to as process analyses or manipulation checks, are analogous to the checks that are sometimes used in laboratory-based studies that determine whether the experimental procedure has had the desired effect (17). For example, cognitive-behavioral approaches put an emphasis on how thoughts, beliefs, and other mental processes influence pain intensity and functional status in individuals with chronic pain. If one were interested in assessing this hypothesized influence, separate measures of mental processes would be given with measures of pain and functioning. Post hoc analyses could then determine magnitude of change in the measures of mental processes, as well as how they are related to main outcome measures.

Domains of Assessment

Behavior can be considered as any action that an organism engages in; this includes activity that can be directly observed by others, but, importantly, also includes that which cannot be directly observed. Therefore, an inclusive formulation of behavior includes thoughts/emotions and physiological sensations and responses, in addition to behavior that can be directly observed (18). This so-called "triple response system" (19) indicates three separate, but intimately related, content areas within which assessment can occur.

The three content areas can be assessed using a variety of data collection methods, including self-report (verbal or nonverbal), direct observation, and automated recording (16), although self-report is by far the most common method, likely because it is the simplest and easiest to accomplish. While verbal/written self-report is sometimes the only practical method of assessing some domains, such as pain intensity, it is necessary to recognize that this method is limited and always an indirect measurement of the domain of interest. For example, it is possible to assess physical functioning via any number of self-report measures (some of which are reviewed below), but responses on these measures are not actual measures of physical activity, but rather measures of *self-reported* physical activity. Self-reports are inherently unreliable, as they can be biased by perceived demands of the situation, memory biases, over reliance on verbal processes, and mistakes in reporting (16). This unreliability does not, of course, preclude their use, although it does indicate that conclusions drawn based on them should be done cautiously.

While the importance and prevalence of self-report measures is well known, overt behavior and physiological responses would ideally be given equal weighting in terms of importance. When possible, assessment should involve multiple methods measuring multiple domains. Given that interdisciplinary treatment programs often offer the services of physical and occupational therapists, it is relatively common to have at least some measures of directly observed physical functioning performed by these treatment providers.

Review of Psychometric Information

The utility of any measurement instrument, self-report or otherwise, depends to a great degree on the reliability and validity of the measure. Although reliability and validity are closely related, there are crucial differences; reliability refers to the agreement between measures taken under *similar* conditions, while validity refers to agreement between measures taken under *dissimilar* conditions or via different methods (20).

In simple terms, a measure's reliability refers to how reproducible any observation or score is when measured in the same way. Therefore, for example, a common measure of depression, the Beck Depression Inventory (BDI) (21), should produce similar scores whether given at different times, split in to different halves, or scored by different people if it is to demonstrate adequate reliability. Adequate reliability is a necessary prerequisite to adequate validity, although it does itself guarantee validity.

Validity, if also defined simply, refers to the adequacy of a measure in measuring the domain of interest (22); in effect, "Are we measuring what we think we are measuring?" Within the behavioral sciences, validity is not often directly measurable, and usually requires that an inference be made based on available data (23). If a series of analyses, again using the BDI, suggests that the measure is correlated strongly with other self-report measures of depression and engagement in "depressed" behavior, as well as being correlated to a lesser degree with more general measures of psychological distress, arguments for its validity in assessing the construct of "depression" are supported.

For a more complete discussion of psychometric properties of measurement, see Nunnally and Bernstein (24). See also Jensen (25) for a concise review of psychometric issues specific to questionnaire validation within the pain literature. With regard to the assessment of treatment outcomes, it is recommended that only measures displaying adequate reliability and validity be selected (unless one is in the process of developing a measure, where of course such information will not be available and such measures should not be used in outcomes analysis until adequate evidence of its psychometric properties has been shown). In the remainder of this chapter, we review some common measurement domains and measures that have established properties.

MEASUREMENT ISSUES

There are a number of resources that can be used to aid in measurement selection; some of them book length [e.g., (26)]. The purpose here is to briefly review the major areas that are often assessed, identify a few well-validated measures, and provide some recommendations. These recommendations are based on our experience with these measures, as well as extant literature and professional consensus. It should also be recognized that measurement development is an active area of research and no doubt the measures reviewed below will be supplanted at some point in the future, as our methods grow more sophisticated.

Measure Selection

Recent analyses of sizeable databases have consistently indicated a few key domains of interest (27–29). These include pain description, emotional distress, and disability/physical functioning. These three domains correspond to a recent consensus statement made by the initiative on methods, measurement, and pain assessment in clinical trials [IMMPACT (30)], as well as domains commonly assessed across published outcomes studies (31). Thus, it seems reasonable to include at least these three domains of measurement in all assessments of treatment outcome. Our focus here is on measures that are accessible to most interdisciplinary clinics; thus the emphasis is on self-report and observed performance. Furthermore, consistent with general clinical practice, where a variety of pain types and complaints are typically seen, we included measures that are intended for general pain complaints, rather than for only specific types or diagnoses of pain.

Pain Description

Measures of pain include not only assessments of quantitative or qualitative pain intensity but also pain interference and pain behavior. These aspects of pain can, and perhaps should, also be assessed with reference to various points in time as well—for instance, average, worst, and least pain over the past week (or any appropriate time period) can often provide useful information that is not captured by measuring current pain alone.

Quantitative and qualitative measures of pain intensity include numeric and descriptive measures, such as numerical rating scales, verbal rating scales, and visual analogue scales [see a comprehensive review by Jensen and Karoly (32)]. Each of these scaling methods has distinct advantages and drawbacks, although it appears that any of them can be used across most situations, especially as they seem to be correlated with one another. The numerical rating scale, in particular, appears to have a number of advantages and few sizable problems (30,33,34).

The most widely used measure of qualitative and affective components of pain is the McGill Pain Questionnaire (35), including its short form (36). The measure was intended to be a more comprehensive assessment of pain and recognizes that pain ratings can be influenced by a variety of emotional, social, and cultural factors, which cannot be adequately captured by any one single rating (37). Both the short and long forms are supported by substantial evidence indicating they are reliable, valid, and sensitive to intervention; the long form has been translated into at least 19 different languages [see (38) for a review of psychometric properties of both forms].

Emotional Distress

Elevated levels of emotional distress are almost invariably a part of the chronic pain experience (39). Specific facets of emotional distress predominantly include depression and anxiety, although anger can be present as well (40).

Depression

Although estimates vary somewhat, it appears that a substantial proportion of those with chronic pain meet diagnostic criteria for a diagnosis of major depressive disorder (41), while the majority of patients experience lesser levels of depressive symptoms (42,43). Therefore, measurement of depressive symptoms is a key target, as these symptoms are often important indicators not only of how patients are feeling emotionally but also how they are functioning in a variety of domains (e.g., sleeping, eating, and social activity). Thus, while it may be helpful to assess depressive symptoms as they relate to diagnostic criteria for a mood disorder, it is of benefit to also take on a broader perspective which includes these other domains of functioning.

The BDI (21) has long been the standard measure, in both general and pain-specific research (44). Some concern has been expressed with regard to the risk of artificially elevated scores in chronic pain patients due to the somatic items of the BDI (45,46); these concerns may be addressed through the flexible use of cutoff scores [e.g., (47)], examination of endorsed item content as it pertains to diagnostic criteria, and caution in interpreting diagnostic status from the measure (48). Even with the caveats regarding potential inflation of scores, the BDI is a widely recognized measure for use in chronic pain and is predictive of many aspects of patient functioning (30). For example, it emerged as the most salient predictor of work status following an interdisciplinary treatment program for chronic pain, when assessed at treatment conclusion as part of a battery of self-report and directly assessed measures of emotional and physical functioning (49).

The Center for Epidemiological Studies-Depression Scale (CES-D) (50) is perhaps almost as well known as the BDI, is a bit shorter, and does not include the somatic items that have led to concerns about scoring with the BDI (47). The CES-D, therefore, is a viable alternative to the BDI.

Finally, we have recently begun to use the British Columbia Major Depression Inventory (BC-MDI) (51). It requires an examination of endorsed items for scoring and interpretation and has demonstrated good sensitivity and specificity with diagnoses of major depressive disorder (51). In addition to assessing symptom severity, the BC-MDI also includes items assessing symptom impact on functioning, which is not included in either the BDI or the CES-D.

Pain-Related Fear/Anxiety

Fear and anxiety related to pain appear to play a crucial role in the functioning of individuals with chronic pain, such that they are frequently associated with other indices of distress, disability, and overall functioning (52). The influence of anxiety and fear on pain is now firmly established, with two well-written reviews published in the late 1990s (53,54) and a more recent edited book on the subject (52). Although interest in this area appears to be a recent phenomenon, Langdon-Brown (55) highlighted the fundamental contribution of fear to the pain experience in a published address to medical students over 70 years ago.

It was common in the past to use general measures of anxiety in chronic pain settings; however, pain-specific measures of fear and anxiety appear to provide more useful information and are more strongly related to the distress and disability experienced by individuals with chronic pain (56). There are four major measures of pain-related fear, each recently reviewed by McNeil and Vowles (57), which include the Pain Anxiety Symptoms Scale (PASS) (58), Fear of Pain Questionnaire-III (FPQ-III) (59), Fear–Avoidance Beliefs Questionnaire (FABQ) (60), and Tampa Scale of Kinesiphobia (TSK) (61). All of these measures have generally demonstrated adequate reliability and validity and appear useful in chronic pain samples; thus, they all meet basic psychometric requirements (57). Test selection can, therefore, primarily depend on which measure, or measures, provide the most relevant information specific to the population or concept of interest. The specific aspects of each measure are briefly reviewed below.

The PASS, including both the long form (58) and short form (62), is designed for use in chronic pain treatment settings. It is a comprehensive measure of cognitive, physiological, and behavioral responses to pain and allows the computation of a total score and four subscale scores (cognitive anxiety, fearful appraisals, physiological responses, and escape/avoidance behaviors). The total score is broadly associated with many aspects of patient functioning (63) and is related to interdisciplinary treatment outcome (64). The four subscales are also useful in the prediction of different aspects of patient functioning (65).

The FPQ-III (59) is designed to be used in acute and chronic pain treatment settings. The item content is, therefore, more general and assesses the degree of fear or anxiety associated with a number of specific painful situations, which are broadly categorized into subscales assessing fear of minor, severe, and medical/dental pain. The measure has demonstrated good psychometric properties (59,66) and has been used in samples of both acute and chronic pain patients (67–69) where the total score has been associated with various measures of patient functioning.

The FABQ (60) is predominantly concerned with beliefs about possible harm arising from physical and work-related situations, which are assessed as separate subscales. Existing literature generally supports the structure of the measure, with the physical subscale being more strongly associated with physical performance, such as flexibility or weight lifting (70,71), while the work subscale is more strongly associated with work disability and restrictions (72,73) and performance on work-related tasks (74).

Finally, the TSK (61) is also designed to assess beliefs about bodily damage arising from physical activity. Various versions of the TSK, with different factor structures, have been used (57). Although there is not yet a clear consensus on which version is most sound, recent confirmatory factor analyses have provided support for a 13-item two-factor model (75,76).

Measures of Functioning

Restoration of functioning that has been lost as a result of chronic pain is often a primary goal of interdisciplinary treatment programs. Functioning is best considered within a broad framework and can include improvements in physical performance, general activity levels (e.g., domestic, recreational, social), work or disability status, health-care use, and medication consumption (77). We have included a number of composite measures in this section to reflect the broad overlap between physical and emotional functioning and other measures of distress (e.g., depression, pain-related fear, etc.). Some of these measures also include items pertaining to pain intensity or emotional functioning and thus can offer an efficient method of assessment, particularly in settings where the completion of more time-consuming batteries is not feasible.

Standardized Self-Report Measures

The Sickness Impact Profile (SIP) (78) is a well-validated and comprehensive measure that has been widely used in rehabilitation settings (79). Although the SIP is lengthy as it contains 136 items, it assesses 12 aspects of daily functioning, many of which are relevant to individuals with chronic pain, and allows calculation of an overall composite score, as well as scores of physical, psychosocial, and "other" disabilities. Computerized scoring is highly recommended as items are individually weighted, which makes hand scoring impractical. A much shortened version of the SIP is the Roland-Morris Disability Scale (80), which contains 20 items and now has evidence for use in a variety of pain conditions (81), not just low back for which it was originally normed.

The West Haven-Yale Multidimensional Pain Inventory (MPI) (82) is another widely used measure which assesses a number of aspects of the pain experience, including pain intensity, affect/distress, and functioning in typical activities. The MPI also includes several useful subscales that assess patient reports of significant other behavior as it relates to the patient's pain. Subscale scores are expressed as *t*-scores (mean of 50; standard deviation of 10) and are based on comparisons with the original normative sample. The MPI has demonstrated utility across a range of pain complaints and conditions (83). It also allows a method of categorizing patients according to key issues of adaptation, for example, patients can be categorized as "adaptive" or "dysfunctional" copers or as "interpersonally distressed." Numerous studies support the utility of these classifications as they pertain to patient functioning (84,85).

There are a few additional questionnaires available. The Medical Outcomes Study Short Form (SF-36) (86) is another widely used measure of functioning. It allows both mental and physical functioning to be assessed and is an international standard when it comes to the quantification of functioning (87). The SF-36 is brief and available in multiple languages, although it is not specific to chronic pain. There is, however, a modified version, the Treatment Outcomes in Pain Survey (88), specifically for use in pain management settings. The Brief Pain Inventory (89) also offers multiple domains of measurement and is relatively brief. Finally, the Pain Outcomes Questionnaire-VA (POQ-VA) (90) assesses functioning across three major domains (pain quality, emotional functioning, and physical functioning) and is intended to be used at multiple assessment points. The POQ-VA has been successfully used in Veterans' Administration hospitals in the United States (90), and the American Academy of Pain Management is currently examining a slightly modified version of the measure, called the Pain Outcomes Profile, in other settings (91).

Measures Involving Direct Observation

Although directly assessed physical functioning has an intuitive appeal as these sorts of tests theoretically introduce a degree of objectivity into the assessment process, they pose a number of problems as well. First, a number of studies have indicated that measures of strength, endurance, and flexibility have only small relations with many aspects of treatment outcome (49,64,92), including return-to-work rates following treatment (49,93,94). For some measures, there is an absence of information with regard to reliability and validity as well. For example, Functional Capacity Evaluations are intended to assess physical capability for certain intensity levels of work (95); however, there is a notable lack of prospective studies demonstrating their predictive value (79). Therefore, careful selection of measures in this domain is an important consideration in order that treatment outcome results can be most appropriately used and to minimize the possibility of confusion.

As one way of addressing the lack of data surrounding measures of physical functioning, Harding et al. (96) assessed the utility of nine physical measures in a sample of 431 patients with diverse types of chronic pain over the course of an interdisciplinary treatment program for chronic pain. The physical measures were completed at pre- and posttreatment, as well as at 1-month follow-up. Analyses of reliability (i.e., interrater, test–retest), validity (i.e., correlations with various subscales of the SIP), and change over the course of treatment were performed. These researchers recommended four tasks, which were found to be the most useful and psychometrically sound. These measures included a 5-minute timed walk, 1-minute stair climbing task, 1-minute sit-to-stand task, and a timed "arm endurance" task requiring patients to extend both arms horizontally and move them in small circles. A subsequent study by Lee et al. (97) provided further support of the timed walk and sit-to-stand tasks; they did not include the stair climbing and arm endurance task. In our clinical experience, we have found these types of tasks to also be of use in that they are responsive to treatment and are generally related to other measures of patient functioning in expected directions [e.g., (98)].

For low back pain only, another option exists as well. Waddell et al., (99) devised a measure, called the Physical Impairment Scale, which was intended to be a reliable assessment of physical functioning in low back pain patients. The measure uses empirically derived cutoff scores for specific physical tasks and allows the calculation of a total score representing global level of physical impairment. It involves seven separate measures of impairment: four involving flexibility (measured in degrees of movement), two involving strength (measured in endurance time), and one assessing the presence or absence of spinal tenderness over a specific area of the lumbar spine. The measure has adequate interrater reliability (99,100), although the spinal tenderness item has been relatively unreliable, with a $\kappa = 0.35$ (100). Additionally, the scale has proven utility in discriminating individuals with and without chronic low back pain (sensitivity 76%; specificity 86%) and explained significant variance in self-reported disability levels (99). Finally, it has been shown to be responsive to intervention (100,101).

Measures of Vocational Status and Health Care Consumption

Although standardized self-report measures and directly observed physical performance are key methods of assessing functioning, the utility of simple frequency reporting should not be discounted. For instance, asking patients about number of recent pain-related interventions, medical visits, and medication consumption can provide valuable information when it comes to assessing treatment outcome. Some of these measures, such as pain-related medical visits and medication use, can directly translate into cost savings for reimbursement sources if they decrease following treatment. Similarly, improved work status (or school status if more developmentally appropriate) offers an outcome variable that is easily understood by interested third parties (e.g., U.S. Workers' Compensation) and provides clear arguments about cost-effectiveness.

Measures of Treatment Process

A consideration of the process, or processes, by which treatment works is clearly important. If we are able to isolate these factors, it is logical to assume that we can then better target them in treatment, which would theoretically lead to improved outcomes. A full review of possible processes by which treatment succeeds or fails is beyond the scope of the present chapter, although some discussion as it pertains to measure selection seems appropriate.

Many interdisciplinary treatment programs are behavioral or cognitive-behavioral in orientation and although the term "cognitive-behavior therapy" can encompass a variety of treatment approaches (46), there are some common features. The principle commonality pertains to the emphasis placed on thoughts, beliefs, emotions, and other mental processes which are considered to play a contributory role in the development and maintenance of suffering (102–104). This assumption has contributed to a number of programs of research, which generally support the contention that these mental processes are important to consider in any treatment program [see (105) for a review]. Thus, the selection of measures directed at these factors seems important.

Recently, cognitive-behavioral approaches have also contributed to a line of research concerned with methods of undermining the many avoidant behavior patterns that contribute to suffering in chronic pain patients. It seems quite natural for pain sufferers to try and avoid the many inherently distressing aspects of chronic pain. This is just normal human behavior—few people are eager to feel physical or emotional pain. The problem arises, of course, when these patterns of avoidant behavior begin to manifest themselves in other realms, such as social, vocational, and family situations, and subsequently contribute to restrictions in living over the long term. These restrictions seem particularly likely to occur when attempts are made to avoid that which is not avoidable, such as one's own thoughts or previous experience.

Therefore, important processes to target for change in treatment also include variables that maintain avoidance behavior when it contributes to suffering in the long term, as well as methods to reengage patients in the important aspects of functioning that support successful living. Approaches that target these key behavioral processes seek to alter the way that difficult or discouraging thoughts, moods, and sensations influence behavior, which may be particularly important when changing them is not possible or when change attempts contribute to further difficulties or suffering (106). An emerging line of research suggests that it is possible to change how individuals interact with these negatively evaluated "private" (i.e., unobservable) experiences in a more adaptive way, such that emotional, physical, social, and work or school-related functioning is improved (98,107–111). The findings of these longitudinal and treatment outcome studies confirm an ongoing series of cross-sectional analyses as well. For example, numerous studies demonstrate that greater acceptance of chronic pain, a goal-directed, willing, and nonstruggling quality of behavior that occurs while in contact with the pain experience (106,112), is associated with improvements in distress, disability, and overall functioning [see (113) for a review].

PRACTICAL CONSIDERATIONS IN THE ASSESSMENT OF TREATMENT OUTCOME

As noted in the early part of this chapter, our focus is not on large *N* analyses. Rather, we assume that for most clinical practices, there is a need to demonstrate efficacy to a funding body, a set of referrers, or for internal audit, where a relatively smaller number of treatment completers will serve as an adequate sample. When it comes to research project design and analysis of this type, there are a few important points to consider.

The first is timing of assessment. At the very least, assessment should take place before and after treatment—there is a very strong argument for also including at least one later follow-up assessment to demonstrate maintenance of treatment gains. Mean follow-up time from Morley et al. (31) in their meta-analysis was 9 months and Peat et al. (114) suggest a follow-up time of at least 6 months; these seem like reasonable time frames that are achievable.

Second, interpretation of scores can at times be problematic. For example, what does a score of 23 on the BDI actually mean? Few measures have empirically derived cutoff scores or published normative data, although some exceptions do exist, for example, the MPI (82). In our clinical practice, we have attempted to overcome this problem by making use of our previously collected assessment data, which serves as a normative sample. Once this sample has been collected, percentile rankings can be derived and score interpretation is then a simple matter of comparing any given individual score with the percentile distribution (i.e., scores around the 50th percentile are the middle of the distribution, and as scores get further from the middle, they are interpreted as more extreme). This, of course, requires that data be collected for a period of time and entered in to some type of "spreadsheet" program (e.g., Microsoft Excel). When normative data are unavailable and there is no time to collect them, it is also possible to contact publishers of research who have used the measure to inquire whether there is a willingness to share normative information.

Third, with regard to data entry, it is not necessary to buy a sophisticated statistical analysis program. Most of the modern spreadsheet programs are adequate for use as databases. Further, most can perform more simple analyses (such as *t*-tests) and can be imported into the more advanced programs, should that be necessary. At times, statistical analyses are not necessary and simple calculations can be sufficient—for instance, percent of treatment completers returning to work or school, change in percentile rank/percent improvement on measures of distress or disability, and decrease in health-care visits are probably more interesting to quality improvement administrators, third-party payers/referral sources than the results of a *t*-test.

Finally, data analysis can often be an intimidating prospect, particularly if one is not familiar with a particular sort of analysis or software package (or if one is far removed from postgraduate training!). If statistical assistance is necessary, consider teaming up with an interested individual at an academic institution, who will generally be thrilled to have an incoming source of data. It is quite possible to have such teamwork lead to published articles, which are usually to the benefit of both parties. All the authors of this chapter have experience with this type of partnership and, as long as the members of the team can agree upon types and purposes of analyses to be performed, it can be a very satisfying way of working. Given the ease with which information can be transmitted anywhere around the world in the present technological period, it no longer appears necessary that the interested academic be at a local institution, as long as patient privacy and confidentiality can be maintained.[a]

CONCLUSIONS

There is no doubt that interdisciplinary treatment programs for chronic pain are successful for the vast majority of patients; success has been more elusive, however, in areas involving public relations, marketing, and reimbursement. The current economic and health-care environment can seem threatening toward this type of treatment. Therefore, individual treatment programs need to begin to take on the responsibility of demonstrating effectiveness for individual programs as one way of educating the relevant parties involved. The purpose of this chapter is to outline one way in which this issue can be addressed. We have presented an approach to measurement selection that relies on careful consideration of what purposes are being served by assessment and on the selection of appropriate and psychometrically sound measures in order to maximize the amount of useful and accurate information that is obtained. It is our hope that this information will be of use to the many practicing clinicians involved in this important method of treatment so that it can continue to be offered to the individual patients whose lives are so often being adversely affected by the presence of chronic pain.

REFERENCES

1. Turk DC. Clinical effectiveness and cost-effectiveness of treatment for patients with chronic pain. Clin J Pain 2002; 18:355–365.
2. British Pain Society. Recommended guidelines for pain management programmes for adults (Provisional copy). Available at www.britishpainsociety.org/pub_professional.htm#pmp; June 2006. Accessed on Nov 16, 2006.
3. Gatchel RJ, Okifuji A. Evidence-based scientific data documenting the treatment and cost-effectiveness of comprehensive pain programs for chronic nonmalignant pain. J Pain 2006; 7:779–793.
4. Weiner RS. The culture of pain. Am J Pain Manage 1993; 3:201.
5. Turk DC, Burwinkle TM. Clinical outcomes, cost-effectiveness, and the role of psychology in treatment for chronic pain sufferers. Prof Psychol Res Pr 2005; 36:602–610.
6. Flor H, Fydrich T, Turk DC. Efficacy of multidisciplinary pain treatment centers: a meta-analytic review. Pain 1992; 49:221–230.
7. Kee WG, Middaugh S, Pawlick K, et al. Cost benefit analysis of a multidisciplinary chronic pain program. Am J Pain Manage 1997; 7:59–62.
8. Jensen IB, Bergström G, Ljungquist T, et al. A 3-year follow-up of a multidisciplinary rehabilitation programme for back and neck pain. Pain 2005; 115:273–283.

[a] The coeditors of this book have been engaged in just this type of clinical research partnership for over 3 years. While surveying the primary editor's pain program for American Academy of Pain Management Pain Program Accreditation, the second editor worked out an agreement with the program manager to collect data to establish the reliability, validity, and sensitivity of the Pain Outcomes Profile (mentioned earlier in this chapter). So far, over 200 patients' data have been analyzed and the results support the reliability and validity of the POP and the effectiveness of the Pinnacle Health Rehab Options chronic pain management treatment program (115–118).

9. Chapman SL. Chronic pain rehabilitation: lost in a sea of drugs and procedures? Am Pain Soc Bull 2000;10. Available at www.ampainsoc.org/pub/bulletin/may00/clin1.htm. Accessed on November 08, 2006.
10. Sanders SH. Chronic pain rehabilitation: should and can it be saved? Am Pain Soc Bull 2001;11. Available at www.ampainsoc.org/pub/bulletin/mar01/clin1.htm. Accessed on November 08, 2006.
11. Kendall PC, Hollon SD, eds. Assessment Strategies for Cognitive-Behavioral Interventions. New York: Academic press; 1981.
12. Nelson RO, Hayes SC. The nature of behavioral assessment. In: Nelson RO, Hayes SC, eds. Conceptual Foundations of Behavioral Assessment. New York: Guilford; 1986:3–41.
13. Hanley GP, Iwata BA, McCord BE. Functional analysis of problem behavior: a review. J Appl Behav Anal 2003; 36:147–185.
14. Galton F. Co-relations and their measurement, chiefly from anthropometric data. Proc Royal Soc London 1890; 45:135–145.
15. Hawkins RP. Selection of target behaviors. In: Nelson RO, Hayes SC, eds. Conceptual Foundations of Behavioral Assessment. New York: Guilford; 1986:331–385.
16. Eifert GH, Wilson PH. The triple response approach to assessment: a conceptual and methodological reappraisal. Behav Res Ther 1991; 29:283–292.
17. Kazdin AE. Research Design in Clinical Psychology. New York: Harper & Row; 1980.
18. Cone JD. The Behavioral Assessment Grid (BAG): A conceptual framework and a taxonomy. Behav Ther 1978; 9:882–888.
19. Lang PJ. Fear reduction and fear behavior: problems in treating a construct. In: Shilien JM, ed. Research in Psychotherapy, Vol. III. Washington, DC: American Psychological Association; 1968.
20. Mischel W. Personality and Assessment. New York: Wiley; 1968.
21. Beck AT, Ward CH, Mendelson M, et al. An inventory for measuring depression. Arch Gen Psychiatry 1961; 4:561–571.
22. Cronbach LJ. Test validation. In: Thorndike RL, ed. Educational Measurement, 2nd edn. Washington, DC: American Council on Education; pp. 443–507.
23. American Psychological Association, American Educational Research Association, National Council on Measurement in Education. Standards for Educational and Psychological Testing. Washington, DC: American Educational Research Association; 1999.
24. Nunnally JC, Bernstein IH. Psychometric Theory, 3rd edn. New York: McGraw-Hill; 1994.
25. Jensen MP. Questionnaire validation: a brief guide for readers of the research literature. Clin J Pain 2003; 19:345–352.
26. Turk DC, Melzack R. Handbook of pain assessment, 2nd edn. New York: Guildford; 2001.
27. DeGagne TA, MIkail SF, D'Eon JL. Confirmatory factor analysis of a four-factor model of chronic pain evaluation. Pain 1995; 60:195–202.
28. Tait RC, Chibnall JT, Duckro PN, et al. Stable factors in chronic pain. Clin J Pain 1989; 323–328.
29. Williams RC. Toward a set of reliable and valid measures for chronic pain assessment and outcome research. Pain 1988; 35:239–251.
30. Dworkin RH, Turk DC, Farrar JT, et al. Core outcome measures for chronic pain clinical trials: IMMPACT recommendations. Pain 2005; 113:9–19.
31. Morley S, Eccleston C, Williams AC de C. Systematic review and meta-analysis of randomised controlled trials of cognitive behaviour therapy and behaviour therapy for chronic pain in adults, excluding headache. Pain 1999; 80:1–13.
32. Jensen MP, Karoly P. Self-report scales and procedures for assessing pain in adults. In: Turk DC, Melzack R, eds. Handbook of Pain Assessment, 2nd edn. New York: Guilford; 2001:15–34.
33. Jensen MP, Karoly P, Braver S. The measurement of clinical pain intensity: a comparison of six methods. Pain 1986; 27:117–126.

34. Paice JA, Cohen FL. Validity of a verbally administered numeric rating scale to measure cancer pain intensity. Cancer Nurs 1997; 20:88–93.
35. Melzack R. The McGill Pain Questionnaire: major properties and scoring methods. Pain 1975; 1:277–299.
36. Melzack R. The short-form McGill Pain Questionnaire. Pain 1987; 30:191–197.
37. Melzack R, Wall PD. The Challenge of Pain, 2nd edn. London: Penguin; 1996.
38. Melzack R, Katz J. The McGill Pain Questionnaire: Appraisal and current status. In: Turk DC, Melzack R, eds. Handbook of Pain Assessment, 2nd edn. New York: Guilford; 2001:35–52.
39. Robinson ME, Riley JL. The role of emotion in pain. In: Gatchel RJ, Turk DC, eds. Psychosocial Factors in Pain: Critical Perspectives. New York: Guilford; 1999:74–88.
40. Fernandez E. Anxiety, Depression, and Anger in Pain: Research Findings and Clinical Options. Texas: Advanced Psychological Resources; 2002
41. Fishbain DA, Goldberg M, Meagher BR, et al. Male and female chronic pain patients categorized by DSM-III psychiatric diagnostic criteria. Pain 1986; 26:181–187.
42. Pincus T, Morley S. Cognitive processing bias in chronic pain: a review and integration. Psychol Bull 2001; 127:599–617.
43. Pincus T, Williams A. Models and measurements of depression in chronic pain. J Psychosom Res 1999; 47:211–219.
44. Beck AT, Steer RA, Garbin M. Psychometric properties of the Beck Depression Inventory: twenty-five years of evaluation. Clin Psychol Rev 1988; 8:77–100.
45. Novy DM, Nelson DV, Berry LA, et al. What does the Beck Depression Inventory measure in chronic pain? A reappraisal. Pain 1995; 61:261–270.
46. Morley S, Williams AC de C, Black S. A confirmatory factor analysis of the Beck Depression Inventory in chronic pain. Pain 2002; 99:289–298.
47. Geisser ME, Roth RS, Robinson ME. Assessing depression among persons with chronic pain using the Center for Epidemiological Studies-Depression Scale and the Beck Depression Inventory: a comparative analysis. Clin J Pain 1997; 13:163–170.
48. Wilson DG, Mikail SF, D'Eon JL, et al. Alternative diagnostic criteria for major depressive disorder in patients with chronic pain. Pain 2001; 91:227–234.
49. Vowles KE, Gross RT, Sorrell JT. Predicting work status following interdisciplinary treatment for chronic pain. Eur J Pain 2004; 8:351–358.
50. Radloff LS. The CES-D scale: a self-report depression scale for research in general populations. Appl Psychol Meas 1977; 1:385–401.
51. Iverson GL, Remick R. Diagnostic accuracy of the British Columbia Major Depression Inventory. Psychol Rep 2004; 95:1241–1247.
52. Asmundson GJG, Vlaeyen JWS, Crombez G, eds. Understanding and Treating Fear of Pain. Oxford: Oxford University Press; 2004.
53. Asmundson GJG, Norton PJ, Norton GR. Beyond pain: the role of fear and avoidance in chronicity. Clin Psychol Rev 1999; 19:97–119.
54. Vlaeyen JWS, Linton SJ. Fear-avoidance and its consequences in chronic musculoskeletal pain: a state of the art. Pain 1999; 85:317–332.
55. Langdon-Brown W. Fear and pain. Lancet 1935; 226:911–912.
56. McCracken LM, Gross RT, Aikens J, et al. The assessment of anxiety and fear in persons with chronic pain: a comparison of instruments. Behav Res Ther 1996; 34:927–933.
57. McNeil DW, Vowles KE. Assessment of fear and anxiety associated with pain: conceptualization, methods, and measures. In: Asmundson GJG, Vlaeyen JWS, Crombez G, eds. Understanding and Treating Fear of Pain. Oxford: Oxford University Press; 2004; 189–211.
58. McCracken LM, Zayfert C, Gross RT. The pain anxiety symptom scale: development and validation of a scale to measure fear of pain. Pain 1992; 50:67–73.
59. McNeil DW, Rainwater AJ. Development of the Fear of Pain Questionnaire-III. J Behav Med 1998; 21:389–409.

60. Waddell G, Newton M, Henderson I, et al. A Fear-Avoidance Beliefs Questionnaire (FABQ) and the role of fear-avoidance in chronic low back pain and disability. Pain 1993; 52:157–168.
61. Kori SH, Miller RP, Todd DD. Kinisophobia: a new view of chronic pain behavior. Pain Manage 1990; Jan/Feb:35–43.
62. McCracken LM, Dhingra L. A short version of the Pain Anxiety Symptoms Scale (PASS-20): preliminary development and validity. Pain Res Manage 2002; 7:45–50.
63. Roelofs J, McCracken LM, Peters ML, et al. Psychometric evaluation of the Pain Anxiety Symptoms Scale in chronic pain patients. J Behav Med 2004; 27:167–183.
64. McCracken LM, Gross RT, Eccleston C. Multimethod assessment of treatment process in chronic low back pain: comparison of reported pain-related anxiety with directly measured physical capacity. Behav Res Ther 2002; 40:585–594.
65. Vowles KE, Zvolensky MJ, Gross RT, et al. Pain-related anxiety in the prediction of chronic low back pain distress. J Behav Med 2004; 27:77–89.
66. Osman A, Breitenstein JL, Barrios FX, et al. The Fear of Pain Questionnaire-III: further reliability and validity with nonclinical samples. J Behav Med 2002; 25:155–173.
67. Hursey KG, Jacks SD. Fear of pain in recurrent headache suffers. Headache 1992; 32:283–286.
68. Sperry-Clark JA, McNeil DW, Ciano-Federoff L. Assessing chronic pain patients: The Fear of Pain Questionnaire-III. In: VandeCreek L, Jackson TL, eds. Innovations in Clinical Practice: A Source book, Vol. 17. Sarasota, FL: Professional Resource Press; 1999:293–305.
69. McNeil DW, Au AR, Zvolensky MJ, et al. Fear of pain in orofacial pain patients. Pain 2001; 89:245–252.
70. Crombez G, Vlaeyen JWS, Heuts PHTG, et al. Pain-related fear is more disabling than pain itself: evidence on the role of pain-related fear in chronic back pain disability. Pain 1999; 80:329–339.
71. Al-Obaidi SM, Nelson RM, Al-Awadhi S, et al. The role of anticipation and fear of pain in the persistence of avoidance behavior in patients with chronic low back pain. Spine 2000; 25:1126–1131.
72. Ciccone DS, Just N. Pain expectancy and work disability inpatients with acute and chronic pain: a test of the fear avoidance hypothesis. J Pain 2001; 2:181–194.
73. Fritz JM, George SZ. Identifying psychosocial variables in patients with acute work-related low back pain: the importance of fear-avoidance beliefs. Phys Ther 2002; 82:973–983.
74. Vowles KE, Gross RT. Work-related beliefs about injury and physical capability for work in individuals with chronic pain. Pain 2003; 101:291–298.
75. Goubert L, Crombez G, Van Damme S, et al. Confirmatory factor analysis of the Tampa Scale for Kinesiophobia. Clin J Pain 2004; 20:103–110.
76. Cook AJ, Brawer PA, Vowles KE. The fear-avoidance model of chronic pain: validation and age analysis using structural equation modeling. Pain 2006; 121:195–206.
77. Sanders SH, Harden RN, Vicente PJ. Evidence-based clinical practice guidelines for interdisciplinary rehabilitation of chronic nonmalignant pain syndrome patients. Pain Pract 2005; 5:303–315.
78. Bergner M, Bobbitt RA, Carter WB, et al. The Sickness Impact Profile: Development and final revision of a health status measure. Med Care 1981; 29:787–805.
79. Battié MC, May L. Physical and occupational therapy assessment approaches. In: Turk DC, Melzack R, eds. Handbook of Pain Assessment, 2nd edn. New York: Guilford; 2001:204–224.
80. Roland M, Morris R. A study of the natural history of low back pain. Part 1: development of a reliable and sensitive measure of disability in low back pain. Spine 1983; 8:141–144.
81. Jensen MP, Strom SE, Turner JA, et al. Validity of the Sickness Impact Profile Roland Scale as a measure of dysfunction in chronic pain. Pain 1992; 50:157–162.
82. Kerns RD, Turk DC, Rudy TE. The West Have-Yale Multidimensional Pain Inventory (WHYMPI). Pain 1985; 23:345–356.

83. Jacob MC, Kerns RD. Assessment of the psychosocial context of the experience of chronic pain. In: Turk DC, Melzack R, eds. Handbook of Pain Assessment, 2nd edn. New York: Guilford; 2001:362–384.
84. Turk DC, Rudy TE. The robustness of an empirically derived taxonomy of chronic pain patients. Pain 1990; 43:27–36.
85. Turk DC, Rudy TE. Classification logic and strategies in chronic pain. In: Turk DC, Melzack R, eds. Handbook of Pain Assessment. New York: Guilford; 1992:409–428.
86. Ware JE, Sherbourne CD. The MOS 36-item Short-Form Health Survey (SF-36). Med Care 1992; 30:473–481.
87. Bullinger M, Alonso J, Apolone G, et al. Translating health status questionnaires and evaluating their quality: The IQOLA project approach. J Clin Epidemiol 1998; 51:913–923.
88. Rogers WH, Wittink HM, Ashburn MA, et al. Using the "TOPS," an outcomes instrument for multidisciplinary outpatient pain treatment. Pain Med 2000; 1:55–67.
89. Cleeland CS, Ryan KM. Pain assessment: global use of the Brief Pain Inventory. Ann Acad Med 1994; 23:129–138.
90. Clark ME, Gironda RJ, Young JW, Jr. Development and validation of the Pain Outcomes Questionnaire-VA [Electronic version]. J Rehabil Res Dev 2003; 40:381–396.
91. Schatman M, Campbell A. Innovations in outcomes assessment in pain management. Pain Pract 2004; 14:6–8.
92. Burton AK, Tillotson KM, Main CJ, et al. Psychosocial predictors of outcome in acute and subchronic low back trouble. Spine 1995; 20:722–728.
93. Fishbain DA, Rosomoff HL, Goldberg M, et al. The prediction of return to the workplace after multidisciplinary pain center treatment. Clin J Pain 1993; 9:3–15.
94. Hildebrandt J, Pfingsten M, Saur P, et al. Prediction of success from a multidisciplinary treatment program for chronic low back pain. Spine 1997; 22:990–1001.
95. King PM, Tuckwell N, Barrett TE. A critical review of functional capacity evaluations. Phys Ther 1998; 78:852–866.
96. Harding VR, Williams AC de C, Richardson PH, et al. The development of a battery of measures for assessing physical functioning of chronic pain patients. Pain 1994; 58:367–375.
97. Lee CE, Simmonds MJ, Novy DM, et al. Self-reports and clinician-measured physical function among patients with low back pain: a comparison. Arch Phys Med Rehabil 2001; 82:227–231.
98. McCracken LM, Vowles KE, Eccleston C. Acceptance-based treatment for persons with complex, long standing chronic pain: a preliminary analysis of treatment outcome in comparison to a waiting phase. Behav Res Ther 2005; 43:1335–1346.
99. Waddell G, Somerville D, Henderson I, et al. Objective clinical evaluation of physical impairment in chronic low back pain. Spine 1992; 17:617–628.
100. Fritz JM, Piva SR. Physical Impairment Index: reliability, validity, and responsiveness in patients with acute low back pain. Spine 2003; 28:1189–1194.
101. Friedrich M, Gittler G, Halberstadt Y, et al. Combined exercise and motivation program: effect on the compliance and level of disability of patients with chronic low back pain. a randomized controlled trial. Arch Phys Med Rehabil 1998; 79:475–487.
102. Turk DC, Rudy TE. Cognitive factors and persistent pain: a glimpse into Pandora's box. Cognit Ther Res 1992; 16:99–112.
103. Smith TW, Follick MJ, Ahern DL, et al. Cognitive distortion and disability in chronic low back pain. Cognit Ther Res 1986; 10:201–210.
104. Matthews A. Towards an experimental cognitive science of CBT. Behav Ther in press.
105. Keefe FJ, Rumble ME, Scipio CD, et al. Psychological aspects of persistent pain: current state of the science. J Pain 2004; 5:195–211.
106. Hayes SC, Strosahl K, Wilson KG. Acceptance and Commitment Therapy: An Experiential Approach to Behavior Change. New York: Guildford; 1999.
107. Dahl J, Wilson KG, Nilsson A. Acceptance and Commitment Therapy and the treatment of persons at risk for long-term disability resulting from stress and pain symptoms: a preliminary randomized trial. Behav Ther 2004; 35:785–802.

108. Kratz AL, Davis MC, Zautra AJ. Pain acceptance moderates the relation between pain and affect in chronic pain patients. Ann Behav Med in press.
109. McCracken LM, Eccleston C. A prospective study of acceptance of pain and patient functioning with chronic pain. Pain 2005; 8:164–169
110. Vowles KE, McCracken LM, Eccleston C. Processes of behavior change in interdisciplinary treatment of chronic pain: contributions of pain intensity, catastrophizing, and acceptance. Eur J Pain in press.
111. Wicksell RK, Melin L, Olsson GL. Exposure and acceptance in the rehabilitation of adolescents with idiopathic chronic pain—A pilot study. Eur J Pain 11:267–274.
112. McCracken LM. Contextual Cognitive-Behavioral Therapy for Chronic Pain. Seattle, WA: IASP Press; 2005.
113. McCracken LM, Vowles KE. Acceptance of chronic pain. Curr Pain Headache Rep 2006; 10:90–94.
114. Peat GM, Moores L, Goldingay S, et al. Pain management follow-ups. A national survey of current practice in the United Kingdom. J Pain Symptom Manage 2001; 21:218–226.
115. Schatman ME, Campbell A. Innovations in outcomes assessment in pain management. Pain Pract 2004; 14:6–8.
116. Schatman ME, Campbell A. Concurrent validity of the pain and physical interference scales of the Pain Outcomes Profile in chronic spinal pain patients. Presented at North American Spine Society, September 27–October 1, 2005, Philadelphia, PA.
117. Campbell A, Schatman ME. Validation of the Pain Outcomes Profile. Presented at The 16th Annual Clinical Meeting of the American Academy of Pain Management, September 23, 2005, San Diego, CA.
118. Campbell A, Schatman ME. New Information on the Use of the Pain Outcomes Profile. Presented at The 17th Annual Clinical Meeting of the American Academy of Pain Management, September 8, 2006, Orlando, FL.

14 Chronic Pain Management Program Accreditation: Providing Standards for Excellence

Alexandra Campbell
The American Academy of Pain Management, Sonora, California, U.S.A.

PROMOTING EXCELLENCE IN INTERDISCIPLINARY PAIN MANAGEMENT

The American Academy of Pain Management (the Academy) was founded in 1988 as a professional membership organization designed specifically to meet the educational and professional needs of clinicians in the emerging discipline of inter- or multidisciplinary pain management. The Academy accomplishes its goals by offering credentialing of pain treatment professionals (1), continuing education, legislative advocacy, pain facility accreditation, and outcomes tools for documenting pain program success. The Academy has become the largest multidisciplinary pain practitioner membership organization in the United States with nearly 5000 members from many different professional disciplines including medical and osteopathic physicians, chiropractic physicians, podiatrists, dentists, psychologists, social workers, acupuncturists, clergy, nurses, pharmacists, physical and occupational therapists, rehabilitation counselors, massage therapists, and others. As one of the Academy founders (2) stated in 1993

> The multidisciplinary team approach, as it has evolved within the context of contemporary pain management has the unique advantage of overlooking paradigmatic blocks, turf barriers, and linear, restricted vision. The multidisciplinary pain management movement is the harbinger of integrated future health care . . . . (p. 201)

The evidence supporting the clinical success and cost-effectiveness of the integrated multidisciplinary approach to pain management continues to mount (3,4) and is discussed in greater detail in Chapter 2 in this volume. The Academy has demonstrated leadership in bringing this approach to the forefront of pain treatment strategies through its approach to pain program accreditation (PPA).

PAIN PROGRAM ACCREDITATION

PPA was created in 1992 (5). Numerous drafts of the accreditation manual and application were scrutinized and refined by the contributions of many clinical and academic professionals through a survey of Academy members conducted by Old Dominion University College of Business and Public Administration, the University of the Pacific School of Pharmacy and the Academy. At the same time, the creation of a National Pain Data Bank (NPDB) was announced for the collection and processing of pain management outcomes information. Credentialed pain professionals located across the country were recruited to receive training in the on-site facility survey process. During the one-day review process, these surveyors are dedicated to helping pain programs "raise the bar" for quality pain management.

The Joint Commission on Accreditation of Healthcare Organizations (JCAHO) adopted standards addressing pain assessment and treatment in 2001 (6), and the Commission on Accreditation of Rehabilitation Facilities (CARF) (7) also incorporates principles of the interdisciplinary approach to pain treatment in their accreditation standards. JCAHO has published valuable resources regarding the improvement of pain management activities in institutional settings (8,9). While JCAHO accredits hospitals and CARF accredits rehabilitative pain programs with specific staffing requirements, the Academy provides accreditation for both large comprehensive multidisciplinary treatment programs and for pain management programs offered by smaller networks of solo practitioners and even for syndrome- or modality-oriented clinics as long as they practice in an interdisciplinary fashion through a well-documented referral process.

One purpose of accreditation through the Academy is to establish credibility for a pain program by demonstrating that patients receive appropriate multidisciplinary services in a safe and effective fashion. PPA standards focus on an organization's ongoing business and personnel management, the physical plant (with an emphasis on safety), and on the clinical services provided to patients. Much of the following material appears in the Academy's Pain Program Accreditation Manual (10) and in three articles (11–13) that are posted on the Academy's Web site.

Two major distinctions are made in the PPA standards. There are *nonclinical standards* and *general clinical standards*, which must be met by all programs, and there are different *classification-specific standards* for specific program models.

NONCLINICAL ACCREDITATION STANDARDS

There are five *nonclinical standards* concerning the organization's purpose and operation. These standards require a mission statement describing the purpose of the organization and the services available; written policies describing the types of patients served and/or the types of conditions addressed; specifically defined (even if broadly) inclusion and exclusion criteria for services (not based on sex, race, color, creed, religion, or national origin); patient education, informational and marketing materials that truthfully describe the personnel, program, and services provided; and practitioners who possess the appropriate training and experience to provide quality treatment.

The intent of the first five standards is to establish a commitment to pain management, to provide services in an ethical manner, and to provide services within a consistent model. When surveying a program, onsite reviewers look for the presence of a mission statement, code of ethics, and patient bill of rights; read written policies about the services provided, patients, or conditions treated; check the truthfulness of marketing and educational materials; check to see if there is evidence of appropriate training and experience for the program pain professionals (usually by reviewing personnel files); and that the program director has the requisite skills to lead a multidisciplinary team. If appropriate, materials for special populations need to be made available to patients (e.g., non-English speaking, visually/hearing challenged). Since the Health Insurance Portability and Accountability Act of 1996

(HIPAA) (14) was signed into law and portions of this law became enforceable in April 2003 (Privacy Rule) and October 2003 (Transactions and Code Sets Rule), pain programs are now asked if they are HIPAA compliant. The surveyor records the answer given by the facility and may look for a Notice of Privacy Policies, but accreditation by the Academy does *not* certify HIPAA compliance. All programs are expected to abide by any and all federal and state/local laws that apply to them. The Academy provides all surveyed facilities with a written notice stating that it abides by HIPAA rules in its dealings with surveyed pain programs and will sign business associate contracts if necessary.

Five more *nonclinical standards* are in place to assess the business practices of the program. These documentation standards require that written administrative and patient-care policies that are reviewed and updated annually; necessary legal documents to engage in practice are available for review; proof of general liability insurance exists for the facility; and that proof of professional liability insurance for all licensed personnel similarly is present. Reviewers determine that the administrative and patient-care policies for the day-to-day operation of the program are adequate, and then check for creation and review dates. Having a system in place to document that staff annually reviews policies and procedures is crucial, in addition to circulating and documenting review of any new policies and procedures that may be instituted between regular annual reviews. See Chapter 12 in this volume for more detailed information on the complexities involved in creating excellent policies and procedures. The exact content of the administrative and patient-care policies is not mandated by PPA in order to allow each unique program the opportunity to develop the policies needed to operate optimally. Surveyors check for current business licenses, certificates of occupancy, Fire Marshall Inspection certificates, professional licenses, and similar documents. Insurance certificates are screened for general liability, Directors and Officers insurance, and professional liability. The intent of this section is to determine whether the pain program is operating lawfully and that adequate patient and staff safeguards exist. Specific insurance limit recommendations are not made, other than regarding professional liability (recommend minimum $500,000/$1,000,000). The reviewer takes into account local variations in the business climate that may affect the types and amounts of insurance policies maintained by the program and its personnel.

Personnel management standards require that there are detailed and specific job descriptions for employees and independent contractors; annual performance evaluations reflecting the job-specific descriptions; written personnel policy; and properly maintained unique personnel files for each employee and independent contractor demonstrating the necessary education, experience, and skills required for work. Surveyors review personnel files to determine whether job-specific descriptions and annual reviews exist for all employees and independent contractors.

Surveyors determine that these descriptions have been updated within the past year. Job descriptions need to be current with respect to duties to accurately reflect performance. Surveyors review personnel files looking for up-to-date resumes or curricula vitae, copies of licenses, documentation of training, and diplomas. To understand employee and employer expectations, surveyors read the program's personnel policy manual. Procedures for resolving grievances, dress codes, duty hours, and assignments are examples of what the standards require. Employee orientation to workplace regulations needs to be documented and should include employees' signatures. Annual documentation of review of personnel policies by all employees is ideal.

Surveyors tour the building and all clinical treatment areas to make a determination about patient and staff safety. The physical plant standards require that the facility (1) be safe for patients and staff by meeting applicable OSHA requirements; (2) is compliant with local codes regarding access for challenged patients consistent with the ADA; (3) has adequate ventilation and is maintained at a comfortable temperature; (4) has written annually updated policies describing the proper handling of waste and the proper handling, storage, and disposal of medications, needles, and soiled linen; (5) maintains electrical equipment free of obvious hazards; (6) has emergency exits that are clearly marked and free of obstructions; (7) has adequate regular and handicapped parking available; (8) has an operating fire detection, warning, and suppression system; (9) has written policies about fire drills and expected employee actions in the event of fire or other emergency situations (e.g., natural disaster, terrorist attack); and (10) complies with local fire codes. Evidence that fire drills and other simulated emergency evacuations are carried out at least annually is important to maintain on file. On-site reviewers must walk throughout the building to determine the overall level of cleanliness; ability of challenged patients to get around in the office; appropriateness of ventilation; and observance of policies about hazardous waste management. Reviewers are asked to imagine themselves in the office during different types of emergency situations including possible natural disasters or terrorist attacks. Could employees and patients get out of the building without assistance? If they had physical or mental challenges, could they still get out of the building? Seeing a current Fire Marshall certificate or similar document usually resolves the issue about compliance with local fire codes. Reviewers want to see smoke detectors, fire extinguishers, and sprinkler systems if required by local codes. Reviewers do not test these items, although they determine whether they are available with inspection dates recorded.

Some may wonder why there are so many standards having little to do with actual patient care. These *nonclinical standards* support ethical business practices, efficiency of practice, and the health, safety, and welfare of employees and patients. Standards have evolved over many years and have been tailored to meet the needs of pain practitioners in a wide variety of practice situations. While many are very specific, some require the judgment of the surveyor to determine compliance. It is the goal of the Academy to improve the programs being surveyed and to provide consultative advice during the accreditation survey process. Rather than merely question the programs and their staff, PPA surveyors strive to gradually raise the overall quality of pain management services in the United States through a collegial process.

GENERAL CLINICAL ACCREDITATION STANDARDS

The NIH Consensus Conference entitled "The Integrated Approach to the Management of Pain" (15) concluded that while there are a multitude of pharmacological and nonpharmacological treatment approaches for pain, "no single treatment modality is appropriate for all or even for most individuals suffering from pain" (p. 12). Hence, the Academy's program standards do not dictate which specific modalities must be present in a treatment program. Typically, though, multi- or interdisciplinary approaches usually incorporate pharmacological, psychological/behavioral, and physical/rehabilitative components, with interventional/surgical and complementary nonallopathic methods (such as acupuncture and massage) possibly being present as well (16). Many published evidence-based guidelines exist that outline standards of treatment for various chronic pain conditions (17,18). These clinical guidelines should be consulted and updates regularly monitored so that appropriate treatment standards are maintained over the years that a pain program is in operation.

In their 2003 survey of the most commonly used techniques for the treatment of chronic pain, Marketdata Enterprises (19) noted a somewhat disturbing trend: the use of nerve blocks increased from 79% of pain practices surveyed in 2001 to 82% in 2003, while physical therapy use dropped from 85% in 2001 to 71% of programs in 2003. The multidisciplinary approach also declined in use from 81% of programs in 2001 to 77% in 2003. This occurred despite the availability of evidence that questions the efficacy of exclusively interventionalist pain-relief strategies and that supports the use of the multidisciplinary approach (20–23), especially when longstanding chronic pain of uncertain pathophysiology is present. Reasons for this alarming reversal of the trend to establish multi- or interdisciplinary pain care include reimbursement issues and economic pressures. See Chapters 2, 3, and 10 in this volume for further in-depth analysis of these problems.

General clinical standards address the core elements of patient care necessary for all pain programs. During an on-site inspection for PPA, after touring the facility and addressing the nonclinical issues, the reviewer focuses on the scope and quality of care being provided. Reviewers will want to know the schedule of team meetings. Usually the facility staff tries to schedule a team meeting for the day of the survey, allowing the reviewer to observe the team operating and interviewing each treatment provider and administrative staff person briefly and informally, to get a sense of how they view the workings of the program. Meeting with individual treatment team members gives the surveyor a chance to assess how the program actually functions on a day-to-day basis. If patients provide permission, the surveyor may speak to one or two of them in order to obtain their impressions of the program. Sometimes staff will provide useful feedback for improving the program that they have not yet had a chance to communicate to management. The surveyor may then share the suggestions for change with upper management during the outbriefing at the end of the survey day. This important meeting also gives the surveyor the chance to communicate the strengths of the program and very often functions as a staff morale booster, increasing the cohesiveness of the team and providing the treatment team as a whole with a set of improvement goals for which to aim.

The chart review is another crucial element of program evaluation. The reviewer needs to examine a sufficient number of clinical records to adequately address the 20 general clinical standards. Usually, at least 10 randomly chosen clinical records, representing both open and closed cases, are reviewed in order to answer the questions raised in the general clinical standards. If full compliance with the general clinical standards is not immediately evident, the reviewer examines five additional records (or more) to resolve his or her concerns. Reviewers may ask the facility representative to show them where in the chart necessary documentation exists that demonstrates how the program is able to meet the general clinical standards. The reviewer notes how many of the charts that are reviewed are in compliance with the standards, and how many are missing required elements.

Necessary elements of the chart include the presence of a well-documented presenting problem with a thorough history and physical. If the referring physician has already done this thorough history and physical, with a more focused problem-oriented assessment done upon admission to the pain program, a copy of the more thorough examination report needs to be obtained by the program.

The needs of the whole patient should be addressed during the initial assessment process and should be verified through adequate documentation of functional and psychosocial status. Patient interviews, examinations, diagnostic laboratory tests, and scores on validated psychosocial assessment instruments should be used to develop a multidimensional conceptualization of the biopsychosocial processes that are contributing to the patient's pain problem. Individualized assessments by providers from different disciplines (when indicated) need to be clearly formulated with working diagnoses and signed notes. Initial therapeutic goals should be formulated in clearly behavioral and specific terms in a treatment plan which the patient agrees to and signs. Over time, charting should reflect progress toward these goals and/or adjustment of the goals themselves. At admission, a discharge plan with measurable goals should be formulated, thereby allowing for the more objective assessment of progress. Expected time frames for improvement and the method for evaluating treatment progress should be clearly spelled out from the beginning of treatment.

All charts need to contain an area for consultations, reports, and results of laboratory tests in addition to ongoing treatment notes from all treatment providers that discuss the relevant clinical information. Written evidence that the different treatment providers within and outside of the facility (as when referrals are made) communicate with each other is a critical charting element. Particularly when invasive procedures are used, documentation of pain levels pre- and postprocedure through the use of a verbal or numerical rating scale provides basic outcomes information. A discharge summary documents the patients' strengths and weaknesses at the time when the bulk of treatment has been delivered and describes any specific limitations and recommendations for activity levels, employment, diet, etc. Referrals to appropriate after-care or follow-up services should be documented. Some programs follow patients indefinitely and do not have clear discharge dates. If patients continue to be seen on a maintenance follow-up basis (e.g., to prevent relapse of chronic pain behaviors), this needs to be appropriately documented as well. Many programs have found it useful to designate a patient as a "program" patient during an initial period of more intensive interdisciplinary treatment, and later, after a significant portion of the expected degree of improvement in pain and functioning has been accomplished, the patient is converted to "clinic" patient status for follow-up medication management or cognitive-behavioral "booster" individual or group support sessions. The patient can be reconverted to "program" status should a major flare-up occur or a new pain problem arise. The documented designation as "program" or "clinic" patient can serve as a cue to all team members to step-up or step-down treatment intensity and documentation and team meeting requirements.

A general consent form for the patient to be treated in the program, in addition to specific consent forms for individual procedures, is required, primarily for the legal protection of the program. The general consent covers the patient who is going through the evaluation process and may have to attend several appointments before a complete treatment plan is generated and initiated. It is also necessary to have unique consent forms for every type of invasive/surgical procedure that patients may receive and which name the procedure, the person performing the procedure, and state that no specific guarantees are being made to the patient about the outcome of the procedure. The patient's name should appear on the consent form and their signature confirms that the patient has been informed of the common risks and benefits of the procedure, has been informed of any treatment alternatives that may be available, and that all of the patient's questions regarding the procedure have been answered to his or her satisfaction. The Academy recommends that all of a patient's questions and the answers given be documented in order to provide extra legal protection for treatment providers. The patient needs to be further informed that consent may be revoked at any time.

Medical Release of Information forms should be specific as to the purpose of the disclosure and be time limited, with separate releases (even if on the same form) for treatment-related information pertaining to mental-health services, substance abuse treatment information, and HIV status. Printed patient materials that explain financial responsibilities and how third-party payers are handled can be helpful in making billing policies clear, especially for those programs in which self-payment may constitute a significant proportion of program revenues.

Provision needs to be made for the secure storage of medical records, preferably in a centralized location. Access to paper or electronic medical records needs to be restricted to appropriate staff, and there should be a designated person who is responsible for maintaining and securing all medical records on a continual basis. HIPAA guidelines give specific recommendations for record and computer security, and these must be followed.

The importance of having a practical, consistent format for the organization of the medical chart cannot be underestimated. The medical record basically "tells the story" of a patient's journey through the treatment program, and it should be able to be understood by the surveyor with little or no direction from staff. Clearly labeled chart tab dividers that separate elements of the chart are commonly used. A system for alerting providers to the presence of any known allergies should be conspicuous. An alert sticker should be placed on the outside of the chart, with the specific allergies listed on the inside cover, in line with health information privacy requirements.

The chart review is not intended to be an onerous process. It is a practical review of treatment records, looking for the elements necessary to accomplish the assessment, complete evaluation, and appropriate treatment of the patient with pain. Obtaining informed consent, permission to release medical records to outside entities, and establishing goals for treatment with the patient are required elements for any successful program.

Several accreditation standards cannot usually be answered in the clinical records, but can be resolved through the examination of other materials. Specialized treatment equipment and all necessary emergency equipment need to be regularly checked and certified by the appropriate state or local authority. Documentation of the certifications may be kept in an easily accessible logbook. 510(k) documents for certain medical devices must also be on file. Documentation that staff has the ongoing training necessary to operate the equipment is necessary (this may be accomplished through training logs and training certificates kept in personnel files).

The final general clinical standard that is applicable to all pain programs addresses the need for the facility to be utilizing some type of outcomes measurement strategy. As this is such an important topic, it will be covered thoroughly later in this chapter.

CLASSIFICATION-SPECIFIC ACCREDITATION STANDARDS

The unique standards for each of the distinct classification types of pain programs will now be discussed. To explain the need for the *classification-specific standards*, a review of the Academy's organizational history regarding accreditation is in order.

Years ago, the leadership of the Academy decided to offer program accreditation to many types and sizes of pain programs, using different designations depending on the type and scope of services offered. It was determined not to be in the interest of the field of pain management, or to the patients served, to exclude any program that was interested in becoming accredited. Instead of only accrediting the larger university and hospital-based programs, the Academy developed a methodology to allow all pain programs to apply for accreditation, whether they were inpatient or outpatient, large or small, or involved only a single practitioner, syndrome, or treatment modality. To meet the diverse needs of the Academy's membership and to be able to provide patient safeguards through the accreditation process, six types of pain programs were identified: major comprehensive multidisciplinary, comprehensive, small, and network multidisciplinary, and syndrome- and modality-oriented. [International Association for the Study of Pain definitions for pain center classification (24) is somewhat different than those of the Academy.]

Each classification of pain program was developed based on specific standards. The most detailed standards were written for the three largest and most complex types of programs. For smaller programs, realistic standards were written in order to motivate solo practitioners and practitioners in syndrome- or modality-oriented programs to address the multidisciplinary needs of patients. A detailed definition of each type of program classification is as follows:

- Major comprehensive multidisciplinary pain program manages various types of painful conditions, conducts education and/or research programs, and involves a minimum of six disciplines operating within the same organization.
- Comprehensive multidisciplinary pain program manages various types of painful conditions, may conduct educational or research programs, and involves a minimum of four disciplines operating within the same organization.
- Small multidisciplinary pain program manages various types of pain conditions and involves a minimum of two disciplines operating within the same organization. It uses consultation and referral as necessary.
- Network multidisciplinary pain program generally involves a solo practitioner or group of clinicians, all of the same discipline, who manage various types of pain conditions by using a network of closely coordinated independent professionals of varying disciplines.

- Syndrome-oriented pain program manages a single type of pain syndrome (e.g., back pain, complex regional pain syndrome, headache, temporomandibular joint dysfunction) using one or more clinicians of the same or different disciplines. It uses consultation and referral as necessary.
- Modality-oriented pain program manages one or more pain syndromes by using a single modality (e.g., acupuncture, biofeedback, counseling, hypnosis, nerve blocks, or transcutaneous electrical nerve stimulation). It uses consultation and referral as necessary.

Unlike CARF (7) accreditation, which requires that all applicant programs have a board-certified medical director and a psychologist on staff, the Academy's system accepts applications from programs that are headed by a qualified multidisciplinary pain practitioner from other disciplines. The Academy will accredit smaller syndrome- or modality-oriented programs provided that the multi- or interdisciplinary treatment philosophy can be demonstrated through appropriate consultation and referral which is adequately documented. The Academy's flexibility regarding program models, affordability of accreditation, orientation toward customer service, and long-term partnerships with accredited programs may partially explain why the number of programs increased by 32% between 2004 and 2006 (from 38 to 50 programs). On the other hand, the number of CARF accredited pain programs dropped by 60% between 1998 and 2005 (from 210 to 84 programs) (25).

MAJOR COMPREHENSIVE, COMPREHENSIVE, AND SMALL MULTIDISCIPLINARY CLINICAL ACCREDITATION STANDARDS

Major comprehensive, comprehensive, and small multidisciplinary programs have the same *classification-specific standards*. Organizational requirements address the purpose and business structure of these larger programs. Documentation of the structure of the governing body, usually in the form of a clear organizational chart, is very helpful to the surveyor, as he or she needs to quickly grasp the lines of communication and authority that exist. This chart should be made available to key employees as well. Minutes of the governing body's meetings should be kept along with a written policy that describes how authority is delegated throughout the organization. Documentation demonstrating commitment to principles of ethical leadership, how policies are determined, and institutional commitment to high-quality patient care are minimal elements that the surveyor will want to ascertain are in place through discussion or viewing of relevant documents. Corporations need to have a written job description for the Chief Executive Officer (CEO) detailing the authority and responsibilities delegated to the CEO by the governing body. The CEO's performance should be evaluated annually by the governing body.

Documentation of the business operations of the larger multidisciplinary programs needs to demonstrate that the financial affairs of the organization are managed on the basis of an annual budget that is approved by the governing body. Evidence of adequate communication between key administrative staff members should be present and may take the form of interoffice memoranda or e-mail, for example.

Clinical operations of large multidisciplinary programs can be complex, but if well thought out policies and procedures are in place and clear to all staff, even the largest programs can operate quite smoothly and efficiently. During the on-site survey, the reviewer will request access to written documentation that identifies a case manager or their equivalent for every client/patient in order to coordinate true interdisciplinary care. Sometimes this is the primary treatment provider and some programs use a patient-care coordinator instead of a nurse case manager. With PPA, there is flexibility regarding this issue and other clinical standards. What is necessary is that the program has an effective way of accomplishing its mission to provide integrated multidisciplinary pain care and that this is clear to the reviewer. Chart notes reflecting that all patients are properly oriented to the program need to be in evidence in addition to documentation of a coordinated team approach to treatment.

Documentation of meetings and case management chart notes indicating how treatment goals are updated and modified by the team and communicated to the patient (with their input and agreement) must be present. Staffings need to take place not less than weekly for clients in daily treatment programs. The case manager is responsible for ensuring that the necessary communication between practitioners takes place, and there needs to be a provider designated to make any final treatment decisions, especially when there is disagreement between practitioners about how to proceed. Documentation needs to demonstrate that care is coordinated. Case conferences address goal setting, discharge planning, ongoing patient care, and modifications to the treatment plan. Tracking and modification of goals (with patient input) must be obvious in the chart. The case manager (or other designee) is also responsible for ensuring appropriate and timely communication between the program and the patient's employer if necessary, with accurate and timely documentation of these contacts and any work-related goals present in the chart. The final duty of the case manager (or other designee) is to ensure that adequate plans are made for discharge. Follow-up appointments, any home-based services needed, along with recommendations and limitations should be documented and present in the discharge summary.

As mentioned above in the section on *nonclinical* accreditation standards, if a major comprehensive, comprehensive, or small multidisciplinary program uses regular consultants or independent contractors to accomplish any treatment components, written agreements between the program director and the consultants/contractors that describe the specific duties and responsibilities of the nonstaff team members should be present. The length of time for which the agreement is in effect should be specified, thereby allowing the agreement to be reviewed and updated regularly. A personnel file should include this agreement, a copy of the consultant/contractor's license to practice, and any other documentation necessary (e.g., DEA certificate, pharmacy registration) for practice in addition to evidence of malpractice insurance in adequate amounts. An annual performance review for the independent contractor or consultant will help ensure that high standards of care are being upheld and will alert management when there is a need to consider altering or ending the relationship.

NETWORK MULTIDISCIPLINARY CLINICAL ACCREDITATION STANDARDS

Network multidisciplinary programs consist of groups of independent practitioners working together in a community to provide interdisciplinary pain care. In most instances, a solo-practice clinician provides leadership for a network multidisciplinary program. This clinician often carries the dual responsibilities of administration and patient care. It is desirable for network multidisciplinary pain program services to be provided by a coordinated interdisciplinary team; however, it is not required that the program actually employs all of the treatment team members. In most network multidisciplinary pain programs, it is common that the other team members are serving as consultants to, or independent contractors for, the primary practitioner providing care. In this case, the standard regarding personnel management for independent contractors described above would apply to this type of program as well.

Organizational and business operation standards for network multidisciplinary and syndrome- or modality-oriented programs are quite similar and are in place to ensure adequate documentation of the governing body or owner/operator's policies and procedures regarding delegation of authority, commitment to ethical leadership, establishment of policy, and maintenance of high-quality patient care. The governing body or person should operate with an annual budget, and communication needs to be adequate between the treatment team members and support staff (usually through documented phone contact, e-mail, and interoffice memoranda).

Clinical standards include documentation of patient orientation and, most importantly, there should be at least monthly treatment conferences (weekly, if possible) attended by team members caring for active patients engaged in regular (possibly daily) treatment. Since this ideal is not always attainable when practitioners do not work in close proximity to each other, telephone contact and other means of communication and record sharing may sometimes have to suffice. Network multidisciplinary programs have to be able to demonstrate to the reviewer that communication between team members occurs and that the documentation of this communication is sufficient to provide truly integrated care. Patients may or may not be involved in the team meetings, and the documentation of the team meetings should be the responsibility of a designated staff member. A central chart needs to demonstrate that individual case management reflects input from the team members and the patient regarding goal setting, discharge planning, patient education, and the modification of goals as treatment progresses.

Like the spokes on a wheel connected to a central hub, the members of a network multidisciplinary pain treatment team have to be strongly connected, in terms of treatment philosophy and communication, to the clinical/administrative center even though they may be located physically at some distance. This innovative practice model may turn out to be one of the more cost-effective program structures.

SYNDROME- AND MODALITY-ORIENTED CLINICAL ACCREDITATION STANDARDS

A solo-practice clinician, carrying the dual responsibilities of administration and patient care, also usually operates syndrome- or modality-oriented pain programs. With respect to patient care, the clinician carries the responsibility for obtaining consultations or referrals when services required by the patient are outside the scope of the clinician's training and experience, and for coordinating these referrals and consultations to effect, as much as possible, a multi- or interdisciplinary treatment approach. Again, in terms of personnel management, consultant agreements are a critical component for the success of this type of program and allow for owner/operator monitoring and quality control.

The syndrome- and modality-oriented program standards covering organization, business practices, and clinical operations are similar to those discussed in the section above for network multidisciplinary programs. In addition, there needs to be evidence that the primary treatment provider makes the necessary referrals and/or seeks consultation when it is clear from the assessment that the patient will benefit from integrated multidisciplinary pain management services outside the scope of training or practical limitation of the primary provider. There should be close communication between the primary provider and any outside consultants and treating providers. This communication must be evident in the medical record, especially in terms of setting and modifying treatment goals.

OUTCOMES MEASUREMENT AND PERFORMANCE IMPROVEMENT

Defining, measuring, and disseminating relevant treatment outcomes information is something even the smallest pain program must do in order to remain viable in today's health-care climate of increased demand for evidence-based practice and cost-containment accountability. Patients, payers, and providers are all stakeholders in the pain management process and are looking for results in terms of specific outcomes variables that are important to them. Reduced pain, functional recovery, reduced need for medication, improved quality of life, and patient satisfaction with treatment are important to patients and providers. Providers, employers, and insurance companies are interested in functional rehabilitation (as evidenced, for example, by return to work) and containing the cost of treatment (as evidenced by settled disability claims and reduced health-care utilization) (20). Every pain management program needs to use outcomes measurement to improve performance and address the needs of stakeholders or it risks losing patients. Programs that successfully use outcomes measurement results in marketing efforts should be more likely to achieve financial profitability. Both JCAHO and CARF have outcomes measurement requirements for the hospitals and pain programs they accredit. The Wisconsin Resource Manual (26), entitled *Building an Institutional Commitment to Pain Management*, outlines the steps necessary to improve pain management in different types of health-care settings based on guidelines published by the Agency for Healthcare Research and Quality (27) and the American Pain Society (28).

Since the Academy accredits different classifications of pain programs, the requirement for outcomes measurement must be realistically assessed within the context of the type of program being reviewed. The goal of adequately assessing treatment success and using the information gained through tracking outcomes to impact treatment quality is best viewed as being on a continuum. This continuum ranges from the use of lengthy, comprehensive multidimensional outcomes assessment instruments or batteries of instruments, to the use of a simple numerical rating scale of pain intensity (obtained whenever the patient is seen or before and after invasive procedures) along with a brief, comprehensive tool that assesses at least the most important aspects of function. Only the larger, comprehensive multidisciplinary pain management programs may have the financial resources and manpower available to employ the more lengthy outcomes measurement systems. However, even smaller programs can be minimally expected to use a brief yet fairly comprehensive system. The Academy's goal is to help all pain programs, regardless of type or size, "raise the bar" for quality care through effectively utilizing multimodal outcomes assessment tools and adequate dissemination techniques. The information gained must be useful to all stakeholders including patients, providers, and payers, and be presented in a clear, concise, understandable format.

In spite of the obvious need for publishable outcomes measurement information to help pain programs continue to exist, the market survey of chronic pain management programs cited above (18) contains a shocking finding. The percentage of pain programs that claimed they could document outcomes data declined from 67% in 2001 to 59% in 2003. The author stated that the main reason for the decline may be an increase in the number of solo anesthesiologists practicing pain management. While 87% of true multidisciplinary pain programs could document outcomes in 2003, only 40% of anesthesia-based intervention-oriented programs could do so. This represents a decline from 1999, when fully 77% of all pain programs surveyed reported that they could document outcomes data. This trend must be reversed for the field of pain management to remain at the forefront of the integrated health-care movement and to continue in its leadership role for the rest of the health-care industry. See Chapter 13 in this volume for a more in-depth discussion of the importance of quality assurance and outcomes assessment in pain management.

The NPDB outcomes measurement system was established by the Academy in the early 1990s, as national policy makers began insisting on the use of standardized outcomes measurement approaches to assess the quality of health care. Use of the NPDB was made a requirement for the Academy's PPA in 1992. The purpose of the NPDB (which included intake, discharge, and follow-up questionnaires) was to provide comparison benchmarks for successful treatment outcomes that could be used by the solo practitioner as well as by the large multidisciplinary treatment program. The NPDB became an important tool in helping pain management programs comply with pain outcomes measurement standards imposed by national accrediting agencies (29). Several reliability and validity studies were conducted that demonstrated adequate psychometric properties of select subscales of the NPDB (30,31). Unfortunately, a major drawback to the use of the NPDB was its length (64 items). Smaller pain programs and solo practitioners found it challenging to allocate the staff for its proper administration, while others were limited by budgetary constraints. In 2001, the mandatory use of the NPDB was removed from the accreditation requirements, and the data bank program was retired in early 2007. Programs are now free to create their own outcomes measurement systems using instruments deemed appropriate for particular practice settings. As discussed above, the decline in the number of practitioners who are incorporating outcomes measures into their pain practices may be due to a lack of clinically useful, validated, *brief, and comprehensive* outcomes measures. In response to the different service delivery models current in the field of pain management, the Academy has published a new brief outcomes measurement tool in an attempt to meet the needs of different types of pain programs.

THE PAIN OUTCOMES PROFILE

Psychometric analysis of certain items from the NPDB revealed those which had the greatest psychometric strength (32). Weaker items were eliminated and several new questions were added to create a brief pain outcomes measurement instrument that the Academy has published under the title "Pain Outcomes Profile" (POP) (33).

The POP is a 20-item self-report questionnaire that uses 11-point, 0 to 10, numerical rating scales to assess a number of relevant dimensions in the pain patient's experience. The POP assesses three domains of a patient's pain experience: pain perception, perceived physical impairment due to pain, and several aspects of emotional functioning. These domains are assessed using two pain intensity scales, three self-report of functional impairment scales, and two scales that address self-reported emotional functioning (resulting in a total of seven scales).

The POP includes 18 items to assess functional outcomes, in addition to two numerical rating scales to assess the patient's experience of *pain intensity right now* and *pain on the average during the last week*. Items on the POP are ordered so that questions from the different content scales appear in a counterbalanced fashion.

There are three scales in the domain of perceived functional impairment due to pain: *mobility*, *activities of daily living* (ADLs), and *vitality*. The *mobility* scale contains four items that rate a patient's perception of pain-related interference with the ability to walk, carry, or handle everyday objects, climb stairs, and the pain-related need for assistive devices (e.g., a walking aid or wheelchair). *ADLs* are assessed with four items that inquire about pain-related interference with the ability to bathe, dress, use the bathroom, and manage personal grooming. The patient's subjective feeling of a lack of *vitality* is assessed with three items rating the ability to perform physical activities, feelings of overall energy, and strength and endurance. Self-reported emotional functioning is assessed with two scales. The *negative affect* scale contains five items asking the patient to rate the degree to which pain affects self-esteem, feelings of depression, feelings of anxiety, ability to concentrate, and feelings of subjective tension. The *fear* scale contains two items that rate how concerned a patient is regarding reinjury due to increasing activity and feelings of safety associated with exercising.

The POP is quickly scored and a cumulative patient scoring record may be placed in the chart. This form allows for tracking of POP scale scores across repeated administrations of the measure (e.g., at intake, several times during active treatment, at discharge).

While not a complete outcomes measurement system, the POP does provide for the assessment of five core functional pain outcomes domains that are of interest to patients, providers, and payers. Other important outcomes that should be assessed include patient satisfaction, disability/litigation status, and medical resource utilization.

POP scores and scores on the other important outcomes variables may be placed into a computer database or even a spreadsheet program such as Excel. Administrative staff should be able to perform at least basic tabulations of changes in scores from the beginning to the end of treatment. Benchmarking outcomes against one's own previous performance by aggregating data for clinically/diagnostically defined subgroups of patients can provide a pain program with a sense of whether clinical quality improvement is occurring over time.

Clark et al. (32) traced the development of the POP (entitled the Pain Outcomes Questionnaire in the VA setting) in a 5-year, cooperative VA Academy project that originated with the NPDB long forms. They concluded that the new brief instrument is reliable, valid, and clinically useful in evaluating the effectiveness of treatment for veterans experiencing chronic noncancer pain. Additional research needs to be completed to validate the measure in different populations of patients with various types of pain diagnoses. The future of multidisciplinary pain management depends on the ability to provide the best combination of treatments for the proper duration and intensity to obtain the most cost-effective results with subgroups of patients (34). The Academy is currently partnering with several independent pain programs across the country (35) and has gathered data to further document the reliability, validity, and sensitivity of the POP (36–38), and to help programs using the POP document and publish treatment successes. In the future, norms should be established with different patient samples. The POP has been translated into Spanish and is available for field testing and research with a Spanish-speaking population.

With the coming shift toward a "person-centered" health system (39), the twenty-first century will hopefully see a much better educated public taking a greater role in health-care decisions, practicing more effective health maintenance behaviors, and gaining a better understanding of health-care financing. As patients become more sophisticated in terms of managing their personal health information, they will begin to demand access to quality ratings of different treatment modalities based on evidence for all health conditions, not just chronic or acute pain. Somewhat akin to the manner in which *Consumer Reports* publishes ratings and information regarding the quality of all kinds of products for the general public, agencies responsible for maintaining standards in health care (e.g., the Agency for Healthcare Research and Quality) may eventually publish treatment success/cost-effectiveness information regarding treatments for many illnesses and disease conditions designed for the general public.

The demand for pain management program outcomes data is not going to decrease. If anything, the need to appropriately disseminate treatment/program quality information will only increase as concepts such as "pay for performance" take root in the American health-care delivery system. This information will need to be presented in different formats for different consumer groups (e.g., the lay public, payers and health-care professionals). Performance improvement and clinical outcomes research should go hand in hand (40). Pain practitioners need to design performance improvement projects that will lead to publication of data in professional or peer-reviewed journals so that the evidence base for successful multidisciplinary pain management will continue to grow. These articles can then be summarized in language appropriate for the general public and disseminated through relevant consumer-health publications. Funding for these activities will undoubtedly be problematic, but strategic research partnerships between membership organizations like the Academy and its accredited programs may lead the way. Linking PPA to clinical quality improvement using the POP may provide one more mechanism for persuading payers that multidisciplinary pain management is beneficial and cost-effective.

STEPS TO GAINING ACADEMY PAIN PROGRAM ACCREDITATION

A PPA brochure, manual order form, and articles describing the standards in detail can be found on the Academy's Web site at www.aapainmanage.org. Once the decision is made to become accredited (after the program has been in operation for at least 6 months), the program director/manager completes the self-assessment found in the manual to determine the extent to which areas of business, clinical or personnel operations already meet the Academy's standards, and which areas need to be improved before submitting the application. Facilities are encouraged to contact the Director of Pain Program Accreditation with any questions or concerns during the application process for clarification. The mission of the Academy is to assist each program in its efforts to raise the bar for quality pain management through the consultative accreditation process. The application and self-assessment are submitted with the appropriate fees along with the required program documents. These consist of the patient history and physical examination forms used, consent for treatment forms (invasive procedure and/or general treatment), program description, mission statement, patient education materials, program brochures, code of ethics and bill of patient rights (both of which can be easily adapted from the Academy's documents), release of information forms, current research protocols (if any), and copies of outcomes measurement and patient satisfaction tools. Resumes or curricula vitae for all licensed professionals and clerical or support staff members who have patient contact are also requested.

Once the completed application and supporting documents have been received and processed, a qualified surveyor, usually working or living geographically near to the facility and having no conflict of interest with the program, is selected by the Director of Pain Program Accreditation to perform the survey. The Academy's highly skilled clinician-surveyors strive to provide expert consultative services to the programs during the one-day review process. Surveyors examine all program documents, previous accreditation reports, supportive materials, and resumes prior to the actual on-site review, thus saving valuable consultation time.

Each pain program accredited by the Academy must pass all of the *general standards* and one of the sets of *classification-specific standards*. The period of accreditation is for 3 years if all of the standards for accreditation are met. If there are any standards not found to be in compliance, remediation is attempted immediately to bring the program into compliance. If this cannot be accomplished fairly quickly, these programs are likely to receive a 1-year provisional accreditation status. Such a program will receive a detailed survey report and must submit a highly specific *action plan* to be completed. To then become fully accredited for the remaining 2 years, these provisionally accredited programs may need to have a second (abbreviated) on-site survey to demonstrate full compliance with the action plan recommendations, unless all deficiencies can be remedied by the creation of new documents which can be faxed/e-mailed to the PPA Director and even, sometimes, through photographs. Over the years that the Academy's PPA service has been available, revisions of the pain program standards and changes in the specific items surveyors assess during their visits to pain programs have improved the overall accreditation process. The process of accreditation has become more standardized, yet it still allows for flexibility in organizational structure. Along with individual practitioner credentialing, continuing education and outcomes measurement to document treatment success, PPA provides treatment organizations as a whole with the final link in the "quality" pain management chain.

FUTURE CHANGES AND ADDITIONS TO PPA STANDARDS

The Academy's accreditation manual is periodically updated and revised in response to advancements in the field of pain management and new legal and ethical requirements that arise. Areas for future revision potentially include:

- critical incident reporting (medication errors, equipment-related and other patient or staff injuries, incidents of workplace violence, etc.)
- better dissemination of outcomes data and incorporation of data into patient education materials
- grievance policies for clients
- background checks for personnel
- risk management policies and procedures

THE VALUE OF PAIN PROGRAM ACCREDITATION

Voluntary accreditation through the Academy demonstrates to peers, payers, and patients that the pain program has submitted to rigorous scrutiny of its policies and procedures, clinical, business, and personnel practices, has met peer-established quality standards, and is committed to excellent patient care and continuous performance improvement. In addition to the invaluable consultation that takes place during the survey process, all accredited pain programs receive an engraved plaque for display in their facility and use of the Academy's accredited pain program logo for marketing purposes. Each facility is listed on the Academy's Web site and is encouraged to supply a detailed program description and photographs of the facility and staff. The Academy receives many calls each week from patients seeking treatment, and while not providing direct referrals to specific programs or practitioners, staff members can direct callers to the Academy Web site to view listings of accredited pain programs and credentialed members. A link directly to the accredited facility's own Web site can also be created if appropriate. If requested, a press release printed on the Academy's letterhead will be provided to any accredited program. Programs are invited to submit updated information to the Director of Pain Program Accreditation for periodic press releases or to revise the program's web page. Assistance locating clinical charting forms, policy and procedure formats, and choosing outcomes measures is also provided by the Director. Several times each year, accredited programs are selected to be featured in *The Pain Practitioner* (41). Along with an article describing the program and its experience of the accreditation process, photographs of the facility and staff are included.

Future services include the availability of the POP Plus (POP+), a computer version of the POP that will give the user instant access to individual patient data graphically displayed and exportable to statistical analysis software for program-wide outcomes assessment. The software may also include a module that will enable physicians to document controlled substance prescribing practices and relevant patient/treatment parameters. A web-based version of the NPDB using the POP questionnaire could be created in the future to make external benchmarking available again. Other products planned for the near future include downloadable samples of charting forms (e.g., discharge summaries, etc.), and a marketing kit that will include a downloadable patient information/education brochure to increase consumers' understanding regarding the benefits of seeking treatment at an Academy accredited pain treatment facility.*

REFERENCES

1. American Academy of Pain Management. Self-Assessment Examination. Sonora, CA: American Academy of Pain Management; 1999.
2. Weiner RS. The culture of pain. Am J Pain Manage 1993; 3(4):201.
3. Flor H, Fydrich T, Turk DC. Efficacy of multidisciplinary pain treatment centers: a meta-analytic review. Pain 1992; 49(2):221.
4. Kee WG, Middaugh S, Pawlick K, et al. Cost benefit analysis of a multidisciplinary chronic pain program. Am J Pain Manage 1997; 7(2):59.
5. Weiner RS. Pain Practitioner: academy to start three new projects. Am J Pain Manage 1992; 2(2):109.
6. Joint Commission on Accreditation of Healthcare Organizations. Comprehensive Accreditation Manual for Hospitals. Oakbrook Terrace, IL: Joint Commission on Accreditation of Healthcare Organizations; 2001.
7. The Commission on Accreditation of Rehabilitation Facilities. Medical Rehabilitation: Standards Manual. Tucson, AZ: The Commission on Accreditation of Rehabilitation Facilities; 2003.
8. Joint Commission on Accreditation of Healthcare Organizations. Improving the Quality of Pain Management through Measurement and Action. Oakbrook Terrace, IL: Joint Commission on Accreditation of Healthcare Organizations; 2003.
9. Joint Commission on Accreditation of Healthcare Organizations. Pain Assessment and Management: An Organizational Approach. Oakbrook Terrace, IL: Joint Commission on Accreditation of Healthcare Organizations; 2000.
10. American Academy of Pain Management. Pain Program Accreditation Manual, 8th edn. Sonora, CA: American Academy of Pain Management; 2007.
11. Cole BE. Pain Program Accreditation: new accreditation standards-part one. Non-clinical accreditation standards. Pain Pract 1999; 9(1):8.
12. Cole BE. Pain Program Accreditation: new accreditation standards-part two. General clinical accreditation standards. Pain Pract 1999; 9(2):4.
13. Cole BE. Pain Program Accreditation: new accreditation standards-part three. Classification specific clinical standards. Pain Pract 1999; 9(3):10.
14. Department of Health and Human Services. The Health Insurance Portability and Accountability Act of 1996 (HIPAA), 1996 edn. Centers for Medicare and Medicaid Services Web site; 1996. Available at www.cms.hhs.gov/hipaa. Accessed on March 24, 2004.
15. National Institutes of Health Consensus Development Conference Statement, 1986 edn. Electronic References: The Integrated Approach to the Management of Pain. NIH Consensus Statement Web site. Available at consensus.nih.gov/cons/055/055_statement.htm; 1986. Accessed on March 24, 2004.
16. National Pharmaceutical Council. Pain: Current Understanding of Assessment, Management, and Treatments. Reston, VA: National Pharmaceutical Council; 2001.

* Portions of this chapter were adapted from: Campbell A, Cole BE. Interdisciplinary pain management programs: the American Academy of Pain Management Model. In: Boswell M, Cole BE, eds. Weiner's Pain Management: A practical guide for clinicians, 7th edn. New York: Taylor & Francis; 2006.

17. Campbell A. Clinical Practice Guidelines: Practical and Ethical Issues in their Development and Implementation. In: Schatman ME, ed. Ethical Issues in Chronic Pain Management. New York: Informa Healthcare; 2007.
18. McCaffery M, Pasero C. Pain Clinical Manual, 2nd edn. St. Louis, MO: Mosby; 1999.
19. Marketdata Enterprises. Pain Management Programs: A Market Analysis. Tampa, FL: Marketdata Enterprises; 2003.
20. Turk DC, Okifuji A. Treatment of chronic pain patients: Clinical outcomes, cost effectiveness, and cost benefits of multidisciplinary pain centers. Crit Rev Phys Med Rehabil 1998; 10:181.
21. Okifuji A, Turk DC. Philosophy and efficacy of multidisciplinary approach to chronic pain management. J Anesth 1998; 12:142.
22. Turk DC, Okifuji A. Multidisciplinary pain centers: boons or boondoggles? J Workers Comp 1997; 6:9.
23. Clark TS. Interdisciplinary treatment for chronic pain: is it worth the money? Baylor Univ Med Ctr Proc 2000; 13:240.
24. International Association for the Study of Pain. Desirable Characteristics for Pain Treatment Facilities. Seattle, WA: International Association for the Study of Pain; 1990.
25. Schatman ME. The demise of the multidisciplinary chronic pain management clinic: bioethical perspectives on providing optimal treatment in an unethical system. In: Schatman ME, ed. Ethical Issues in Chronic Pain Management. New York: Informa Healthcare; 2006.
26. Gordon DB, Dahl JL, Stevenson KK, eds. Building an Institutional Commitment to Pain Management: The Wisconsin Resource Manual, 2nd edn. Madison, WI: University of Wisconsin Board of Regents; 2000.
27. Agency for Healthcare Research and Quality. Management of Cancer Pain; 1994 edn. Rockville, MD: AHRQ Department of Health and Human Services; 1994. Publication No. 94-0592.
28. American Pain Society. Quality improvement guidelines for the treatment of acute and cancer pain. Jr Am Med Assoc 1995; 274(3):1874.
29. Cole BE. Ease and satisfaction for use of the National Pain Data Bank and Pain Program Accreditation. Am J Pain Manage 2000; 10(3):134.
30. Clark ME, Gironda RJ. Concurrent validity of the National Pain Data Bank: preliminary results. Am J Pain Manage 2000; 10:25.
31. Gironda RJ, Azzarello L, Clark ME. Test-retest reliability of the National Pain Data Bank v. 2.0. Am J Pain Manage 2002; 12:24.
32. Clark ME, Gironda RJ, Young RW, Jr. Development and validation of the Pain Outcomes Questionnaire-VA. J Rehabil Res Dev [serial online]. 2003; 40(5):381.
33. American Academy of Pain Management. Pain Outcomes Profile: Instruction Manual. Sonora, CA: American Academy of Pain Management; 2004.
34. Chapman SL. Chronic pain rehabilitation: lost in a sea of drugs and procedures? American Pain Society Bulletin [serial online] 2000; 10(3).
35. Schatman M, Campbell A. Innovations in outcomes assessment in pain management. Pain Pract 2004; 14(1):6–8.
36. Campbell A, Schatman M. Validation of the Pain Outcomes Profile. Presented at The 16th Annual Clinical Meeting of the American Academy of Pain Management, San Diego, CA, September 23, 2005.
37. Schatman M, Campbell A. Concurrent validity of the pain and physical interference scales of the Pain Outcomes Profile in chronic spinal pain patients. Presented at North American Spine Society, Philadelphia, PA, September 27–October 1, 2005.
38. Campbell A, Schatman M. New Information on the Use of the Pain Outcomes Profile. Presented at The 17th Annual Clinical Meeting of the American Academy of Pain Management, Orlando, FL, September 8, 2006.
39. Innovators and visionaries: strategies for creating a person-centered health system. FACCT-Foundation for Accountability. Available at www.facct.org; 2003. Accessed on March 30, 2004.

40. Campbell A. Linking Pain Practice Standards with Outcomes Measurement: Improving Treatment Quality through Clinical Pain Research. Presented at Agency for Healthcare Research and Quality Conference: Translating Research in Policy and Practice, Washington, DC, July 11, 2006.
41. Campbell A. American Academy of Pain Management Pain Program Accreditation. Pain Pract 2005; 15(4):62–69.

15 Multidisciplinary Chronic Pain Treatment: Minimizing Financial Risk

Ronald J. Kulich
Massachusetts General Hospital Pain Center, Wang Ambulatory Care Center; Department of General Dentistry, Tufts School of Dental Medicine; and Departments of Psychiatry and Anesthesia, Harvard Medical School, Boston, Massachusetts, U.S.A.

Michael Adolph
Pain and Palliative Medicine Service, James Cancer Hospital and Solove Research Institute, Ohio State University Medical Center, Columbus, Ohio, U.S.A.

INTRODUCTION: REIMBURSEMENT FOR MULTIDISCIPLINARY TREATMENT

Clinicians often lament the changes in reimbursement for health-care services, and report fond memories of the ability to provide multidisciplinary treatment in the late 1970s through the mid-1980s. Proponents of comprehensive multidisciplinary chronic pain management extol the virtues of their approach, and authors in this book argue convincingly about positive outcome data. Arguments support its cost-effectiveness, particularly in view of long-term outcomes. However, discordant stakeholder interests continue to fuel financial conflicts between health insurance plans (HIPs) and pain therapy clinicians. Discordant stakeholder interests, rather than failed clinical outcomes, have led to a decline in the staff-model multidisciplinary pain rehabilitation center (Table 1). The successful pain therapy program will consider discordant stakeholder goals when designing and implementing strategic plans for clinical and business operations.

This chapter will propose measures to optimize business operations for the multidisciplinary pain management program. We will describe the unique features of patient populations with chronic pain that affect business relationships. Additionally, we will encourage the pain therapy clinician to continue to advocate for patients and families experiencing chronic pain. Finally, we will explore the underlying nature of discordant stakeholder interests and how they affect business relationships with HIPs.

To define terms in simple language for this chapter, an HIP is *any corporation that receives health-care premium revenues and pays health-care insurance claims.* A managed care organization (MCO) is any corporation that *exerts control over patient workflows and cash flows* to clinicians and health-care service corporations (such as hospitals and ambulatory care centers), for any purpose (such as quality management or cost containment). Thus, an HIP may also be an MCO. Alternatively, for example, an HIP may outsource all or portions of medical management, quality management, or claims administration to an MCO or other entity, if it serves the HIP's business interests. Both HIPs and MCOs are also referred to as insurance "carriers" in this document. A health maintenance organization (HMO) is an MCO

TABLE 1 Annual Number of CARF-Accredited Interdisciplinary Pain Rehabilitation Programs for 2001–2006

Year	Number of programs
2001	171
2002	126
2003	128
2004	128
2005	129
2006	118

Source: Commission on Accreditation of Rehabilitation Facilities, Research Division, personal communication, January 2007.

that has legal obligations to perform services such as screening, and exerts the most control over patient workflow and provider services as compared to other MCO hybrids (1).

Shortly before the publication of *Managed Care and Pain* by the American Pain Society (APS) in 2000 (2), HIPs expanded their market share of workers' compensation, Medicare, and Medicaid subscribers. Unambiguous trends are now evident, and in retrospect were heralded by health-plan leaders at APS roundtable discussions in 2000.

This chapter offers that actuarial concerns, not clinical outcomes, primarily drive decisions for an innovation to be adopted, sustained, or rejected by HIP leaders. Even superlative clinical outcomes may not serve the financial interests of certain stakeholders, such as health plans and their employer-clients. Now more than ever, careful oversight of business functions will help the pain clinician deliver clinical services within a financially viable program.

IMPROVING FINANCIAL RISK

Carrier Negotiating Strategies

Well-conceived and well-planned chronic pain rehabilitation clinics may fail if negotiating strategies suffer. For an existing program, a good place to start negotiating is with plans whose contracts, policies, or procedures (including payment and nonpayment of claims) are found by the clinic to be unacceptable. To limit disruptions, existing practices might consider renegotiating with one plan at a time, starting with the lowest-paying plan. The process of developing these components is thoroughly covered in other sources (1,3,4). A few general principles will be emphasized here.

Prior to entering into negotiations, a program representative should meet with health-plan representatives and explore the needs and expectations of the health plan for the specialty care that the program provides. The health plan's interests, for example, employer satisfaction, streamlining referrals, data management, or government-mandated quality outcomes should be determined. Multidisciplinary chronic pain management can be expensive, and a negotiating strategy should not only include support for outcomes and costs, but also additional components the health plan may want to explore through mutual negotiations.

For example, disease-management corporations have negotiated their services with health plans through a return-on-investment (ROI), or a before-and-after costs per member, basis (5). Disease-management approaches range from value-added nurse triage telephone systems to case management, to utilization management by physicians (6).

The leverage of a chronic pain program and the plan's market share will play important roles in the conduct and outcomes of contract negotiations. Successful negotiations are achieved only if the program has the leverage to negotiate or renegotiate a contract. Before entering into carrier negotiation, a program should assess its amount of leverage. Negotiating discounted fee-for-service MCO contracts is quite different from negotiating capitation contracts. Tinsley describes six strategies for leveraging negotiations in discounted fee-for-service contracts (4): *numbers, geography, lack of competition, quality, patient volume, and threatening termination.* A *numbers* strategy is employed by networking in a group program, IPA, PHO, or provider network. Ultimately, if a payer knows that it has alternate same-service pain programs for its subscribers in the coverage area, it is unlikely to concede any terms in negotiation. Enthusiasm for a numbers strategy should be tempered by a working knowledge of antitrust principles.

Leverage in *geography* may be present if the pain program's absence will create a geographic "hole" in the MCO network, whereby members cannot find providers. Subscribers complain loudly to employers and MCOs when forced to drive excessive distances to receive the same care another program provides. The MCO recognizes that if complaints continue without remedy, then employers will change to a different plan with broader geographic coverage. Mapping locations of one's offices, competitor's offices, and health-plan coverage areas is the initial step in evaluating geographic leverage. Mapping local major employers should be considered, as well. Because local employers emphasize access, some health plans fear that a gap in their provider panel leads large employers to consider dropping the health plan.

A chronic pain management program may have competitive leverage in negotiations if there is a *lack of competition* in a health plan's service area. Are there other comprehensive pain programs in the plan's service area? Defining one's competition, the services they provide, and how a program differentiates its services in its geographic region will help with assessment of competitive leverage. If a payer is unable to sign the program into its network, services will be paid as charged, and the health plan's costs for the specialty will rise.

While a lack of competition constitutes a powerful form of leverage, the most powerful form of leverage in MCO contract negotiations, according to Tinsley (4) (p. 49), is finding leverage in *quality*. However, clinical quality data may not represent marketable leverage for chronic pain rehabilitation centers, given the historical data. MCOs recognize that health care is provided in different ways by different providers. Data can be presented to demonstrate the quality a program provides in terms of financial indicators (e.g., cost per patient by diagnosis code, pharmacy costs, reduced hospital admissions, etc.), clinical outcomes (please refer to Chapter 13 in this volume for a detailed analysis of this issue), or utilization outcomes (e.g., procedures performed as a percentage of total office encounters, or comparing a program against national or regional published or health-plan utilization data).

If a pain management program finds that 20% of its total managed care revenue (actual collections) is from a single MCO plan, then the program is treating a substantial number of the MCO's patients. Should this be the case, the health plan will likely be invested in maintaining positive relationships and provider status for the pain program, and perhaps consent to negotiations based upon *patient volume* leverage. Alternatively, if a program sends out patient surveys and presents favorable patient satisfaction data with the original surveys to the MCO, patient volume leverage exists. Finally, an increase in referrals over time to a chronic pain management program for plan subscribers is helpful data to demonstrate that patients and primary-care physicians (PCPs) are satisfied with provided services.

There are circumstances in which *threatening MCO contract termination* (by certified letter with a stated date of execution) will force a recalcitrant MCO to the negotiating table. This maneuver must be carefully calculated, as well as its potential consequences. If a plan calls a termination "bluff," will the program have future opportunity or need to get back into the MCO network? Regardless, the high cost of doing business with some plans may warrant contract termination from time to time. Being concerned with patient advocacy, a chronic pain management program will carefully communicate concerns to covered patients prior to contract termination. If an MCO feels that the pain program is valuable to the network, it will resume talks prior to the termination date.

Capitation is a separately negotiated contractual arrangement wherein insurance risk is transferred from the HMO to the providers (1). A multidisciplinary pain program does not submit fees for service in such cases, but rather negotiates a per-member-per-month (PMPM) dollar figure, receiving monthly revenues for the entire population in order to meet its pain management needs. In this type of arrangement, a pain clinician may be in a risk pool with area PCPs or in a specialty risk pool; in a specialty risk pool the patient population may be larger, yet PMPM figures generally parallel PMPM figures for PCP programs in the region. Inherent to assuming maximal risk is the need for substantial cash reserves upon which to draw when monthly PMPM revenues do not meet expenses for services rendered. In 2002, Banja addressed the reality that many provider groups "may be dangerously undercapitalized despite their risk exposure," meriting "regulatory attention" (7). Examples of capitation "nightmares" were plentiful in the 1990s for a variety of reasons, particularly in California; accordingly a capitation approach to reimbursement for multidisciplinary chronic pain management programs cannot necessarily be advocated.

For example, between the periods 1990–1993 and 1997–1999 in California, the HMO capitation PMPM rate for PCPs decreased from $45 to $29. However, clinicians continued in capitation arrangements for fear of losing monthly revenue streams needed to provide care. Page and colleagues pointed out that providers became overly dependent on monthly revenues from HMOs, trimming their program overheads to dangerous levels, and refusing to say no in contract negotiations (8). These worst case scenarios prompted one author to comment that the "fundamental moral lesson for ... group programs points to the need for extremely astute risk calculations coupled with the moral courage to decline contracts whose terms are unreasonable" (9).

Substantial obstacles to negotiating the financing of multidisciplinary pain rehabilitation may confront even the best-prepared program. Most HIPs have separate divisions for prior-authorization of medical and mental-health care that require considerable coordination and application to both divisions. Well-organized programs that require coordination and continuity of care to achieve favorable outcomes may find it difficult to stop patient progress, file additional MCO paperwork, await approval for five more physical therapy visits, the completion of four more psychology sessions, and approval for group therapy which was denied in the first place.

Effectively Managing the Revenue Cycle

Historically, the health-care "revenue cycle" began with a service and ended with a mutually agreeable payment, in a reasonable time frame. Presently, obtaining reimbursement for health-care services often appears more complex than delivering the services themselves. Nevertheless, carefully managing the flow of payments from HIPs has become an increasingly necessary task. The goal is to verify that the proper payment is received in the proper time from the proper payer, by each transaction, and in aggregate by health plan. The revenue cycle is highly influenced by negotiations and contracting, but requires diligent reconciliation of claims paid and claims denied. The pain rehabilitation program is forced to do business with a variety of payers: HMOs, commercial insurance, governmental organizations, etc. Despite the diversity of payers, Shapiro contends they hold one objective in common: delaying payment for services rendered as long as possible (10).

In business dealings with MCOs, there are many more process steps in the revenue cycle, and therefore more potential for error (11). The early detection of adverse changes in aggregate reimbursement trends is the key to managing a pain program's revenue cycle (12). This process is affected by contracting (in which reimbursement, utilization, and clinical expectations are set), proceeds through patient encounters, and terminates with an effort to reconcile payments (or payment denials) with negotiated amounts and negotiated time frames for prompt payment. For example, adjudicating denied claims is a key focus in reconciling the reimbursement portion of the revenue cycle (13).

We recommend that a multidisciplinary chronic pain management program establishes a *revenue cycle team*. Such a team should include clinicians, patient accounts personnel, the program manager, and registration representatives. A common mistake is to delegate oversight of the revenue cycle solely to financial/patient accounts personnel. Clinician involvement is critical because payment denials are often based upon quality, utilization, or medical necessity criteria. We believe that the clinician at the bedside is a better captain of quality, utilization, or medical necessity than is a distant MCO claims administrator. Cross-functional teams composed of representatives from clinical and financial areas will systematically tackle recurrent breakdowns detected in the revenue cycle (14). The team should meet monthly, review financial reports and trended data, and design "drill-down" focused studies of each adverse trend. Within a 1–3-month period, adverse trends may be recognized. Once an adverse trend is identified, payment denials are codified by reason, and trended further for the revenue cycle team to review. The team then designs an action plan for time-dependent escalated communications with health-plan representatives in order to reconcile unpaid claims in a timely fashion. Early detection of denied claims, and early intervention, will help to prevent major adverse financial consequences of continuing to deliver unpaid services with the pain management program's resources (in effect, insuring the plan's covered lives).

For example, a health plan's definition of "medical necessity" may change, and a program may not become aware of the change until claims are denied.

Unknown to a midwestern program, an MCO adopted recently published third-party criteria to determine medical necessity for ambulatory services, and proceeded to deny previously approved services. The program identified a problem only after an increase in denied claims from the plan had occurred. Requests for communication with the plan's local representatives were scheduled, eventually occurring 1–2 months from the initial problem detection. The local plan representative met with the program, heard its concerns, but acknowledged that he had no authority in the areas of contracting, claims, or arbitration. A month after the meeting, the representative requested claims data from the program on each claim denied. After 8 more months had passed, the plan informed the program that the claims were denied due to the change in the medical necessity policy, which the plan felt authorized to unilaterally enact based upon broad utilization management language in the managed-care contract. "We sent a letter to all providers informing of our adoption of [third-party] criteria before the policy was implemented," wrote the representative. Only after the plan received a certified letter threatening civil legal action for breach of contract, did a representative with negotiating and reconciliation authority contact the program to reach an agreeable disposition on the denied claims. A mutually agreeable disposition occurred 16 months after the trend was initially detected.

A simple approach to managing populations of transactions that result in ebbs and flows of revenues into a financially sustainable chronic pain management program might include:

1. assignment of revenue-cycle team-member responsibility,
2. delineation of the scope of revenue cycle for the program (e.g., designing a detailed process map),
3. identification of at-risk steps in the revenue cycle for failure,
4. identification of indicators ("metrics") related to important aspects of managing a program's revenue cycle,
5. establishing thresholds for evaluation,
6. collecting and organizing data at planned intervals,
7. evaluating the effectiveness of the process when indicated by the chosen threshold,
8. taking actions for improvement when opportunities for improvement or problems are identified (thereby avoiding "paralysis by analysis"),
9. assessing effectiveness of the actions,
10. communicating relevant information to organization-wide personnel for continuous performance improvement of the revenue cycle.

Outstanding claims should be monitored for their status every 30 days (13). Problem payers slow to process or reimburse claims are a major focus of the revenue cycle team. If a contracted period for payment, for example 60 days, is routinely exceeded, the plan may be in breach of contract, and escalated communications with plan representatives are initiated. If a claim is denied, then a program must submit an entirely new claim; this creates extra work and further payment delays. Reasons for payment denials are codified and tracked by patient accounts personnel, with monthly reports evaluated by the revenue cycle team. Payment denials are trended, and an adverse trend stimulates a focused monthly review. Beyond appeals (each appeal is ideally sent with a letter signed by a clinician), communications with plan representatives are also stimulated when a pattern of adverse claims behaviour is detected. Copies of communications are kept on file to evaluate an HIP's performance in claims reconciliation, with an eye to future contract renegotiations.

Graphically analyzing claims data will help the revenue-cycle team recognize areas of weakness and opportunity (15). Identified trends in superficial reports should encourage a prompt drill-down analysis for subsequent action plans by the revenue-cycle team. Reconciliation and measurement of revenue processes should also include internal patient information flow processes. After all, a program's use of resources has an overall effect on the revenue cycle. For example, an excessive delay between initial consultation and insurance approval was noted by one program, as pending approvals grew. Evaluation of internal insurance preauthorizing processing agents identified a fourfold difference in time-to-approval. Further analysis demonstrated that insurance approval agents were more successful at achieving insurance approval if the agent had a history of more direct experience in the health-care field.

Which plans deserve closer scrutiny? Checking the numbers acquired by a pain management program's revenue-cycle team, as described above, is foundational. In general, though, Schlesinger and colleagues surveyed over 1600 physicians for health-plan trustworthiness in business relationships and were able to identify trends by health-plan ownership type (16). *For-profit plans* affiliated with multistate corporations were consistently reported by affiliated physicians to engage in behaviors associated with reduced trustworthiness, as compared to local nonprofit plans. *Nonprofit plans affiliated with multistate corporations* had more physician-reported behaviors associated with trustworthiness than did for-profit corporate plans on multiple outcomes, but appeared less trustworthy than *locally controlled nonprofit plans.* The extent of ownership-related differences declined as the market share of nonprofit plans increased: in some measures, ownership-related variations in trustworthiness were entirely absent when nonprofits enrolled over 30% of the local health-plan market. The authors concluded that the combination of *for-profit ownership and multistate corporate control* consistently reduced physician-reported measures related to the trustworthiness of health plans. Given that this is the fastest growing form of managed care, the authors expressed concerns about policymakers preserving a market niche for nonprofit plans as a means "[to restore] trust in the health care system" (16).

Establishing Personal Relationships: Carrier Representatives and Carrier Influencers

Relationships with carrier representatives and entities that influence carriers help multidisciplinary chronic pain management programs maintain positive business relationships, and to reconcile business difficulties when reinforcement of contractual payments is necessary. Routine follow-up with third party payers is an important tool for accomplishing timely claims resolution and ensuring adherence to contractual terms. Shapiro (10) details the following methods:

1. Developing relationships with appropriate individuals associated with the carriers—direct contact may be made concerning large balances, or complex cases.
2. Periodically scheduling meetings with representatives from those carriers with whom a provider has significant volume.
3. Identifying contact personnel to directly fax original claims that are denied, as well as follow-up notices, in order to expedite and verify receipt.

4. Identifying contact personnel to send selected claims by certified mail—this can be done for exceptionally large claims or as a routine when submitting to a particularly troublesome carrier.
5. Keeping a database for each plan with the appropriate health-plan contacts, their positions, duties, superiors, and contact information—being kind yet clear in all communications.
6. Most importantly, continually emphasizing to all health-plan personnel the importance of providing assistance in obtaining a timely payment from the carrier.

From a practical standpoint, population data supportive of efficacy and improved outcomes may be insufficient to achieve adequate financial reimbursement if one is in the position of maintaining solvent multidisciplinary pain management services. In pursuing a successful financial strategy, clinicians with the proclivity to develop multidisciplinary pain services might first harken back to their behavioral science roots. Adequate financial reimbursement should be viewed as a behavior a program should choose to reinforce. Individuals, as well as corporate health-care entities, generally might be assumed to respond to some positive consequence. Indeed, they may behave in a manner to terminate some negative state (negative reinforcement). Overall corporate "rewards" might include increasing revenue or reducing costs, increasing market share, reducing staff turnaround, embellishing their corporate image, improving efficiency, or even eliminating overly costly components of the business. Indeed, from an insurance carrier's perspective, certain subject populations present a financial risk that would appear untenable, such as the chronic pain population.

An initial step toward improving reinforcement for any chronic pain treatment must involve some assessment of the carrier's needs, as well as addressing its concern regarding risks. Additionally, individuals and other entities also may have a direct impact on reimbursement. The individual goals of an adjuster or corporate medical director may have as much of an impact on financial reimbursement as any established corporate policy, clinical pathway, or company-endorsed program guideline. Indeed, experience may demonstrate that carrier administrators sometimes resort to the company guideline as simply a strategy for declining coverage and thereby denying payment. Similarly, the true "customer" from the carrier perspective is often the employer, i.e., the purchaser of large group policies. Patients routinely switch carriers, a financial reprieve for the for-profit managed care entity when a patient becomes disabled, unemployed, and switches to a Medicare or Medicaid plan. In contrast, the MCO may take greater notice when the employer begins complaining about the adequacy of clinical services.

In brief, there appears to be a narrow range of reinforcers for the various entities that control financial reimbursement. Employees desire a reasonably priced health-care product, and one that results in some level of employee satisfaction. Benefits officers and company administrators are often responsive when their carrier declines particular clinical services for a valued employee. The concern may heighten when corporate officers are treated shabbily in their interaction with the company's insurer. In turn, the carriers expect to "control" and minimize costs, maintain their customer base, and provide the appropriate services under their contract. Further, they desire predictability and uniformity with respect to treatment services. As will soon be described, long-term health-care outcomes for patients may be less of an immediate concern.

Comments from medical directors and executives from the 2000 APS Managed Care Roundtable were definitive in their request for uniform guidelines. Notwithstanding the efforts of noble individuals in the pain field, conflicting definitions of "interdisciplinary" or "multidisciplinary" and the lack of uniform guidelines continue to plague programs that do business with MCOs. Again, an illustrative comment from a past medical director of Tufts Health Plan in New England in reference to a hospital-based in-patient multidisciplinary program states that "they never saw a disciplinary they didn't like . . ." (RJ Kulich, personal communication). Most agreed that the academic societies or credentialing societies (Committee on Accreditation of Rehabilitation Facilities, American Academy of Pain Management) have failed to provide uniform guidelines. Assuming the absence of this uniformity and no agreed-upon treatment pathways, each multidisciplinary program must stand on its own with respect to promulgating a guideline and convincing the carrier that its product meets the specific carrier's needs.

Judiciously Screening for "Best Fit" Patients

Traditionally, pain rehabilitation programs have been referred many "worst case" patients with disability and chronic pain. Indeed, adverse selection is both a concern for an MCO as well as a for a multidisciplinary chronic pain management program. Considering the rationale of selecting patients who will clearly benefit from the extensive resources provided in a multidisciplinary pain management program, it is reasonable to prescreen patients who are most likely to benefit from enrollment and most likely to complete the program. While there are no uniform guidelines for identifying "best fit" patients, the program with a strategy for triaging patients to appropriate levels of care will demonstrate due diligence to health-plan negotiators.

For example, Tollison and Kriegel list broad program inclusion criteria: (1) pain for at least 6 months, (2) pain not due to active disease process attributed to potentially correctable medical or psychiatric illness, (3) patient and family agree to active participation in the program, (4) no evidence of severe psychological/psychiatric disturbance, and (5) clinical staff agreement that the patient is motivated to reduce pain and disability (17). To help clarify expectations and identify motivated patients, Kulich developed the "Functional Restoration Treatment Agreement" (18). This multidisciplinary patient-specific document is developed, reviewed, and signed by the patient after initial consultation. The document helps delineate individualized realistic treatment goals and target dates for outcomes within biopsychosocial and functional domains.

Other investigators have identified factors that adversely impact favorable outcomes. For example, McGeary and colleagues found that extremely high (8 to 10 of 10) pretreatment pain ratings were associated with poor outcomes after a structured pain rehabilitation therapy program, including posttreatment lost productivity, high utilization of health care, and cost shifting of state Workers' Compensation payments to federal resources (19).

Hildebrandt and colleagues evaluated 90 disabled patients with back pain who underwent multidisciplinary rehabilitation, with end points of return-to-work and the reduction of pain intensity (20). Predictors of success included self-evaluation for predicting return-to-work, the length of absence from work, application for pension, and a decrease in disability following treatment (20).

Patients referred for multidisciplinary treatment continue to represent a complicated heterogeneous population from many perspectives, with access-to-care and reimbursement-for-services being well-known hurdles. In general, patients with persistent pain are underemployed or unemployed in many cases. They immediately represent a suboptimal payer mix. While the presence of any chronic medical condition has an impact on compliance, the higher incidence of comorbid psychiatric and substance abuse problems in patients with chronic pain further complicate care and reimbursement for care. Notwithstanding the best treatment "contract," many of these patients have higher no-show rates, are often impaired with respect to advocating for their care, and show relatively poorer outcomes. Perhaps further complicating the issue, many patients already are involved in various litigation efforts, often complicating reimbursement and compromising the patient's ability to achieve treatment success. From a positive perspective, there is an increasing societal recognition that these patients require care, and *comprehensive multidisciplinary* care.

POSTMORTEM: THE DECLINE OF THE COMPREHENSIVE MULTIDISCIPLINARY CHRONIC PAIN REHABILITATION PROGRAM

> *The present danger lies in the fact that a major subset of patients whose lives and function have been the most pervasively affected by pain are losing the opportunity to participate in the precise mode of treatment (i.e., comprehensive interdisciplinary pain rehabilitation) that has been proven to be the most effective in helping them improve their ability to function and their productivity. Unfortunately, the reasons for this have more to do with politics, profit, and the structure of current insurance than with evidence-based quality care* (21).
>
> *Stanley L Chapman, APS Bulletin, 2000*

The business objectives of HIPs are met by successfully applying actuarial principles. A clear understanding of the underlying considerations may help in strategic management for a multidisciplinary chronic pain program, particularly in relationship to organizational threat analysis (22), contract negotiations (1,4), contingency planning (23), patient advocacy, and political activism (24).

What are the business principles that govern the pain clinician's arrangements with HIPs? Behind every HIP is an actuary (25). An actuary computes premium rates, dividends (revenues), and risks and calculates corresponding premium levels, according to probabilities based on statistical norms (26). While pain clinicians base their practices on sound biomedical principles and proven innovations, the HIP focuses its business upon actuarial assumptions (27). These are statistical assumptions that an actuary uses in determining expected costs and revenues of an insurance plan in a population, including carve-outs for items like pain therapy. Financial stability for an HIP derives from a larger population of well "patients" (members/subscribers), whose premium revenues cover health-care costs for the unwell; typically an approximate ratio of 80% well to 20% unwell is sought by a managed care plan (28). While chronic pain therapy programs concentrate on patients, the HIP must have an acceptable and predictable mix of well members (well subscribers) and patients (unwell subscribers). *Any unpredictable burden of unwell patients to an HIP drives up premiums and threatens an HIP's competitiveness and financial stability.* This is a particular problem with provider-sponsored health plans, which tend to view members as patients and misunderstand that a health plan requires more members than patients to be financially sound (29).

Payer Attitudes Toward Chronic Disease, Out-Patient Populations, and Chronic Pain Management

As business entities, a primary objective of an HIP is to maximize shareholder wealth, i.e., maximizing the value achieved by HIP stockholders (30,31). By the 1990s, HIPs succeeded in raising profits for themselves and lowering premiums to employers by reducing health-care utilization in high-cost settings (such as applying case management to hospital inpatients and precertifying acute-care hospitalizations and procedures). *The Managed Health Care Handbook* (fourth edition), a 1400-page major health insurance industry textbook, describes this approach on page 1375 in this manner: *"Sutton's Law, 'Go where the money is!' . . . is a good law to use when determining what needs attention in a managed care plan"* (28). These initial cost-cutting measures achieved value for their shareholders and for their employer-clients. An HIP that makes a concerted effort to manage care, costs, and quality by allocation, case management, precertification, claims analysis, and contracting is considered an MCO.

However, chronic pain, largely an outpatient disease-management problem, is a moving target for HIPs. While MCOs would prefer generalists, i.e., the "cheapest alternative" (28) to manage chronic pain, generalists favor referring patients with chronic pain to specialist programs, and do so repeatedly. As such, it proves more difficult for established HIP cost-cutting measures to strike. Mining MCO claims data to identify the chronic pain population is also difficult. Claims analysis for chronic pain patients, a primary tool used by the HIP to manage care, is limited by 1) the complete absence of ICD-9 codes reflecting pain syndromes (now available since October 2006, 'however'), and 2) by HIPs routinely denying evaluation and management claims submitted by PCPs when coded for pain symptoms by anatomic site. In contrast, it is a simple matter to detect ICD-9 codes for diabetes mellitus and asthma in claims data, prompting case managers to enroll patients in appropriate disease-management programs. HIPs may also choose to outsource disease-management functions for specific diagnoses in order to maintain competitiveness in a given market. Disease-management corporations provide HIPs not only with outsourced care for chronic illness and high-risk conditions but also with data.

The challenge of chronicity in disease management raises further questions: isn't a multidisciplinary chronic pain management program providing disease management of chronic pain? The difference may be that patients in HIPs ultimately leave the HIP and therefore leave the HIP-partnered disease-management program. Disenrollment rates, a parameter generally applied to assess subscriber satisfaction with an HIP, have gained recent focus as HIPs evaluate both competitiveness and effectiveness, particularly with respect to chronic disease management. Are patients enrolled in an HIP long enough to benefit from disease management? After all, effective disease-management programs warrant a long-term focus. Compounding this temporal aspect of chronic pain management, the typical HIP carries disenrollment rates of over 16% of subscribers per year (32); this figure can be compared to the 29% of 6400 nonelderly, privately insured telephone survey respondents who switched from HMO to HMO in the Community Tracking Study household survey of 37,000 U.S. citizens (33), and the 42% of Medicare patients who disenrolled from HMOs in the 1990s (prompting federal legislature to protect the HIP financial interests) (34). Outcomes from meta-analyses of over 65 multidisciplinary pain programs in 1992 and 1998 reveal stable improvements at an average 95 weeks follow-up (35,36). So, what is the benefit for HIPs? These data suggest that, while an HIP may finance a successful multidisciplinary pain rehabilitation program for a given patient, the HIP does not reap the future benefit of a reasonably well and functional patient in its future risk pool—representing an actuarial loss to the HIP.

Do patients change HIPs voluntarily or involuntarily? The most common reasons for HMO switching in the Community Tracking Study were "employer changed offerings" (36%) and "job change" (32%) (33). The former change suggests employer economic interests, while the latter is less well defined. It would appear that subscribers leave HIPs largely due to conditions beyond the subscribers' control, unless an HIP substantially raises its premium, or employers raise the subscribers' copays for a given HIP. A disease management program is a short-term HIP solution to manage retained chronically unwell patients. Proliferation of disease-management programs is on the rise, largely due to HIPs outsourcing business to disease-management companies. Over 40% of all employers and 60% of large employers offered employees at least one form of disease-management program in 2005 (37). This proliferation suggests that at least in the short term, both employers and HIP are achieving some measurable ROI for disease-management programs, though the data for patients with chronic pain is limited. Unfortunately, disease-management program methods and outcomes are proprietary information and may not be available for public scrutiny. We are aware that HIPs recognize that predictive actuarial models are lacking to help reliably underwrite chronic illnesses requiring disease management, and that they have turned to trade organizations to help with the process (38).

How does an HIP's actuary describe patients with chronic pain? Chronic pain patients demonstrate high current health-care resource utilization (39), high predicted future health care utilization, anticipated adverse claims histories, are frequently noncompliant, and are prone to select plans that serve their best interests (consumerism)—all major risk factors for adverse financial consequences to the experienced actuarial insurance underwriter (40,41). Proctor and colleagues studied over 1300 patients with chronic disabling work-related musculoskeletal conditions treated with rehabilitation. They found that 25% of patients pursue new health-care services after completing a course of treatment and that this subgroup accounts for a significant proportion of lost worker productivity, unremitting disability payments, and excess health-care consumption (42). Impending distress for an HIP executive is an extreme form of consumerism potentially programmed by unwell patients: "*adverse selection.*" Adverse selection drives individuals or employer groups that had previously foregone insurance or could not afford insurance to elect to enroll, or maintain enrollment, in an insurance plan because they perceive that it is to their economic benefit to do so. As such, adverse selection results in a subscriber population with a deviation from the statistically expected probability norm for well and unwell members, thus making financial predictions less reliable. The scenario of a sustained program, such as multidisciplinary chronic pain management, that encourages adverse selection is not just a bad dream for health plan. A health plan's nightmare is the "insurance death spiral," i.e., unexpected adverse selection and corresponding high premium rates that create unrecoverable underwriting losses that exceed competitively priced premium revenue, rendering the HIP financially insolvent (28). Even the federal government has given considerable attention to the concept of adverse selection as an actuarial assumption when considering its potential impact on the costs of Medicare Part D prescription benefits (43).

As a consequence, within the limits of various state laws, a carrier may actively pursue policies that minimize "adverse selection" in their covered subscriber population. To illustrate, the APS Managed Care Roundtable generated a telling quote from a managed care executive: "Probably the worst thing in the world we (HIPs) want to do is create the best program on the block for pain management and be the only guy on the block with it, because we'll get adverse selection" (2). Gray cautioned that, "because premiums reflect the cost of an average patient, HMOs have great incentives to avoid enrolling potentially high cost patients and, even worse, to displease high-cost patients among existing enrollees. Even a report that 90–95 percent of enrollees are satisfied could conceal indifference to the needs of the few patients who are particularly vulnerable and need costly services" (44). Kulich advocated legislative activism and also recommended that pain specialists get involved in HMO ethics committees to help safeguard patients against obstructive HMO practices that adversely impact patient care (45). For example, the HMO practice of supporting carve-outs to non-CPP providers for services such as mental health (46), while financially advantageous to MCOs, has a negative impact on overall patient outcomes (47,48). (Please refer to Chapter 3 in this volume for a detailed analysis of the clinical implications of "carving out" specific elements of a multidisciplinary chronic pain management program.) Excessively stringent HIP standards for fully approving medically recognized, evidenced-based multidisciplinary care have also been promulgated in the field of obesity surgery by MCOs (49,50). Interestingly, in other specialties some authors have proposed that patients denied comprehensive program services by health plans may serve as "randomized" control groups for evaluating outcomes of study interventions (51).

The chronic pain patient is considered unwell by HIPs. It is precisely the population of subscribers with chronic diseases that HIPs are struggling to deal with today. After successful efforts to produce cost savings in acute-care hospitals, to the point of reactionary tort litigation by health-care systems, HIPs must focus on chronic diseases to sustain their profits and prove their continued value to their clients: employers, the government, and worker's compensation.

Health plans are also cognizant of the financial underwriting cycle that governs the ebb and flow of premiums and after-tax profits for HIPs, though in recent years this financial cycle has become less predictable (52). The chronic pain patient population does not fit the HIP description of a component of a "strategic [MCO] portfolio" (28). As the health-care system becomes less predictable, HIP thought leaders are viewing future business projections through the lens of *chaos theory*, and perhaps tending to be more risk averse, akin to "driving the nitroglycerine truck on a foggy night" (28).

A response by some MCOs has been to establish their own *in-house pain facilities*, or at least, recruit a specialist who can minimize the financial exposure for the carrier. One of the medical directors of an in-house behavioral program commented that the "My (MCO) hired me to keep patients away from the local interdisciplinary inpatient facility" (RJ Kulich, personal communication). She offered an outpatient time–limited behavioral group program, unidisciplinary in focus. Her ultimate replacement was an oncologist who provides screening and pharmacotherapy, as well as a part-time staff anesthesiologist who provides interventional procedures. It is also interesting to note that this particular HIP has one of the highest ratings of patient satisfaction in the country, perhaps underscoring the issue of the satisfaction of particular vulnerable subgroups potentially being concealed when a generally healthy HIP population is assessed.

With the change in market forces, staff-model HIPs are markedly more scarce. Many consider this fortunate. As a result, carriers now find themselves in the position in which they must deal with clinicians who offer services to a range of HIPs. Hence, there may be a growing financial opportunity for multidisciplinary chronic pain management programs, or at least for those that are run efficiently and cost-effectively. For more information on this topic, please refer to Chapter 16 in this volume, which discusses the success of Kaiser Permanente in providing multidisciplinary chronic pain management services within the context of managed care.

Now that the floor on reducing inpatient costs has approached, HIP leaders and their employer-clients may not realize similar cost-cutting success with the challenges of chronic diseases. Perhaps chronic pain is a condition that, like much of U.S. health care, has a limited relationship between improved quality, better health, and lower costs (53).

INTERDISCIPLINARY TREATMENT: CHALLENGES IN NEW ENGLAND

The Tufts Associated Health Plan, Massachusetts offers a broad array of pain therapies. A behavioral group program offered multidisciplinary outpatient treatments, and anesthesiology-based interventions were developed on a fee-for-service basis, but clinicians' services were reimbursed through specialty-specific submitted claims. Multidisciplinary behaviorally oriented pain therapy services were developed by faculty at the affiliated academic teaching hospital. Behavioral outcome measures included the Multidimensional Pain Inventory, formal functional capacity assessment, and SF-36/SF-12 (18). Similar to the predicament at other academic medical centers, substantial administrative support is required to justify a pain program's variable bottom-line revenue production when viewed as a free-standing cost center. For example, if the behavioral pain therapy program is perceived as not only an important component of comprehensive care but also as a source of referrals to procedure-generating specialists at the institution, then internal administrative demands may be satisfied. Nevertheless, a tension exists to justify internal financial end points to academic medical center administrators while balancing the need to defend a cost-efficient program that is pleasing to HMO leaders. While behavioral health outcomes measurements such as the SF-36 have proven too insensitive to detect differences in multidisciplinary pain therapy from controls, other measures studied and validated at the Tufts-New England Medical Center Program such as the Treatment Outcomes in Pain Survey (TOPS) have demonstrated the benefits of multidisciplinary chronic pain management.

The multidisciplinary pain therapy program stands squarely in the aim of HIP cost-cutting measures. Competition in Massachusetts has led to an environment increasingly focused on academic health systems (54). There are four medical schools and six academic health centers in the state. Massachusetts' hospitals are ahead of their peers in generating performance improvements, while maintaining inpatient costs to within 11% of the adjusted national average. Three HIPs control 75% of the health plan market: Blue Cross and Blue Shield of Massachusetts, Tufts Associated Health Plan, and Harvard Pilgrim Health Care. All HIPs are aware that costs in academic medical centers and major teaching hospitals exceed those of community nonteaching hospitals (55). All HIPs are also aware that outpatient visits per 1000 in Massachusetts are 180% higher than the national average (54). More than 65% of employers favor recent state legislation for mandated pay-for-performance and support public information on provider performance.

CASE MODELS FOR POSSIBLE SUCCESS

An early champion of interdisciplinary pain management, John Loeser, asked the question in 2002: Will pain be abolished, or just pain management specialists? He comments further, "This is not a trivial question when one is addressing ... a pain association .... However, from the perspective of a Nation's health-care delivery system, the advent or demise of pain specialist is not likely to be noticed ..." (56,57).

Reimbursement "issues" and payer attitudes with respect to multidisciplinary pain management have a long and rather checked history. As with many clinical services in the 1970s and early 1980s, carriers simply reimbursed the bills as they arrived. Inpatient programs abounded, many 6 weeks in duration. While some offered the Seattle model focusing on operant pain behavior and return-to-work, some pursued a "pain relief" model involving all possible forms of intervention. Assessments by consultants were extensive. For example, one program offered a 5–6-hour neuropsychological assessment battery upon admission. A pain psychologist in New England continued the program on an outpatient basis for years after the inpatient facilities closed, perhaps under the innocent assumption that the Wechsler Intelligence Scale and other instruments had some impact on treatment planning for their multidisciplinary services. While some programs screened patients based upon prognostic indices, acceptance rates for many programs were inexplicably high. Outcome goals varied among programs.

Perhaps in response to multidisciplinary chronic pain management, Thomas Mayer charted a course with "Functional Restoration," in which he intentionally distinguished his product from the services being offered by multidisciplinary pain treatment programs (58). Mostly multidisciplinary, outpatient, operant, and having a major focus on return-to-work, worker compensation adjusters warmed to his services. Patients were judiciously screened, and some argued that this resulted in the initially high return-to-work rates. Indeed, franchise-like Functional Restoration programs abounded in the late 80s, concurrent with competition from "Work Hardening" programs that were decidedly less than multidisciplinary. It appeared that there was one point during the mid-1980s during which no community hospital was without a program of its own. Standardization suffered, staff expertise varied despite a plethora of "certifications," most franchise programs closed, and the remaining physical therapy programs paid scant lip service to any multidisciplinary focus. This history is well known to senior adjusters who work with industrial accident clients. As one managed care administrator states, "... being totally candid, there's a lot of suspicion among physician executives that there's chicanery in the field. We not long ago found that we were sending a patient to a pain center and he was getting magnet therapy . . ." (RJ Kulich, personal communication).

In the period 1995–2001, a collaborative approach with Tufts Health Plan and pain rehabilitation programs grew from the concept of "stepwise carrier approvals." Weekly telephone case review conferences between comprehensive pain program clinicians and the Tufts Health Plan medical director served to update the health plan on patients' progress in the inpatient pain rehabilitation unit. In turn, the health plan medical director would approve or deny additional coverage for the next week's level of care based upon the patient's clinical response. The model was conceived by Joe Gerstein, MD, the health plan medical director, who was also a practicing pain specialist and addictionologist. The success of this HIP-pain program collaboration was therefore heavily dependent upon a "champion" for chronic pain rehabilitation *within the health plan itself.* This approach served as an intermediate option between global payments (not palatable to health plans) and fragmented payments (not agreeable to pain programs with a multidisciplinary approach).

STRATEGIES FOR REVERSING THE PRESENT TREND

Innovations, such as multidisciplinary pain therapy in the U.S. health-care system, may meet resistance in the process of diffusing through a social system (59); sources of resistance to innovations include economic factors (59). The innovation of multidisciplinary chronic pain rehabilitation failed to diffuse throughout managed care medicine and its contractual relationships because of real or potential threats to HIP profitability. Each comprehensive pain program must build its own case in negotiations with MCOs on the basis of leverage, outcomes, best evidence, and cost-effectiveness, considering the business, quality, utilization, and cost goals of the MCO.

Collaborating with MCOs to develop disease-management measures is an appealing avenue for MCOs. For example, if a chronic pain program works with a health plan to construct health-care delivery models for a plan's chronic pain patients, the health plan may ascribe considerable value-added services to its dealings with the pain program. A pain program negotiations team could help an MCO evaluate per-patient costs of chronic pain on the basis of proposed improvements in (1) aggregate annual existing per-patient costs, (2) distributions of per-patient utilization and costs by encounter and episode type, or (3) distribution of costs by comorbid conditions (60). Naturally, subsequent contractual interventions proposed by the program would serve as an important part of the solution to the plan's chronic pain population, built upon a sustainable business case, (61–63) for a prime target for disease management, in the MCOs view: chronic pain patients (46). Plocher states that a positive ROI in disease management should be driven by a business plan and must be realized "within fewer than three years" (64).

Clinical research, including new study designs such as group randomized trials (GRTs) (65), may meet the needs of both MCOs and comprehensive pain programs in answering population-based questions like "which interventions work best in what time frame, are the most cost-effective, and in which subset or diagnoses of the chronic pain population?" Most randomized studies involve randomization of individuals into intervention arms and do not account for an intraclass correlation over time, thereby ignoring variability due to patient interaction, patient similarities, or geographic similarities such as a clinic unit. Conversely, the unit of randomization with a GRT is a clinic, worksite, town, or workers' compensation population, or chronic low back pain population, for example, which represent a social group with interaction effects (66). Behavioral interventions, group interventions, complex surveys, and patient groups with the same incentives lend themselves well to evaluation by GRT, particularly with respect to surveillance study over time (67,68).

Many patients and family members do have the capacity to act as advocates for access and reimbursement, and advocacy organizations can play a role in reversing the current trend. When given some degree of direction from well-informed staff at a multidisciplinary chronic pain management program, there are countless examples in which individual patient advocacy with an elected representative, state insurance commissioner, or employer resulted in approval of pain services. Patient advocacy (69,70), grassroots coalitions, ballot initiatives (propositions, bills, and laws), and litigation are avenues that may warrant additional strategic planning for professional societies with an interest in carrier coverage for comprehensive multidisciplinary chronic pain management programs. Unlike other areas in medicine, there is a substantial evidence-based argument to support the fight. This evidence basis is well documented in Chapter 2 in this volume. Now that federal and state governments are customers for managed care corporations, however, the battle for coverage of evidenced-based pain programs may face additional formidable obstacles.

Unfortunately, state or federal legislation specifically mandating that MCOs must cover comprehensive pain program services may be the irreducible force that changes the current position of MCOs. While patients with chronic pain are prevented from receiving evidence-based comprehensive multidisciplinary pain program services, how strong is the cost-effectiveness argument of the HIP? After all, the cost-effectiveness mantra of MCOs is not borne out in their payment of CEO salaries and benefits. As Pollack and Slass note (Tables 2 and 3),

> Publicly traded for-profit managed care and insurance companies are considerably more cost conscious when they oppose the establishment of consumer rights than when they approve compensation for their top executives. For publicly traded managed care companies, remuneration in annual compensation and unexercised stock options for top executives routinely reaches millions of dollars. Indeed, for some companies, such remuneration reaches tens of millions of dollars. The managed care and insurance industry's protestations about costs appear to be highly selective. While they argue that they will need to raise premiums to be able to provide basic protections for managed care consumers, their top executives make millions of dollars each year (71).

SUMMARY

As is discussed in other chapters in this volume as well as in the recent works of Schatman (72,73), the health insurance industry's emphasis on cost-containment and profitability poses a serious risk to the future of multidisciplinary chronic pain management—despite the plethora of high-quality research supporting its clinical efficacy and cost-efficiency. Other authors who contributed to this volume have presented myriad reasons for the perpetuation of the comprehensive approach to

TABLE 2 The 25 Highest Paid HMO Executives 1996 Annual Compensation Exclusive of Unexercised Stock Options.

Executive/plan	Annual compensation ($)
1. Stephen Wiggins, CEO, Oxford Health Plans, Inc.	29,061,599
2. Wilson Taylor, Chairman and CEO, CIGNA Corporation	11,568,410
3. David Snow, Executive Vice President, Oxford Health Plans, Inc.	10,403,451
4. Robert Smoler, Executive Vice President, Oxford Health Plans, Inc.	10,085,972
5. William Sullivan, President, Oxford Health Plans, Inc.	7,823,076
6. Joseph Sebastianelli, President, Aetna, Inc.	7,394,506
7. Michael Cardillo, Executive Vice President, Aetna, Inc.	7,069,969
8. Leonard Schaeffer, Chairman and CEO, WellPoint Health Networks, Inc.	7,010,698
9. George Jochum, President and CEO, Mid-Atlantic Medical Services, Inc.	6,526,065
10. Ronald Compton, Chairman and CEO, Aetna, Inc.	5,813,287
11. Wayne Smith, Former President, Humana, Inc.	5,166,575
12. James Stewart, Executive Vice President, CIGNA Corporation	4,832,799
13. Richard Huber, Vice Chairman, Aetna, Inc.	4,801,841
14. Roger Taylor, Executive Vice President, PacifiCare Health Systems, Inc.	4,103,864
15. Daniel Crowley, CEO and President, Foundation Health Corporation	3,849,023
16. Gerald Isom, President, Property and Casualty, CIGNA Corporation	3,778,293
17. Alan Hoops, President and CEO, PacifiCare Health Systems, Inc.	3,221,602
18. Daniel Kearney, Executive Vice President, Aetna, Inc.	3,189,272
19. D. Mark Weinberg, Executive Vice President, WellPoint Health Networks, Inc.	3,009,944
20. Donald Levinson, Executive Vice President, CIGNA Corporation	2,985,017
21. Ronald Williams, Executive Vice President, WellPoint Health Networks, Inc.	2,827,381
22. Allen Wise, Executive Vice President, United HealthCare Corporation	2,697,751
23. Jeffrey Elder, Senior Vice President, Foundation Health Corporation	2,235,783
24. H. Edward Hanway, President CIGNA HealthCare, CIGNA	2,217,711
25. Kirk Benson, President and COO, Foundation Health Corporation	2,104,414
Total 1996 annual CEO compensation	$153,778,303

Source: Ref. 71.

TABLE 3 The 10 HMO Executives with the Largest Unexercised Stock Option Packages in 1996.

Executive/plan	Stock option package ($)
1. Stephen Wiggins, CEO, Oxford Health Plans, Inc.	82,799,000
2. William McGuire, CEO, United HealthCare Corporation	50,042,237
3. David Snow, Executive Vice President, Oxford Health Plans, Inc.	23,888,000
4. William Sullivan, President, Oxford Health Plans, Inc.	20,408,000
5. Alan Hoops, President and CEO, PacifiCare Health Systems, Inc.	15,338,120
6. Robert Smoler, Executive Vice President, Oxford Health Plans, Inc.	14,015,000
7. Wilson Taylor, Chairman and CEO, CIGNA Corporation	12,057,758
8. Samuel Miller, Executive Vice President, United Wisconsin Services, Inc.	9,340,174
9. Wayne Smith, Former President, Humana, Inc.	9,170,060
10. Ronald Compton, Chairman and CEO, Aetna, Inc.	8,466,861
Total 1996 HMO CEO unexercised stock option packages	245,525,210

Source: Ref. 71.

chronic pain. Unfortunately, the health insurance community does not appear to be particularly motivated to see the science flourish, despite the fact that it constitutes the closest thing to a "cure" for chronic pain. Patient quality of life, unfortunately, is seen as less important to third-party payers than is the bottom line.

As a result of the "penny-wise and pound-foolish" approach of the insurance industry, the majority of the comprehensive multidisciplinary chronic pain management programs in the United States have been forced to close their doors over the past decade (72,73) Those that have survived, and will survive, are the ones that are able to understand the *business ethos* of the health insurance industry and function in their interactions with third-party payers as *businesses*. Business operations of chronic pain management programs must be optimized, minimizing financial risk to those who operate these much-needed clinics. By aggressively negotiating with insurance carriers, effectively managing revenue cycles, establishing functional yet positive relationships with more pragmatic third-party payers, and judiciously screening patients to ensure continued cost-effectiveness of treatment, multidisciplinary chronic pain management programs will be able to remain financially viable and continue to restore quality of life to the patients to whom they provide treatment. Failure to minimize financial risk factors, on the other hand, will result in the optimal treatment for chronic pain going the way of the dinosaur.

REFERENCES

1. Studin I. Marketing to managed care organizations. In: Lande SD, Kulich RJ, eds. Managed Care and Pain. Glenview, IL: American Pain Society; 2000:71–86.
2. Lande SD, Kulich RJ. Managed Care and Pain. Glenview, IL: American Pain Society; 2000.
3. Varga CA. Starting a pain clinic. In: Boswell MV, Cole BE, eds. Weiner's Pain Management: A Practical Guide for Clinicians, 7th edn. Boca Raton, FL: CRC Press; 2006:1531–1540.
4. Tinsley R. Managed Care Contracting: Successful Negotiation Strategies. Chicago, IL: American Medical Association; 1999.

5. Plocher DW. Disease management and return on investment. In: Kongstvedt PR, Plocher DW, eds. Best Practices in Medical Management. Gaithersburg, MD: Aspen Publishers; 1998.
6. Kongstvedt PR, Plocher DW: Best Practices in Medical Management. Gaithersburg, MD: Aspen Publishers; 1998.
7. Banja J. Bad Ethics, bad business. Part II: ethical considerations for achieving economic stability in physician group practices. J Quality Health Care 2002; 1:12–15.
8. Page L. Capitation at the crossroads: the trend back to fee for service. Am Med News 2001; 44:17.
9. Banja J. Bad ethics, bad business. Part I: ethical considerations for achieving economic stability in physician group practices. J Quality Health Care 2002; 1:6–11.
10. Shapiro DE. Ensuring cash flow. In: DeKaye AP, ed. The Patient Accounts Management Handbook. Gaithersburg, MD: Aspen Publishers; 1997:167–182.
11. Schneider RJ, Mandelbaum SP, Graboys K, et al. Process-centered revenue-cycle management optimizes payment process. Healthc Financ Manage 2001; 55:63–66, 68–69.
12. Berger S. Managing the revenue cycle. Patient Acc 2003; 26:4–5.
13. Davison J, Lewis M. Working with Insurance and Managed Care Plans: A Guide for Getting Paid. Los Angeles, CA: PMIC; 1999.
14. LaForge RW, Tureaud JS. Revenue-cycle redesign: honing the details. Healthc Financ Manage 2003; 57:64–71.
15. DeKaye AP. Measuring monthly performance. In: DeKaye AP, ed. The Patient Accounts Management Handbook. Gaithersburg, MD: Aspen Publishers; 1997.
16. Schlesinger M, Quon N, Wynia M, et al. Profit-seeking, corporate control, and the trustworthiness of health care organizations: assessments of health plan performance by their affiliated physicians. Health Serv Res 2005; 40:605–645.
17. Tollison CD, Kriegel ML. Interdisciplinary Rehabilitation of Low Back Pain. Baltimore, MD: Williams & Wilkins; 1989.
18. Kulich R. Functional restoration treatment agreement. In: Wittink H, Hoskins Michel T, eds. Chronic Pain Management for Physical Therapists, 2nd edn. Boston, MA: Butterworth-Heinemann; 2002:157–158.
19. McGeary DD, Mayer TG, Gatchel RJ. High pain ratings predict treatment failure in chronic occupational musculoskeletal disorders. J Bone Joint Surg Am 2006; 88:317–325.
20. Hildebrandt J, Pfingsten M, Saur P, et al. Prediction of success from a multidisciplinary treatment program for chronic low back pain. Spine 1997; 22:990–1001.
21. Chapman S. Chronic pain rehabilitation: lost in a sea of drugs and procedures? Am Pain Soc Bull 2000; 10:8–9.
22. Thompson AA, Strickland AJ. Strategic Management: Concepts and Cases. Boston, MA: McGraw-Hill/Irwin; 2003.
23. Donaldson L. The Contingency Theory of Organizations. Thousand Oaks, CA: Sage Publications; 2001.
24. Turk D. Progress and directions for the agenda for pain management. Am Pain Soc Bull 2004; 14:3–13.
25. Cigich S. Actuarial services in an integrated delivery system. In: Kongstvedt P, ed. The Managed Health Care Handbook, 4th edn. Gaithersburg, MD: Aspen Publishers; 2001:971–976.
26. Pickett JP: The American Heritage Dictionary. New York: Dell Publishing; 2001.
27. Tindall WN. A guide to Managed Care Medicine. Gaithersburg, MD: Aspen Publishers; 2000.
28. Kongstvedt PR. The Managed Health Care Handbook. Gaithersburg, MD: Aspen Publishers; 2001.
29. Kongstvedt PR. Common operational problems in managed health care plans. In: Kongstvedt PR, ed. The Managed Health Care Handbook, 4th edn. Gaithersburg, MD: Aspen Publishers; 2001:886–903.
30. Friedman M. The social responsibility of business is to increase its profits. The New York Times Magazine. New York: The New York Times Company; September 13, 1970.

31. Emery DR, Finnerty JD, Stowe JD. Principles of Financial Management. Upper Saddle River, NJ: Prentice Hall; 1998.
32. Group Health Association of America: HMO Industry Profile, 1994 edn. Washington, DC: GHAA; 1994.
33. Cunningham PJ, Kohn L. Health plan switching: choice or circumstance? Health Aff (Millwood) 2000; 19:158–164.
34. No author listed. Watch out for Medicare HMO disenrollment as high as 42%. Public Sect Contract Rep 1997; 3:13–15.
35. Flor H, Fydrich T, Turk DC. Efficacy of multidisciplinary pain treatment centers: a meta-analytic review. Pain 1992; 49:221–230.
36. Turk DC. Efficacy of multidisciplinary pain centers: an antidote to anecdotes. Baillieres Clin Anaesthesiol 1998; 12:103–119.
37. Blumenthal D. Employer-sponsored insurance-riding the health care tiger. N Engl J Med 2006; 355:195–202.
38. Graziano C. DMAA Details Progress on Predictive Modeling "Buyer's Guide." Society of Actuaries/DMAA Predictive Modeling and Risk Adjustment Seminar, Chicago, IL, 2006.
39. Blyth FM, March LM, Brnabic AJ, et al. Chronic pain and frequent use of health care. Pain 2004; 111:51–58.
40. Lippe G. Operational underwriting in managed care organizations. In: Kongstvedt PR, ed. The Managed Health Care Handbook, 4th edn. Gaithersburg, MD: Aspen Publishers; 2001:997–999.
41. Lande S. The Problem of pain in managed care. In: Lande SD, Kulich RJ, eds. Managed Care and Pain. Glenview, IL: American Pain Society; 2000:15–36.
42. Proctor TJ, Mayer TG, Gatchel RJ, et al. Unremitting health-care-utilization outcomes of tertiary rehabilitation of patients with chronic musculoskeletal disorders. J Bone Joint Surg Am 2004; 86-A:62–69.
43. Centers for Medicare & Medicaid Services (CMS) H: Medicare Program; Medicare Prescription Drug Benefit, 42 CFR Parts 400, 403, 411, 417, and 423. Fed regist 1995; 70:4221–4497.
44. Gray BH. Trust and trustworthy care in the managed care era. Health Aff (Millwood) 1997; 16:34–49.
45. Kulich RJ. Comprehensive HMO legislation: an opportunity for better access. Am Pain Soc Bull 1999; July/August 9(4):5–9.
46. Biskupiak JE, Chofoff P, Nash D. Disease management in managed care organizations. In: Todd WE, Nash DB, eds. Disease Management: A Systems Approach to Improving Patient Outcomes. Chicago, IL: American Hospital Publishing; 1997.
47. Gatchel RJ, Polatin PB, Noe C, et al. Treatment- and cost-effectiveness of early intervention for acute low-back pain patients: a one-year prospective study. J Occup Rehabil 2003; 13:1–9.
48. Keel PJ, Wittig R, Deutschmann R, et al. Effectiveness of in-patient rehabilitation for sub-chronic and chronic low back pain by an integrative group treatment program (Swiss Multicentre Study). Scand J Rehabil Med 1998; 30:211–219.
49. Hall MA. Health insurers' medical necessity determinations for bariatric surgery. Surg Obes Relat Dis 2005; 1:86–90.
50. Murphy-Barron CM. Can we design a fair benefit for bariatric surgery? Manag Care 2006; 15:35–36, 39–40.
51. Choban P, Lu B, Flancbaum L. Insurance decisions about obesity surgery: a new type of randomization? Obes Surg 2000; 10:553–536.
52. Teugels JL, Sundt B. Encyclopedia of Actuarial Science. Hoboken, NJ: Wiley; 2004.
53. Galvin RS, Delbanco S. Between a rock and a hard place: understanding the employer mind-set. Health Aff (Millwood) 2006; 25:1548–1555.
54. Mechanic RE. What will become of the medical mecca? Health care spending in Massachusetts. Health Aff (Millwood) 2003; 22:130–141.
55. Mechanic R, Coleman K, Dobson A. Teaching hospital costs: implications for academic missions in a competitive market. JAMA 1998; 280:1015–1019.

56. Loeser JD. The future. Will pain be abolished or just pain specialists? Minn Med 201; 84:20–21.
57. Loeser JD. Pain and suffering. Clin J Pain 2000; 16:S2–S6.
58. Mayer T, Tabor J, Bovasso E, et al. Physical progress and residual impairment quantification after functional restoration. Part I: lumbar mobility. Spine 1994; 19:389–394.
59. Rogers E. Diffusion of Innovations. New York: Free Press; 2003.
60. Kipp RA, Towner WC, Levin HA. Financial and actuarial issues. In: Todd WE, Nash DB, eds. Disease Management: A Systems Approach to Improving Patient Outcomes. Chicago, IL: American Hospital Publishing; 1997.
61. Cicala RS, Wright H. Outpatient treatment of patients with chronic pain: an analysis of cost savings. Clin J Pain 1989; 5:223–226.
62. Simmons JW, Avant WS, Jr, Demski J, et al. Determining successful pain clinic treatment through validation of cost effectiveness. Spine 1988; 13:342–344.
63. Caudill M, Schnable R, Zuttermeister P, et al. Decreased clinic use by chronic pain patients: response to behavioral medicine intervention. Clin J Pain 1991; 7:305–310.
64. Plocher DW. Fundamentals and core competencies of disease management. In: Kongstvedt PR, ed. The Managed Health Care Handbook, 4th edn. Gaithersburg, MD: Aspen Publishers; 2001:402–412.
65. Simpson JM, Klar N, Donnor A. Accounting for cluster randomization: a review of primary prevention trials, 1990 through 1993. Am J Public Health 1995; 85:1378–1383.
66. Varnell SP, Murray DM, Janega JB, et al. Design and analysis of group-randomized trials: a review of recent practices. Am J Public Health 2004; 94:393–399.
67. Loyd R, Fanciullo GJ, Hanscom B, et al. Cluster analysis of SF-36 scales as a predictor of spinal pain patients response to a multidisciplinary pain management approach beginning with epidural steroid injection. Pain Med 2006; 7:229–236.
68. Fanciullo GJ, Hanscom B, Weinstein JN, et al. Cluster analysis classification of SF-36 profiles for patients with spinal pain. Spine 2003; 28:2276–2282.
69. American Pain Foundation. http//www.painfoundation.org. Accessed 12/1/2006.
70. Partners Against Pain. Your Around-the-Clock Resource for Pain Management. Available at http://www.partnersagainstpain.com/painadvocacycommunity/ Accessed 12/1/2006.
71. Pollack R, Slass L. Premium Pay: Corporate Compensation in America's HMOs. Washington, DC: Families USA Foundation; 1998:24.
72. Schatman M. The demise of the multidisciplinary chronic pain management clinic: Bioethical perspectives on providing optimal treatment when ethical principles collide. In: Schatman M, ed. Ethical Issues in Chronic Pain Management. New York: Informa Healthcare; 2007:43–62.
73. Schatman M. The demise of multidisciplinary pain management clinics? Pract Pain Manage 2006; 6:30–41.

16 Chronic Pain Management in the Era of Managed Care

Bill H. McCarberg
Kaiser Permanente San Diego and University of California, San Diego, San Diego, California, U.S.A.

INTRODUCTION

Persistent and recurring pain is a significant problem for a substantial proportion of the world's population. Worldwide surveys (1–4) conducted in 1998 of over 197,000 adults established that 28% of the sample had experienced pain in the lower back, 16% severe headache, and 15% pain in the neck region in the prior 3 months (5). A third of the adults reported a limitation due to pain that affected their ability to walk, climb steps without resting, or engage in other activities of daily living.

Prevalence of chronic pain is difficult to determine and varies depending on how syndromes are defined. In the United States, estimates are reported to be as high as 30–60 million people. The largest categories of chronic pain syndromes, including musculoskeletal disorders, show that the vast majority of patients have symptoms that are not related to identifiable pathology but to locations, such as low back, headache, or widespread pain (e.g., fibromyalgia syndrome) (6). In 1995, a national survey of pain specialists demonstrated that 2.9 million Americans are treated annually by health-care professionals specializing in chronic pain (7). This number would be much larger if it included primary-care providers or visits to practitioners of complementary and alternative medicine. The survey also did not take into account patients who self-medicated with over-the-counter preparations.

Chronic pain management remains an elusive and frustrating goal despite growing knowledge about the pathophysiology of pain. Patients seek cure based on physical abnormalities. Health-care providers look for pathology that is often not discoverable.

Even more perplexing to physicians is the variability among pain patients. Physical abnormalities are not predictive of pain severity or dysfunction (8). Large numbers of patients experience pain over long periods of time, and yet their life functioning is not changed in major ways. Conversely, there are other patients with similar structural abnormalities who suffer substantially more and cannot maintain their usual levels of activity (9). Despite similar pathology, these patients engage in behaviors that are maladaptive, anticipate more distress, amplify sensations associated with pain, spend more time resting, and complain of less ability to control pain (10,11).

An analgesic medication (hydrocodone/acetaminophen) is the most widely prescribed medication in the United States (12). The number of people taking non-prescription analgesics far exceeds these figures. There are currently over 176 non-prescription products containing analgesics either alone or in combination with other medications available for purchase by the U.S. public (13). Three quarters of

American adults included in the Third National Health and Nutrition Examination survey consumed nonprescription analgesic medication and 9% prescription analgesic medication in the month prior to the survey (14).

HISTORICAL PERSPECTIVE

The United States remains the only industrialized country where employers have taken on the burden of health-care financing. In an attempt to attract workers in a tight labor market after World War II, health insurance was offered (15). This system was cost-effective when foreign competition was limited and the cost of health care was low. Prior to 1965, there was little price competition among health-care providers, and the predominant type of insurance coverage was low dollar comprehensive coverage with free choice of providers and only minor differences in out of pocket fees. It was virtually impossible to create market pressure based on price. Total health spending was only 6.1% of the gross national product (GNP) in 1965 and had not risen much since 1950.

Medicare and Medicaid were introduced and by 1970 health-care expenditures reached 7.6% of GNP, growing 25% faster than the rest of the economy. Employers were paying a higher percentage of the nation's heath-care bill reaching 20% in 1970. The federal government, which makes the health-care laws and purchases health care for Medicare and Medicaid, implemented steps in the 1970s to save money which were largely related to hospital costs: encouraging outpatient surgery, second opinions for surgery, and restricted payments. There was still very little price competition.

In 1983, California's Medicaid program negotiated directly with hospitals; physicians could only use a limited number of the 500 hospitals in the state. This was the first effort at competitive pricing followed later in the 1980s by California Blue Cross/Blue Shield organizing preferred providers. Patients were restricted to a limited number of physicians (preferred providers) who were paid a reduced service fee. The patients benefited by reduced prices, the providers had an endless supply of patients, and the insurance company controlled costs. This was the first example of discounted fee-for-service. The era of managed care had begun.

Cost could be managed through a variety of mechanisms:

- evaluate the risk group costs and predict yearly costs in the future
- limit risk by accepting only healthy populations
- dilute risk by enrolling large numbers of patients
- shift costs by charging some patients more to cover underpaying patients (uninsured)
- preventative care
- implement best practice guidelines

All of these strategies worked but health-care costs were still increasing by nearly 10% until the 1990s when capitation and risk sharing occurred. This has led to cost controls for the first time (Fig. 1) and created an environment of public hostility and distrust.

Employers and the federal government remain the major purchaser of health care. Employees view insurance contributions as a supplement to, rather than a substitute for, cash compensation. Health insurance puts American companies at a substantial disadvantage against foreign competitors who do not have this added

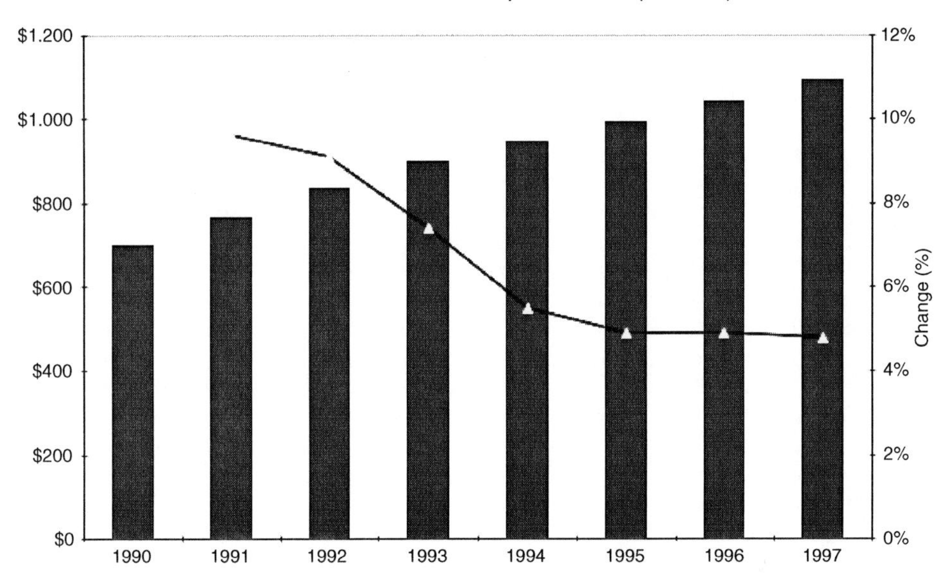

FIGURE 1 National health-care expenditure. From Health Care Financing Administration.

expense. At the same time, our citizens increasingly believe they have a right to unrestricted access to ever more convenient, personalized, and high-quality services.

Managing care by controlling costs led employers, insurers, and some physician organizations to develop managed care as a private sector alternative to governmental regulation. By persuading patients to switch to managed care, providers and employers achieved short-term gains, with an unprecedented slowdown in cost inflation during the 1990s (16). Narrow physician panels, gatekeeping, utilization review, and capitation were all financially very successful but cultural and political disasters. The backlash has led to a renouncing of managed care by insurers and employers. Managed care sought to restrain rising costs through volume price discounts from physicians, gatekeeper restraints on specialty consultations, drug formularies, and prior authorization of tests and admissions (17). Consumers experienced barriers to access, administrative complexity, and frustrated unhappy caregivers.

Presently, employers are retreating from managed care constraints while simultaneously restricting coverage and benefits. Enrollment is shifting from tightly managed health maintenance organization products to lightly managed alternatives. At the same time, employees are being asked to pay a greater share of the health insurance premium, with a consequent unprecedented rise in the number of individuals who are offered but decline employment-based coverage (18). The increase in copayments and benefit exclusions was only muted by the imperative to retain employees, but many firms are waiting for a loosening of labor markets to increase cost sharing and reduce benefits. The trend is to offer information, options, and partial financial support, but otherwise to get out of the decision-making position in health care.

PAIN MANAGEMENT

Despite the much published demise of managed care, cost control and management of the health-care dollar are more critical today than ever before. Health maintenance organizations are not vilified in the newspaper as they were 5 years ago, but costs are once again becoming a factor in health-care decisions. The nation lacks the economic resources to remain competitive and continue to finance health care. Yet we remain no closer to solving the problem of resource allocation because initiatives aimed at controlling health-care costs remain exceedingly unpopular.

Health-care costs comprise the single greatest expense in this country, with 15.3% of the GNP devoted to health care in 2003 (19). Legislation that increases costs, through expansion of coverage, benefits, and access is politically fashionable yet constitutes economic malfeasance. Criticizing managed care and calling for universal health care for all Americans, while popular, is financially perilous and a simplistic solution. Managed care was viewed as a medical program to make insurers and health plans wealthy and it occasionally did. We all must take responsibility for the inevitable rise in health-care costs. The concern is that the country will not be able to support paying for the care of its citizens.

As insurers and employers are looking for means to control costs, pain is being recognized as a driver of much of the health-care utilization. The silent epidemic of the undertreatment of pain is also viewed as a cause of the rapid escalation of cost that goes largely unrecognized.

In 1992, Fishman studied a large managed care organization (MCO) in the Pacific Northwest and followed costs of care for 18 of the most common conditions seen in primary care (20). Four of these conditions were described as painful: neck pain, back pain, facial pain, and headache (arthritis excluded). The cost of treating the 18 conditions was compared to the health-care expenditures for a comparable population without the conditions. Stroke had the highest annual cost per diagnosis at $13,139 followed by HIV-AIDs ($10,246), dementia ($9,824), and cancer ($8,992). The painful conditions yielded relatively low annual costs: back and neck pain ($4,226), facial pain ($4,088), and headache ($4,989). Despite the low costs, the conditions described as painful were highly prevalent. Multiplying cost and prevalence, the expense of managing all covered lives can be estimated. In this managed care population, combining the four painful complaints, pain ranked number 1 of the 18 conditions at an annual cost of $198 million followed by heart disease ($170 million), hypertension ($112 million), respiratory disease ($90 million), diabetes ($86 million), cancer ($55 million), stroke ($38 million), and HIV-AIDs ($4 million).

Care management plans often exist for other less costly conditions which include case management, algorithms, physician education, and patient support groups. Very little emphasis is placed on the conditions described as painful despite large allocation of health care dollars.

Managed Care and Pain

In 2004, 74 managed care administrators were surveyed to discover how pain was viewed in their organizations (21). The MCOs ranged in size from 2200 to 25 million covered lives. The health plans represented a variety of types:

- 52% network plans
- 33% independent practice association (IPA)

- 8% group plans
- 7% staff plans

When asked what painful conditions were seen as most difficult for their providers, back pain, headache, and fibromyalgia syndrome were identified. These conditions mirror the enrollment in many specialized pain clinics throughout the United States. Seventy-five percent felt that pain programs and guideline development would be instrumental in quality care and controlling cost, yet 66% did not have such programs and 59% had no guidelines disseminated to their primary-care providers. Most believed that rehabilitation programs were more effective by a large percentage than surgery or anesthetic procedures, yet more readily reimbursed for procedures. Eighty-four percent stated that self-management was a critical aspect in chronic pain care, but only 11% indicated that their organization did a good job of educating patients about their chronic pain problems.

Several MCOs had specialized programs:

- Excellus Health Plan in Rochester, New York, developed community wide clinical guidelines for pain management. These guidelines were disseminated to the relevant health-care providers along with educational programs for proper pain care. Single page handouts showed how to assess pain, available treatment options, and how to set goals with patients. The training of the providers also included case and disease management programs.
- Health Net of San Diego, California, instituted a patient-directed care management program for chronic pain. Patients were instructed on how to ask appropriate questions about their low back, hip, and other joint pain at each physician visit. Nurse health coaches were available by phone to offer medication information and advice. A trifold patient-directed pharmacy handout outlined the use of opioids and adjunctive analgesics. A description of symptoms, possible diagnoses, appropriate examinations, tests, and recommended treatments are made available to patients.
- Three Rivers Health Plan in Pittsburgh, Pennsylvania, developed a polypharmacy reporting procedure to inform the primary treatment provider about opioid prescriptions from multiple sources.
- Fallon Community Health Plan Worcester, Massachusetts, used quantity limits and prior authorization for opioid prescriptions to control utilization.

Managed Care Organizations

Managed care comes in a variety of plan types that can have a significant effect on the care provided to a patient. In a staff model, providers are salaried by the health plan. Treatment among providers may vary but care is more often standardized. All providers in a group attend the same meetings, sit on care committees, and develop treatment options together as a group. There is likely only one formulary in a staff model MCO. Military medicine is largely a staff model with the physicians following federal guidelines and a government formulary.

In contrast, an IPA is a group of providers practicing alone or in a group and its members are only related by the fact that they all receive reimbursement from the health plan. Doctors may belong to many IPAs thereby having multiple health plans that oversee the care of a patient panel. These providers must be aware of the reimbursement restrictions of multiple payers and may have to consider 10 or more formularies when prescribing medications. Determining the best care options for a disease like diabetes or low back pain and disseminating this to the relevant providers is easier to accomplish in the staff model MCO, compared to the loosely knit IPA.

KAISER PERMANENTE CALIFORNIA

Kaiser Permanente is a health maintenance organization largely found in California and is operating under a group model with salaried partner providers. Within California, Kaiser is divided between northern and southern regions. There is interaction between the two groups, but each operates independently. Northern California Kaiser started a cognitive-behavioral approach with group visits for pain management in the late 1970s. A similar program started in Southern California Kaiser in the mid 1980s, which also uses a cognitive-behavioral strategy.

The steps necessary to develop a pain management program in the setting of managed care are similar to those addressing any large organizational problem and have been described in other settings including the automobile industry, quality issues in customer service, etc. As illustrated in the above survey (21), MCOs have tried a variety of methods to improve pain care. Educating providers, utilizing case managers, and enforcing quantity limits were all used. Health Plan Employer Data and Information Set (HEDIS) is attempting to improve pain care by monitoring the use of the inappropriate pain medication propoxyphene.

According to the survey of 74 administrators described above, the power structure of MCOs recognizes the problem (e.g., under treatment of pain) and understands some of the solutions (e.g., patient education), yet does not take the necessary steps to change provider behavior. The fact that all organizations are not taking the same steps or adopting an effective approach to improve pain care suggests that these administrators are not sure how to address the problem or do not think that pain is a significant cost or ethical issue. Sometimes, the complexity of an organization makes a solution very difficult to initiate and maintain.

Starting a pain program within managed care can be a challenge and I will use my experience with Southern California Kaiser as an example. This model has been repeated successfully in other areas across the United States and is not unique to Southern California; however, the steps taken to implement a program will vary in MCOs that are network based or in IPA models due to the different types of relationships among the providers.

STEPS TO DEVELOPING A PAIN MANAGEMENT PROGRAM

A brief look at how I started a pain program in a large health maintenance organization will demonstrate some of the steps needed for successful implementation of a program. These steps have been enumerated and discussed in detail elsewhere (22) and will just be examined related to starting a pain program.

- find a pain champion
- organize a team including various disciplines
- perform a needs assessment
- develop a plan to address the needs

- build consensus
- implement the plan
- monitor effectiveness

Find a Pain Champion

It is important that the pain champion be recognized in the organization and respected among peers. Developing a program often starts with the recognition of a pain problem and the champion is identified due to interest in the topic. For example, when the Joint Commission on Accreditation of Healthcare Organizations (JCAHO) instituted pain assessment criteria, a problem surfaced in the hospitals accredited by JCAHO: complying with the new pain standards. Hospitals likely had many pain-related problems which were never addressed; JCAHO's pain standards became the rallying point for improvement.

A pain champion usually emerges as an organization commits resources to the new problem. As with any model endorsing behavior change, resistance will surface. The pain champion will have to commit time, energy, and perhaps take their reputation to the project. Appointing a committee may produce manuals and printouts, but a champion is needed to accomplish significant organizational change. As the champion, I had the vision and was willing to volunteer all my free time to the project, a commitment I needed to make. Identifying the champion may be difficult but is essential given the consensus building necessary in managed care.

Organize a Team Including Various Disciplines

Many groups work together to provide successful medical care. Sometimes the interaction can produce conflict if care groups do not agree on treatments. A group of doctors mandating a specific treatment will be ineffective if the nursing staff does not agree to the new intervention. Important in the later step of consensus building is having different disciplines discuss the problems together. Everyone on the care team is affected by patients in pain, from the doctors and nurses to the hospital administrators and clergy. Frequently included on a pain team are doctors, nurses, pharmacists, and other disciplines depending on the pain area being addressed. I was particularly interested in chronic pain, much of which is musculoskeletal; therefore, my team had providers from medicine, nursing, pharmacy, physical therapy, anesthesia, physical medicine, and psychiatry. At the initial meeting, I organized the heads of departments and the hospital administrator to develop support from these groups as well.

Perform a Needs Assessment

An identified problem often leads an organization to put resources behind a pain program. In my institution, I was the main motivator for better pain management. The medical group administrators did not feel that pain needed to be addressed. Getting support for this project included demonstrating that there was a need. From the primary-care viewpoint, pain was a problem in some patients. Referrals to specialists and standard treatment resulted in most patients returning to near normal function, but a small group of patients continued to suffer. These patients often presented back to primary care with no clear guidance on what could be done to manage the continued pain complaint. My motivation in accepting the pain champion role was to help primary care with the chronic pain patient.

Part of the needs assessment included collecting information on the magnitude of the chronic pain problem, documenting the cost of fragmented care and communicating the high level of dissatisfaction of patients and providers. Administrators pay attention to cost and satisfaction and became strong supporters of the process once this information was presented.

Finding out what the MCO, with all its parts, identifies as the pain problem is just as important. One may identify postoperative pain as the major undertreated pain problem, but this may not be important to some providers. Perhaps the emergency department and the organization view emergency room visits with readmissions after surgery as more important. If the readmissions result from inadequate postoperative pain control, both issues can be addressed together. A pain champion with a pet project may address one small issue unsuccessfully unless a larger needs assessment is undertaken.

Develop a Plan to Address the Needs

Developing a plan to ameliorate the identified needs can be time consuming and often involves redefining the problem. We determined that chronic back pain was a major problem, yet with more study, it was clear that many parts of the organization were already involved in the care of patients with this problem. We originally decided to address the problem by organizing a specialty clinic for chronic back pain patients. After further investigation, we realized that many if not most of our chronic pain patients, including cancer patients, shared similar characteristics: high levels of pain, disturbed sleep, cognitive distortions, deconditioning, depression, anxiety, etc. The problem was redefined by not limiting care to a small subset of patients. Instead of creating yet another narrowly focused subspecialty clinic, we decided to group all the chronic pain patients together. Patient-focused pain management skills education could be taught effectively to a larger group using fewer resources.

Build Consensus

Even the best plan will fail without agreement among those individuals who must implement the plan. In 1988, a well-conceived, researched guideline was developed for the evaluation and management of low back pain in Canada (23). The development group was well-respected leaders in the medical community. The guidelines, although published and distributed, were never adopted since the primary stakeholders were not consulted during guideline development. The Veterans Administration adopted the principle of treating pain levels as a vital sign in their hospitals before JCAHO mandated measuring pain. Despite this wonderful idea, pain outcomes did not change (12). Were the nurses who recorded pain scores and doctors who had to act on the scores involved in the pain management decisions?

In our organization, consensus building was a continuous process and lasted 3 years. When a specific problem was identified, stakeholders were consulted if they were not on the team. When a plan to address the problem was identified, stakeholders again were informed and allowed time to focus on their concerns. All the stakeholders were not on the development team due to the potential size of the team. It was not necessary to have all interested parties at every meeting. When it was time for implementation of the plan, everyone who could be involved in the rollout was already aware of the plan and had agreed to the implementation process.

Implement the Plan

Depending on the model developed to address the problem, implementation will vary. Our team decided to start a cognitive-behavioral group. Referrals were identified from a clinic staffed by a neurologist and psychiatrist where patients were already being followed for chronic pain. Patient evaluations were reviewed, medication was optimized, and patients who met strict inclusion/exclusion criteria were referred for group treatment. Implementation is the most visible step in the initiation of a new program, yet the steps leading up to implementation are critically important for the success of a pain program.

Evaluation

Evaluating the program is the ultimate arbiter of success. Publishing a guideline is certainly important, but determining whether guideline implementation leads to desired changes in provider behaviors is critical. Steps can be taken to improve the model and plan if the evaluation shows results that were not anticipated. When the Veterans Administration found good compliance to measuring pain but no change in high pain scores, what was the next step? Deciding to make pain the fifth vital sign was not the problem, nor was the implementation of the vital sign since good record keeping was confirmed. Awareness of high pain scores should have lead to steps to lower these scores, but this did not happen. The process was good, the plan was good, but the results were not. What steps should be taken next?

In our program, there was concern about large numbers of referrals to the pain program. Estimates from surveys noted that 35,000 patients could potentially have been referred. Our model included screening and strict inclusion/exclusion criteria. After 12 months, 50 patients had been referred to the program. It was discovered that patients did not need screening since they had had many workups prior to referral. Excluding patients because of diagnosis (e.g., cancer, fibromyalgia syndrome, etc.) or litigation status made no difference in outcomes. When all departments including primary care were invited to refer patients, numbers increased by 10-fold, yet were manageable for 10 years of the study.

The pain problem being studied often is dynamic, and plans to resolve programmatic issues have to change as the problem changes or as new problems are recognized. For example, the ordering of MRIs for musculoskeletal low back pain was perceived as a financial drain by the administration at Kaiser. Many evidence-based guidelines have been developed pertaining to imaging studies and back pain. The MCO republished and distributed the guidelines. No change in MRI ordering occurred. It was discovered that most of the studies came from primary care, which led to an educational initiative focused at these providers. No change occurred. Prescreening for authorization of the procedure was the next plan. Before data could be collected, membership complaints increased dramatically. A prime motivator for excessive use of MRIs was patient expectation and demand. The primary care providers were placed in an awkward position; they are patient advocates and are evaluated on patient satisfaction, yet must deny a procedure which patients have come to expect. The pain problem started from a quality and financial perspective but was discovered to be more complicated, involving member satisfaction and erroneous beliefs about the benefits of imaging. The solutions were well planned and implemented but without any impact. The problem needed to be redefined and this was only discovered through the process of program evaluation.

The preceding steps illustrate how chronic pain was approached in a MCO representing 500,000 patients. After many failed attempts at change, a highly effective and popular program was developed. This approach uncovered problems, biases, and practice styles leading to undertreated pain. Through persistence, a structured approach to pain management was found to be highly effective as measured by patient and provider satisfaction, high numbers of referrals from primary and specialty care, continued support from administration, improved pain scores and functional outcomes, and lower health-care costs.

Every organization will have a different approach to the numerous identified pain problems. Simple steps may be effective. If the use of meperidine is recognized as a problem, removing it from the formulary may have a dramatic effect on prescribing behavior. More often, the pain issues in an organization are deep seated and complex. Removing meperidine could result in safety issues if the orthopedic surgeons do not know how to use alternative postoperative medications; therefore adequate continuing education for providers is crucial. Primary care may substitute hydromorphone intramuscularly in migraine patients in the urgent-care setting with unsatisfactory results as well. Patient satisfaction could be a concern if meperidine were widely used and accepted by the patients. Taking the simple, quick solution can be tempting but may have unanticipated results and make the pain team and pain champion feel disenfranchised and isolated.

CONCLUSIONS

Retreating from the issues surrounding costs of pain care is hazardous to society as a whole. Politically, popular proposals for comprehensive, universal health care have been unsuccessful despite the assurances given during election seasons. Consumer-driven health-care decision making is currently trendy but fraught with problems. Consumers will face significant obstacles in understanding the quality and even the comparative price of health insurance. The new paradigm is particularly difficult for those most needy, the impoverished, and poorly educated. Consumers demand more information about health-care costs. Transparency will make difficult the pooling of risk from healthy citizens and those who have chronic pain or redistribution of income from rich to poor that otherwise results from the collective purchasing and administration of health insurance.

Medical costs are arising and are expected to consume 18.7% of the GNP within 10 years (19). With an aging society, a population that will experience more pain, a larger voting block will also be the chief consumer of health care. There has been rhetoric connected to these costs including insurance greed, pharmaceutical excesses, governmental corruption, yet the answer is more likely complex and multifaceted. Medical care is expensive. New technology, championed by all, has a price. Breakthrough medications are prohibitively expensive to discover unless profits can offset multiple failed drug trials.

Undertreated pain is a disgrace in an advanced society with the best health care in the world. We are a wealthy nation, yet our poor, indigent, elderly, mentally challenged, and racial minorities are the most likely to suffer unrelieved pain. The evaluation and management of pain is perhaps the most costly of the medical conditions being followed in primary care (20). The restraint on inflation in health-care costs only occurred in the 1990s with the widespread introduction of managed care.

Our nation lacks the financial resources to provide all pain services to all individuals. The question concerns at what level and by whom difficult decisions will be made. The United States appears to be no closer to resolving the problem of resource allocation than it ever has been. The fundamental flaw of managed care was that it sought to navigate the tensions between limited resources and unlimited expectations behind the scenes. Cost-control was achieved with a political and cultural backlash.

If the war on pain is to be successful, a new approach is needed. Instead of maligning managed care, perhaps the restraints employed should be reexamined. A consumer-centered health-care system will have incomplete information on quality, inadequate spreading of insurance risk, and insufficient financial subsidies for the poor. If our country cannot afford an MRI or spinal cord stimulator for everyone with low back pain, who should have this imaging study or receive this interventional procedure? An open, accountable system recognizing the inevitability of resource allocation is needed. There are multiple examples of such medical care structures operating efficiently in the United States, for example, in the Kaiser Permanente system. The tragedy of untreated pain coupled with spiraling costs will lead to another crisis. Disregarding the problems is currently fashionable because of the political disaster that could befall any attempt for change. We cannot afford to wait and managed care offers our best hope.

REFERENCES

1. Verhaak P, Kerssens J, Dekker J, et al. Prevalence of chronic benign pain disorder among adults: a review of the literature. Pain 1998; 77:231–239.
2. Volinn E. The epidemiology of low back pain in the rest of the world. A review of surveys in low- and middle-income countries. Spine 1997; 22:1747–1754.
3. Lousberg R. Chronic pain. Multiaxial diagnostics and behavioral mechanisms. Thesis, University of Maastricht, 1994.
4. Beregman S, Herrstrom P, Hogstrm K, et al. Chronic musculoskeletal pain, prevalence rates and sociodemographic associations in a Swedish population study. J Rheumatol 2001; 28:1369–1377.
5. Stang P, Von Korff M, Galer BS. Reduced labor force participation among primary care patients with headache. J Gen Intern Med 1998; 13:296–302.
6. Joranson DE, Lietman R. The McNeil National Pain Survey. New York: Louis Harris; 1994.
7. Marketdata Enterprises. Chronic Pain Management Programs: A Market Analysis. New York: Valley Stream; 1995.
8. Flor H, Turk DC. Chronic back pain and rheumatoid arthritis: predicting pain and disability from cognitive variables. J Behav Med 1988; 11:251–265.
9. Sanders SH, Brena SF, Spier CJ, et al. Chronic back pain patients around the world: cross-cultural similarities and differences. Clin J Pain 1992; 8:317–323.
10. Reesor KA, Craig KD. Medically incongruent chronic back pain physical limitations, suffering, and ineffective coping. Pain 1988; 32:35–45.
11. Pinsky J. Chronic pain syndromes and their treatment. In: Brodwin MG, Tellez F, Brodwin SK, eds. Medical, Psychosocial and Vocational Aspects of Disability. Athens, GA: Elliott & Fitzpatrick; 1993; 179–194.

12. Mularski RA, White-Chu F, Overbay D, et al. Measuring Pain as the 5th Vital Sign Does Not Improve Quality of Pain Management. J Gen Intern Med 2006; 21(6):607–612.
13. Physicians' Desk Reference, Toronto, Canada: Thomson Corporation; 2005.
14. Paulose-Ram R, Hirsch R, Dillon C, et al. Prescription and non-prescription analgesic use among the US adult population: results fro the third National Health and Nutrition Examination Survey (NHANES III). Pharmacoepidemiol Drug Saf 2003; 112:315–326.
15. Starr P. The Social Transformation of American Medicine. New York: Basic Books; 1983.
16. Levit J, Cowan D, Lazenby H, et al. Health spending in 1998: signals of change. Health Aff (Millwoood) 1999; 19:124–138.
17. Zelman W, Berenson R. The Managed Care Blues and How to Cure Them. Washington, DC: Georgetown University Press; 1998.
18. Thorpe K, Florence C. Why are workers uninsured? Employer-sponsored health insurance in 1997. Health Aff (Millwood) 1999; 18:213–218.
19. National Coalition on Health Care. Available at http://64.233.161.104/search?q = cache:U_xRYfphv3YJ:www.nchc.org/facts/cost.shtml+health+care+costs+gross+national+product&hl = en. Accessed on December 21, 2005.
20. Fishman P, Von Korff M, Lozano P, et al. Chronic care costs in managed care. Health Aff (Millwood) 1997; 16(3):239–247.
21. Turk D, McCarberg B, Kelly N. Chronic pain care trends: perspectives from managed care, providers, and employers. Washington DC: Kikaku America International 2006.
22. Gordon DB, Dahl JL, Stevenson KK. Building an Institutional Commitment to Pain Management: The Wisconsin Resource Manual for Improvement, 2nd edn. Madison, WI: Wisconsin Cancer Pain Initiative 2000.
23. Spitzer W, Leblanc F, Dupuis M, et al. Scientific approach to the assessment and management of activity-related spinal disorders. A monograph for clinicians. Report of the Quebec Task Force on Spinal Disorders. Spine 1987; 12 (Suppl):S1–S59.

Index